Searchlights on Health: Light on Dark Corners
By B.G. Jefferis and J.L. Nichols

Knowledge is Safety.

1. The old maxim, that "Knowledge is power," is a true one, but there is still a greater truth: "KNOWLEDGE IS SAFETY." Safety amid physical ills that beset mankind, and safety amid the moral pitfalls that surround so many young people, is the great crying demand of the age.[4]

2. **Criticism.**—While the aim of this work, though novel and to some extent is daring, it is chaste, practical and to the point, and will be a boon and a blessing to thousands who consult its pages. The world is full of ignorance, and the ignorant will always criticise, because they live to suffer ills, for they know no better. New light is fast falling upon the dark corners, and the eyes of many are being opened.

3. **Researches of Science.**—The researches of science in the past few years have thrown light on many facts relating to the physiology of man and woman, and the diseases to which they are subject, and consequently many reformations have taken place in the treatment and prevention of diseases peculiar to the sexes.

4. **Lock and Key.**—Any information bearing upon the diseases of mankind should not be kept under lock and key. The physician is frequently called upon to speak in plain language to his patients upon some private and startling disease contracted on account of ignorance. The better plan, however, is to so educate and enlighten old and young upon the important subjects of health, so that the necessity to call a physician may occur less frequently.

5. **Progression.**—A large, respectable, though diminishing class in every community, maintain that nothing that relates exclusively to either sex should become the subject of popular medical instruction. But such an opinion is radically wrong; ignorance is no more the mother of purity than it is of religion. Enlightenment can never work injustice to him who investigates.

6. **An Example.**—The men and women who study and practice medicine are not the worse, but the better for such knowledge; so it would be to the community in general if all would be properly instructed on the laws of health which relate to the sexes.

7. **Crime and Degradation.**—Had every person a sound understanding on the relation of the sexes, one of the most fertile sources of crime and degradation would be removed. Physicians know too well what sad consequences are constantly occurring from a lack of proper knowledge on these important subjects.

8. **A Consistent Consideration.**—Let the reader of this work study its pages carefully and be able to give safe counsel and advice to others, and remember that purity of purpose and purity of character are the brightest jewels in the crown of immortality.

[5]

The Beginning of Life.
Beginning Right.

1. **The Beginning.**—There is a charm in opening manhood which has commended itself to the imagination in every age. The undefined hopes and promises of the future—the dawning strength of intellect—the vigorous flow of passion—the very exchange of home ties and protected joys for free and manly pleasures, give to this period an interest and excitement unfelt, perhaps, at any other.

[6]

2. **The Growth of Independence.**—Hitherto life has been to boys, as to girls, a dependent existence—a sucker from the parent growth—a home discipline of authority and guidance and communicated impulse. But henceforth it is a transplanted growth of its own—a new and free power of activity in which the mainspring is no longer authority or law from without, but principle or opinion within. The shoot which has been nourished under the shelter of the parent stem, and bent according to its inclination, is transferred to the open world, where of its own impulse and character it must take root, and grow into strength, or sink into weakness and vice.

3. **Home Ties.**—The thought of home must excite a pang even in the first moments of freedom. Its glad shelter—its kindly guidance—its very restraints, how dear and tender must they seem in parting! How brightly must they shine in the retrospect as the youth turns

from them to the hardened and unfamiliar face of the world! With what a sweet, sadly-cheering pathos they must linger in the memory! And then what chance and hazard is there in his newly-gotten freedom! What instincts of warning in its very novelty and dim inexperience! What possibilities of failure as well as of success in the unknown future as it stretches before him!

4. **Vice or Virtue.**—Certainly there is a grave importance as well as a pleasant charm in the beginning of life. There is awe as well as excitement in it when rightly viewed. The possibilities that lie in it of noble or ignoble work—of happy self-sacrifice or ruinous self-indulgence—the capacities in the right use of which it may rise to heights of beautiful virtue, in the abuse of which it may sink to the depths of debasing vice—make the crisis one of fear as well as of hope, of sadness as well as of joy.

5. **Success or Failure.**—It is wistful as well as pleasing to think of the young passing year by year into the world, and engaging with its duties, its interests, and temptations. Of the throng that struggle at the gates of entrance, how many may reach their anticipated goal? Carry the mind forward a few years, and some have climbed the hills of difficulty and gained the eminence on which they wished to stand—some, although they may not have done this, have kept their truth unhurt, their integrity unspoiled; but others have turned back, or have perished by the way, or fallen in weakness of will, no more to rise again; victims of their own sin.

6. **Warning.**—As we place ourselves with the young at the opening gates of life, and think of the end from the [7]beginning, it is a deep concern more than anything else that fills us. Words of earnest argument and warning counsel rather than of congratulation rise to our lips.

7. **Mistakes Are Often Fatal.**—Begin well, and the habit of doing well will become quite as easy as the habit of doing badly. "Well begun is half ended," says the proverb; "and a good beginning is half the battle." Many promising young men have irretrievably injured themselves by a first false step at the commencement of life; while others, of much less promising talents, have succeeded simply by beginning well, and going onward. The good, practical beginning is, to a certain extent, a pledge, a promise, and an assurance of the ultimate prosperous issue. There is many a poor creature, now crawling through life, miserable himself and the cause of sorrow to others, who might have lifted up his head and prospered, if, instead of merely satisfying himself with resolutions of well-doing, he had actually gone to work and made a good, practical beginning.

8. **Begin at the Right Place.**—Too many are, however, impatient of results. They are not satisfied to begin where their fathers did, but where they left off. They think to enjoy the fruits of industry without working for them. They cannot wait for the results of labor and application, but forestall them by too early indulgence.

SOLID COMFORT AND GOOD HEALTH.
Health a Duty.

Perhaps nothing will so much hasten the time when body and mind will both be adequately cared for, as a diffusion of the belief that the preservation of health is a duty. Few seem conscious that there is such a thing as physical morality.

Men's habitual words and acts imply that they are at liberty to treat their bodies as they please. Disorder entailed by disobedience to nature's dictates they regard as grievances, not as the effects of a conduct more or less flagitious. Though the evil consequences inflicted on their descendents and on future generations are often as great as those caused by crime, they do not think themselves in any degree criminal.

It is true that in the case of drunkenness the viciousness of a bodily transgression is recognized; but none appear to infer that if this bodily transgression is vicious, so, too, is[8]every bodily transgression. The fact is, all breaches of the law of health are physical sins.

When this is generally seen, then, and perhaps not till then, will the physical training of the young receive all the attention it deserves.

Purity of life and thought should be taught in the home. It is the only safeguard of the young. Let parents wake up on this important subject.

2

Value of Reputation.

1. Who Shall Estimate the Cost.—Who shall estimate the cost of a priceless reputation—that impress which gives this human dross its currency—without which we stand despised, debased, depreciated? Who shall repair it injured? Who can redeem it lost? Oh, well and truly does the great philosopher of poetry esteem the world's wealth as "trash" in the comparison. Without it gold has no value; birth, no distinction; station, no dignity; beauty, no charm; age, no reverence; without it every treasure impoverishes, every grace deforms, every dignity degrades, and all the arts, the decorations and accomplishments of life stand, like the beacon-blaze upon a rock, warning the world that its approach is dangerous; that its contact is death.

2. The Wretch Without It.—The wretch without it is under eternal quarantine; no friend to greet; no home to harbor him, the voyage of his life becomes a joyless peril; and in the midst of all ambition can achieve, or avarice amass, or rapacity plunder, he tosses on the surge, a buoyant pestilence. But let me not degrade into selfishness of individual safety or individual exposure this individual principle; it testifies a higher, a more ennobling origin.

3. Its Divinity.—Oh, Divine, oh, delightful legacy of a spotless reputation: Rich is the inheritance it leaves; pious the example it testifies; pure, precious and imperishable, the hope which it inspires; can there be conceived a more atrocious injury than to filch from its possessor this inestimable benefit to rob society of its charm, and solitude of its solace; not only to out-law life, but attain death, converting the very grave, the refuge of the sufferer, into the gate of infamy and of shame.

4. Lost Character.—We can conceive few crimes beyond it. He who plunders my property takes from me that which can be repaired by time; but what period can repair a ruined reputation? He who maims my person effects that which medicine may remedy; but what herb has sovereignty over the wounds of slander? He who ridicules my poverty or reproaches my profession, upbraids me with that which industry may retrieve, and integrity may purify; but what riches shall redeem the bankrupt fame? What power shall blanch the sullied show of character? There can be no injury more deadly. There can be no crime more cruel. It is without remedy. It is without antidote. It is without evasion.

Influence of Associates.

If you always live with those who are lame, you will yourself learn to limp.—FROM THE LATIN.

If men wish to be held in esteem, they must associate with those who are estimable.—LA BRUYERE.

GATHERING WILD FLOWERS.

1. By What Men Are Known.—An author is known by his writings, a mother by her daughter, a fool by his words, and all men by their companions.

2. Formation of a Good Character.—Intercourse with persons of decided virtue and excellence is of great importance in the formation of a good character. The force of example is powerful; we are creatures of imitation, and, by a necessary influence, our tempers and habits are very much formed on the model of those with whom we familiarly associate. Better be alone than in bad company. Evil communications corrupt good manners. Ill qualities are catching as well as diseases; and the mind is at least as much, if not a great deal more, liable to infection, than the body. Go with mean people, and you think life is mean.

3. Good Example.—How natural is it for a child to look up to those around him for an example of imitation, and how readily does he copy all that he sees done, good or bad. The importance of a good example on which the young may exercise this powerful and active element of their nature, is a matter of the utmost moment.

4. A True Maxim.—It is a trite, but true maxim, that "a man is known by the company he keeps." He naturally assimilates by the force of imitation, to the habits and manners of those by whom he is surrounded. We know persons who walk much with the lame, who have learned to walk with a hitch or limp like their lame friends. Vice stalks in the streets unabashed, and children copy it.

5. **Live with the Culpable.**—Live with the culpable, and you will be very likely to die with the criminal. Bad company is like a nail driven into a post, which after the first or second blow, may be drawn out with little difficulty; but being once driven in up to the head, the pinchers cannot take hold to draw it out, which can only be done by the destruction of the wood. You may be ever so pure, you cannot associate with bad companions without falling into bad odor.

6. **Society of the Vulgar.**—Do you love the society of the vulgar? Then you are already debased in your sentiments. Do you seek to be with the profane? In your heart you are like them. Are jesters and buffoons your choice friends? [12]He who loves to laugh at folly, is himself a fool. Do you love and seek the society of the wise and good? Is this your habit? Had you rather take the lowest seat among these than the highest seat among others? Then you have already learned to be good. You may not make very much progress, but even a good beginning is not to be despised.

7. **Sinks of Pollution.**—Strive for mental excellence, and strict integrity, and you never will be found in the sinks of pollution, and on the benches of retailers and gamblers. Once habituate yourself to a virtuous course, once secure a love of good society, and no punishment would be greater than by accident to be obliged for half a day to associate with the low and vulgar. Try to frequent the company of your betters.

8. **Procure no Friend in Haste.**—Nor, if once secured, in haste abandon them. Be slow in choosing an associate, and slower to change him; slight no man for poverty, nor esteem any one for his wealth. Good friends should not be easily forgotten, nor used as suits of apparel, which, when we have worn them threadbare, we cast them off, and call for new. When once you profess yourself a friend, endeavor to be always such. He can never have any true friends that will be often changing them.

9. **Have the Courage to Cut the Most Agreeable Acquaintance.**—Do this when you are convinced that he lacks principle; a friend should bear with a friend's infirmities, but not with his vices. He that does a base thing in zeal for his friend, burns the golden thread that ties their hearts together.

Self-Control.

"Honor and profit do not always lie in the same sack."—GEORGE HERBERT.

"The government of one's self is the only true freedom for the individual."—FREDERICK PERTHES.

"It is length of patience, and endurance, and forebearance, that so much of what is called good in mankind and womankind is shown."—ARTHUR HELPS.

1. **Essence of Character.**—Self-control is only courage under another form. It may also be regarded as the primary essence of character. It is in virtue of this quality that Shakespeare defines man as a being "looking before and after." It forms the chief distinction between man and the mere animal; and, indeed, there can be no true manhood without it.

THE RESULT OF BAD COMPANY.

2. **Root of all the Virtues.**—Self-control is at the root [14]of all the virtues. Let a man give the reins to his impulses and passions, and from that moment he yields up his moral freedom. He is carried along the current of life, and becomes the slave of his strongest desire for the time being.

3. **Resist Instinctive Impulse.**—To be morally free—to be more than an animal—man must be able to resist instinctive impulse, and this can only be done by exercise of self-control. Thus it is this power which constitutes the real distinction between a physical and a moral life, and that forms the primary basis of individual character.

4. **A Strong Man Ruleth His Own Spirit.**—In the Bible praise is given, not to a strong man who "taketh a city," but to the stronger man who "ruleth his own spirit." This stronger man is he who, by discipline, exercises a constant control over his thoughts, his speech, and his acts. Nine-tenths of the vicious desires that degrade society, and which, when indulged, swell into the crimes that disgrace it, would shrink into insignificance before

the advance of valiant self-discipline, self-respect, and self-control. By the watchful exercise of these virtues, purity of heart and mind become habitual, and the character is built up in chastity, virtue, and temperance.

5. **The Best Support.**—The best support of character will always be found in habit, which, according as the will is directed rightly or wrongly, as the case may be, will prove either a benignant ruler, or a cruel despot. We may be its willing subject on the one hand, or its servile slave on the other. It may help us on the road to good, or it may hurry us on the road to ruin.

6. **The Ideal Man.**—"In the supremacy of self-control," says Herbert Spencer, "consists one of the perfections of the ideal man. Not to be impulsive, not to be spurred hither and thither by each desire that in turn comes uppermost, but to be self-restrained, self-balanced, governed by the joint decision of the feelings in council assembled, before whom every action shall have been fully debated, and calmly determined—that it is which education, moral education at least, strives to produce."

7. **The Best Regulated Home.**—The best regulated home is always that in which the discipline is the most perfect, and yet where it is the least felt. Moral discipline acts with the force of a law of nature. Those subject to it yield themselves to it unconsciously; and though it shapes and forms the whole character, until the life becomes crystallized in habit, the influence thus exercised is for the most part unseen, and almost unfelt.[15]

8. **Practice Self-denial.**—If a man would get through life honorably and peaceably, he must necessarily learn to practice self-denial in small things as well as in great. Men have to bear as well as to forbear. The temper has to be held in subjection to the judgment; and the little demons of ill-humor, petulance, and sarcasm, kept resolutely at a distance. If once they find an entrance to the mind, they are apt to return, and to establish for themselves a permanent occupation there.

9. **Power of Words.**—It is necessary to one's personal happiness, to exercise control over one's words as well as acts: for there are words that strike even harder than blows; and men may "speak daggers," though they use none. The stinging repartee that rises to the lips, and which, if uttered, might cover an adversary with confusion, how difficult it is to resist saying it! "Heaven, keep us," says Miss Bremer, in her 'Home', "from the destroying power of words! There are words that sever hearts more than sharp swords do; there are words the point of which sting the heart through the course of a whole life."

10. **Character Exhibits Itself.**—Character exhibits itself in self-control of speech as much as in anything else. The wise and forbearant man will restrain his desire to say a smart or severe thing at the expense of another's feeling; while the fool blurts out what he thinks, and will sacrifice his friend rather than his joke. "The mouth of a wise man," said Solomon, "is in his heart: the heart of a fool is in his mouth."

11. **Burns.**—No one knew the value of self-control better than the poet Burns, and no one could teach it more eloquently to others, but when it came to practice, Burns was as weak as the weakest. He could not deny himself the pleasure of uttering a harsh and clever sarcasm at another's expense. One of his biographers observed of him, that it was no extravagant arithmetic to say that for every ten jokes he made himself a hundred enemies. But this was not all. Poor Burns exercised no control over his appetites, but freely gave them the rein:

"Thus thoughtless follies laid him low,
And stained his name."

LOST SELF-CONTROL.

12. **Sow Pollution.**—Nor had he the self-denial to resist giving publicity to compositions originally intended for the delight of the tap-room, but which continued secretly to sow pollution broadcast in the minds of youth. Indeed, notwithstanding the many exquisite poems of this writer, it is not saying too much that his immoral writings have done far more harm than his purer writings have done good; and [16]it would be better that all his writings should be destroyed and forgotten, provided his indecent songs could be destroyed with them.

13. **Moral Principle.**—Many of our young men lack moral principle. They cannot look upon a beautiful girl with a pure heart and pure thoughts. They have not manifested or

practiced that self-control which develops true manhood, and brings into subordination evil thoughts, evil passions, and evil practices. Men who have no self-control will find life a failure, both in a social and in a business sense. The world despises an insignificant person who lacks backbone and character. Stand upon your manhood and womanhood; honor your convictions, and dare to do right.

14. **Strong Drink.**—There is the habit of strong drink. It is only the lack of self-control that brings men into the depths of degradation; on account of the cup, the habit of taking drink occasionally in its milder forms—of playing with a small appetite that only needs sufficient playing with to make you a demon or a dolt. You think you are safe; I know you are not safe, if you drink at all; and when you get offended with the good friends that warn you of your danger, you are a fool. I know that the grave swallows daily, by scores, drunkards, every one of whom thought he was safe while he was forming his appetite. But this is old talk. A young man in this age who forms the habit of drinking, or puts himself in danger of forming the habit, is usually so weak that it doesn't pay to save him.

[17]

Habit.

It is almost as difficult to make a man unlearn his Errors as his Knowledge.—COLTON.

There are habits contracted by bad example, or bad management, before we have judgment to discern their approaches, or because the eye of Reason is laid asleep, or has not compass of view sufficient to look around on every quarter.—TUCKER.

1. **Habit.**—Our real strength in life depends upon habits formed in early life. The young man who sows his wild oats and indulges in the social cup, is fastening chains upon himself that never can be broken. The innocent youth by solitary practice of self-abuse will fasten upon himself a habit which will wreck his physical constitution and bring suffering and misery and ruin. Young man and young woman, beware of bad habits formed in early life.

2. **A Bundle of Habits.**—Man, it has been said, is a bundle of habits; and habit is second nature. Metastasio entertained so strong an opinion as to the power of repetition in act and thought, that he said, "All is habit in mankind, even virtue itself." Evil habits must be conquered, or they will conquer us and destroy our peace and happiness.

3. **Vicious Habits.**—Vicious habits, when opposed, offer the most vigorous resistence on the first attack. At each successive encounter this resistence grows fainter and fainter, until finally it ceases altogether and the victory is achieved. Habit is man's best friend and worst enemy; it can exalt him to the highest pinnacle of virtue, honor and happiness, or sink him to the lowest depths of vice, shame and misery.

4. **Honesty, or Knavery.**—We may form habits of honesty, or knavery; truth, or falsehood; of industry, or idleness; frugality, or extravagance; of patience, or impatience; self-denial, or self-indulgence; of kindness, cruelty, politeness, rudeness, prudence, perseverance, circumspection; in short, there is not a virtue, nor a vice; not an act of body, nor of mind, to which we may not be chained down by this despotic power.

5. **Begin Well.**—It is a great point for young men to begin well; for it is the beginning of life that that system of conduct is adopted which soon assumes the force of habit. Begin well, and the habit of doing well will become quite easy, as easy as the habit of doing badly. Pitch upon that course of life which is the most excellent, and habit will render it the most delightful.

[18]

A Good Name.

1. **The Longing for a Good Name.**—The longing for a good name is one of those laws of nature that were passed for the soul and written down within to urge toward a life of action, and away from small or wicked action. So large is this passion that it is set forth in poetic thought, as having a temple grand as that of Jupiter or Minerva, and up whose marble steps all noble minds struggle—the temple of Fame.

2. **Civilization.**—Civilization is the ocean of which the millions of individuals are the rivers and torrents. These rivers and torrents swell with those rains of money and home and fame and happiness, and then fall and run almost dry, but the ocean of civilization has gathered up all these waters, and holds them in sparkling beauty for all subsequent use. Civilization is a fertile delta made by the drifting souls of men.

3. **Fame.**—The word "fame" never signifies simply notoriety. The meaning of the direct term may be seen from its negation or opposite, for only the meanest of men are called infamous. They are utterly without fame, utterly nameless; but if fame implied only notoriety then infamous would possess no marked significance. Fame is an undertaker that pays but little attention to the living, but who bedizens the dead, furnishes out their funerals and follows them to the grave.

4. **Life-Motive.**—So in studying that life-motive which is called a "good name," we must ask the large human race to tell us the high merit of this spiritual longing. We must read the words of the sage, who said long centuries ago that "a good name was rather chosen than great riches." Other sages have said as much. Solon said that "He that will sell his good name will sell the State." Socrates said, "Fame is the perfume of heroic deeds." Our Shakspeare said, "He lives in fame who died in virtue's cause."

5. **Influences of Our Age.**—Our age is deeply influenced by the motives called property and home and pleasure, but it is a question whether the generation in action to-day and the generation on the threshold of this intense life are conscious fully of the worth of an honorable name.

6. **Beauty of Character.**—We do not know whether with us all a good name is less sweet than it was with our fathers, but this is painfully evident, that our times do not sufficiently behold the beauty of character—their sense does not [19]detect quickly enough or love deeply enough this aroma of heroic deeds.

7. **Selling Out Their Reputation.**—It is amazing what multitudes there are who are willing to sell out their reputation, and amazing at what a low price they will make the painful exchange. Some king remarked that he would not tell a lie for any reward less than an empire. It is not uncommon in our world for a man to sell out all his honor and hopes for a score or a half score of dollars.

8. **Prisons Overflowing.**—Our prisons are all full to overflowing of those who took no thought of honor. They have not waited for an empire to be offered them before they would violate the sacred rights of man, but many of them have even murdered for a cause that would not have justified even an exchange of words.

9. **Integrity the Pride of the Government.**—If integrity were made the pride of the government, the love of it would soon spring up among the people. If all fraudulent men should go straight to jail, pitilessly, and if all the most rigid characters were sought out for all political and commercial offices, there would soon come a popular honesty just as there has come a love of reading or of art. It is with character as with any new article—the difficulty lies in its first introduction.

10. **A New Virtue.**—May a new virtue come into favor, all our high rewards, those from the ballot-box, those from employers, the rewards of society, the rewards of the press, should be offered only to the worthy. A few years of rewarding the worthy would result in a wonderful zeal in the young to build up, not physical property, but mental and spiritual worth.

AN ARAB PRINCESS.

11. **Blessing the Family Group.**—No young man or young woman can by industry and care reach an eminence in study or art or character, without blessing the entire family group. We have all seen that the father and mother feel that all life's care and labor were at last perfectly rewarded in the success of their child. But had the child been reckless or indolent, all this domestic joy—the joy of a large group—would have been blighted forever.

12. **An Honored Child.**—There have been triumphs at old Rome, where victors marched along with many a chariot, many an elephant, and many spoils of the East; and in all times money has been lavished in the efforts of States to tell their pleasure in the name of some general; but more numerous and wide-spread and beyond expression, by chariot or cannon or drum, have been those triumphal [20]hours, when some son or daughter has

7

returned to the parental hearth beautiful in the wreaths of some confessed excellence, bearing a good name.

13. Rich Criminals.—We looked at the utter wretchedness of the men who threw away reputation, and would rather be rich criminals in exile than be loved friends and persons at home.

14. An Empty, or an Evil Name.—Young and old cannot afford to bear the burden of an empty or an evil name. A good name is a motive of life. It is a reason for that great encampment we call an existence. While you are building the home of to-morrow, build up also that kind of soul that can sleep sweetly on home's pillow, and can feel that God is not near as an avenger of wrong, but as the Father not only of the verdure and the seasons, but of you. Live a pure life and bear a good name, and your reward will be sure and great.

[21]
The Mother's Influence.

Mother, O mother, my heart calls for you,
Many a Summer the grass has grown green,
Blossomed and faded, our faces between;
Yet with strong yearning and passionate pain,
Long I to-night for your presence again.—*Elizabeth Akers Allen.*
A mother is a mother still,
The holiest thing alive.—*Coleridge.*
There is none,
In all this cold and hollow world, no fount
Of deep, strong, deathless love, save that within
A mother's heart.—*Mrs. Hemans.*
And all my mother came into mine eyes,
And gave me up to tears.—*Shakespeare.*

A PRAYERFUL AND DEVOTED MOTHER.

1. Her Influence.—It is true to nature, although it be expressed in a figurative form, that a mother is both the morning and the evening star of life. The light of her eye is always the first to rise, and often the last to set upon man's day of trial. She wields a power more decisive far than syllogisms in argument or courts of last appeal in authority.

2. Her Love.—Mother! ecstatic sound so twined round our hearts that they must cease to throb ere we forget it; 'tis our first love; 'tis part of religion. Nature has set the mother upon such a pinnacle that our infant eyes and arms are first uplifted to it; we cling to it in manhood; we almost worship it in old age.

3. Her Tenderness.—Alas! how little do we appreciate a mother's tenderness while living. How heedless are we in youth of all her anxieties and kindness! But when she is dead and gone, when the cares and coldness of the world come withering to our hearts, when we experience for ourselves how hard it is to find true sympathy, how few to love us, how few will befriend us in misfortune, then it is that we think of the mother we have lost.

4. Her Controlling Power.—The mother can take man's whole nature under her control. She becomes what she has been called, "The Divinity of Infancy." Her smile is its sunshine, her word its mildest law, until sin and the world have steeled the heart.

[22]
5. The Last Tie.—The young man who has forsaken the advice and influence of his mother has broken the last cable and severed the last tie that binds him to an honorable and upright life. He has forsaken his best friend, and every hope for his future welfare may be abandoned, for he is lost forever. If he is faithless to mother, he will have but little respect for wife and children.

6. Home Ties.—The young man or young woman who love their home and love their mother can be safely trusted under almost any and all circumstances, and their life will not be a blank, for they seek what is good. Their hearts will be ennobled, and God will bless them.

Home Power.

"The mill-streams that turn the clappers of the world arise in solitary places."—
HELPS.

"Lord! with what care hast Thou begirt us round!
Parents first season us. Then schoolmasters
Deliver us to laws. They send us bound
To rules of reason."—GEORGE HERBERT.

HOME AMUSEMENT.

1. **School of Character.**—Home is the first and most important school of character. It is there that every human being receives his best moral training, or his worst, for it is there that he imbibes those principles of conduct which endure through manhood, and cease only with life.

2. **Home Makes the Man.**—It is a common saying, "Manners make the man;" and there is a second, that "Mind makes the man;" but truer than either is a third, that "Home makes the man." For the home-training includes not only manners and mind, but character. It is mainly in the home that the heart is opened, the habits are formed, the intellect is awakened, and character moulded for good or for evil.

3. **Govern Society.**—From that source, be it pure or impure, issue the principles and maxims that govern society. Law itself is but the reflex of homes. The tiniest bits of opinion sown in the minds of children in private life afterwards issue forth to the world, and become its public opinion; for nations are gathered out of nurseries, and they who hold the leading-strings of children may even exercise a greater power than those who wield the reins of government.

4. **The Child Is Father of the Man.**—The child's character is the nucleus of the man's; all after-education is but superposition; the form of the crystal remains the same. Thus the saying of the poet holds true in a large degree, "The child is father of the man;" or as Milton puts it, "The childhood shows the man, as morning shows the day." Those impulses to conduct which last the longest and are rooted the deepest, always have their origin near our birth. It is then that the germs of virtues or vices, of feelings or sentiments, are first implanted which determine the character of life.

5. **Nurseries.**—Thus homes, which are nurseries of children who grow up into men and women, will be good or bad according to the power that governs them. Where the spirit of love and duty pervades the home, where head and heart bear rule wisely there, where the daily life is honest and virtuous, where the government is sensible, kind, and loving, then may we expect from such a home an issue of healthy, useful, and happy beings, capable as they gain the requisite strength, of following the footsteps of their parents, of walking uprightly, governing themselves wisely, and contributing to the welfare of those about them.

6. **Ignorance, Coarseness, and Selfishness.**—On the other hand, if surrounded by ignorance, coarseness, and selfishness, they will unconsciously assume the same character, and grow up to adult years rude, uncultivated, and all the more dangerous to society if placed amidst the manifold temptations of what is called civilized life. "Give your child to be educated by a slave," said an ancient Greek, "and, instead of one slave, you will then have two."

7. **Maternal Love.**—Maternal love is the visible providence of our race. Its influence is constant and universal. It begins with the education of the human being at the outstart of life, and is prolonged by virtue of the powerful influence which every good mother exercises over her children through life. When launched into the world, each to take part in its labors, anxieties, and trials, they still turn [25]to their mother for consolation, if not for counsel, in their time of trouble and difficulty. The pure and good thoughts she has implanted in their minds when children continue to grow up into good acts long after she is dead; and when there is nothing but a memory of her left, her children rise up and call her blessed.

8. **Woman, above All Other Educators**, educates humanly. Man is the brain, but woman is the heart of humanity; he its judgment, she its feeling; he its strength, she its grace,

9

ornament, and solace. Even the understanding of the best woman seems to work mainly through her affections. And thus, though man may direct the intellect, woman cultivates the feelings, which mainly determine the character. While he fills the memory, she occupies the heart. She makes us love what he can make us only believe, and it is chiefly through her that we are enabled to arrive at virtue.

9. **The Poorest Dwelling**, presided over by a virtuous, thrifty, cheerful, and cleanly woman, may thus be the abode of comfort, virtue, and happiness; it may be the scene of every ennobling relation in family life; it may be endeared to man by many delightful associations; furnishing a sanctuary for the heart, a refuge from the storms of life, a sweet resting-place after labor, a consolation in misfortune, a pride in prosperity, and a joy at all times.

10. **The Good Home Is Thus the Best of Schools**, not only in youth but in age. There young and old best learn cheerfulness, patience, self-control, and the spirit of service and of duty. The home is the true school of courtesy, of which woman is always the best practical instructor. "Without woman," says the Provencal proverb, "men were but ill-licked cubs." Philanthropy radiates from the home as from a centre. "To love the little platoon we belong to in society," said Burke, "is the germ of all public affections." The wisest and best have not been ashamed to own it to be their greatest joy and happiness to sit "behind the heads of children" in the inviolable circle of home.

[26]

To Young Women.
MEDITATION.

1. **To Be a Woman**, in the truest and highest sense of the word, is to be the best thing beneath the skies. To be a woman is something more than to live eighteen or twenty years; something more than to grow to the physical stature of women; something more than to wear flounces, exhibit dry goods, sport jewelry, catch the gaze of lewd-eyed men; [27]something more than to be a belle, a wife, or a mother. Put all these qualifications together and they do but little toward making a true woman.

2. **Beauty and Style** are not the surest passports to womanhood—some of the noblest specimens of womanhood that the world has ever seen have presented the plainest and most unprepossessing appearance. A woman's worth is to be estimated by the real goodness of her heart, the greatness of her soul, and the purity and sweetness of her character; and a woman with a kindly disposition and well-balanced temper is both lovely and attractive, be her face ever so plain, and her figure ever so homely; she makes the best of wives and the truest of mothers.

3. **Beauty Is a Dangerous Gift.**—It is even so. Like wealth, it has ruined its thousands. Thousands of the most beautiful women are destitute of common sense and common humanity. No gift from heaven is so general and so widely abused by woman as the gift of beauty. In about nine cases in ten it makes her silly, senseless, thoughtless, giddy, vain, proud, frivolous, selfish, low and mean. I think I have seen more girls spoiled by beauty than by any other one thing. "She is beautiful, and she knows it," is as much as to say that she is spoiled. A beautiful girl is very likely to believe she was made to be looked at; and so she sets herself up for a show at every window, in every door, on every corner of the street, in every company at which opportunity offers for an exhibition of herself.

4. **Beware of Beautiful Women.**—These facts have long since taught sensible men to beware of beautiful women—to sound them carefully before they give them their confidence. Beauty is shallow—only skin deep; fleeting—only for a few years' reign; dangerous—tempting to vanity and lightness of mind; deceitful—dazzling often to bewilder; weak—reigning only to ruin; gross—leading often to sensual pleasure. And yet we say it need not be so. Beauty is lovely and ought to be innocently possessed. It has charms which ought to be used for good purposes. It is a delightful gift, which ought to be received with gratitude and worn with grace and meekness. It should always minister to inward beauty. Every woman of beautiful form and features should cultivate a beautiful mind and heart.

5. **Rival the Boys.**—We want the girls to rival the boys in all that is good, and refined, and ennobling. We want them to rival the boys, as they well can, in learning, in

understanding, in virtues; in all noble qualities of mind and heart, but not in any of those things that have caused them, justly or unjustly, to be described as savages. We want [28]the girls to be gentle—not weak, but gentle, and kind and affectionate. We want to be sure, that wherever a girl is, there should be a sweet, subduing and harmonizing influence of purity, and truth, and love, pervading and hallowing, from center to circumference, the entire circle in which she moves. If the boys are savages, we want her to be their civilizer. We want her to tame them, to subdue their ferocity, to soften their manners, and to teach them all needful lessons of order, sobriety, and meekness, and patience, and goodness.

6. **Kindness.**—Kindness is the ornament of man—it is the chief glory of woman—it is, indeed, woman's true prerogative—her sceptre and her crown. It is the sword with which she conquers, and the charm with which she captivates.

7. **Admired and Beloved.**—Young lady, would you be admired and beloved? Would you be an ornament to your sex, and a blessing to your race? Cultivate this heavenly virtue. Wealth may surround you with its blandishments, and beauty, and learning, or talents, may give you admirers, but love and kindness alone can captivate the heart. Whether you live in a cottage or a palace, these graces can surround you with perpetual sunshine, making you, and all around you, happy.

8. **Inward Grace.**—Seek ye then, fair daughters, the possession of that inward grace, whose essence shall permeate and vitalize the affections, adorn the countenance, make mellifluous the voice, and impart a hallowed beauty even to your motions. Not merely that you may be loved, would I urge this, but that you may, in truth, be lovely—that loveliness which fades not with time, nor is marred or alienated by disease, but which neither chance nor change can in any way despoil.

9. **Silken Enticements of the Stranger.**—We urge you, gentle maiden, to beware of the silken enticements of the stranger, until your love is confirmed by protracted acquaintance. Shun the idler, though his coffers overflow with pelf. Avoid the irreverent—the scoffer of hallowed things; and him who "looks upon the wine while it is red;" him too, "who hath a high look and a proud heart," and who "privily slandereth his neighbor." Do not heed the specious prattle about "first love," and so place, irrevocably, the seal upon your future destiny, before you have sounded, in silence and secrecy, the deep fountains of your own heart. Wait, rather, until your own character and that of him who would woo you, is more fully developed. Surely, if this "first love" cannot endure a short probation, fortified by "the [29]pleasures of hope," how can it be expected to survive years of intimacy, scenes of trial, distracting cares, wasting sickness, and all the homely routine of practical life? Yet it is these that constitute life, and the love that cannot abide them is false and must die.

[30]
Influence of Female Character.
ROMAN LADIES.

1. **Moral Effect.**—It is in its moral effect on the mind and the heart of man, that the influence of woman is most powerful and important. In the diversity of tastes, habits, inclinations, and pursuits of the two sexes, is found a most beneficent provision for controlling the force and extravagance of human passion. The objects which most strongly seize and stimulate the mind of man, rarely act at the same time and with equal power on the mind of woman. She is naturally better, purer, and more chaste in thought and language.

2. **Female Character.**—But the influence of female character on the virtue of men, is not seen merely in restraining and softening the violence of human passion. To her is mainly committed the task of pouring into the opening mind of infancy its first impressions of duty, and of stamping on its susceptible heart the first image of its God. Who will not confess the influence of a mother in forming the heart of a child? What man is there who can not trace the origin of many of the best maxims of his life to the lips of her who gave him birth? How wide, how lasting, how sacred is that part of a woman's influence.

3. **Virtue of a Community.**—There is yet another mode, by which woman may exert a powerful influence on the virtue of a community. It rests with her in a pre-eminent degree, to give tone and elevation to the moral character of the age, by deciding the degree of virtue that shall be necessary to afford a passport to her society. If all the favor of woman were

given only to the good, if it were known that the charms and attractions of beauty, and wisdom, and wit, were reserved only for the pure; if, in one word, something of a similar rigor were exerted to exclude the profligate and abandoned of society, as is shown to those who have fallen from virtue,—how much would be done to re-enforce the motives to moral purity among us, and impress on the minds of all a reverence for the sanctity and obligations of virtue.

4. **The Influence of Woman on the Moral Sentiments.**—The influence of woman on the moral sentiments of society is intimately connected with her influence on its religious character; for religion and a pure and elevated morality must ever stand in the relation to each other of effect and cause. The heart of a woman is formed for the abode of sacred truth; and for the reasons alike honorable to her character and to that of society. From the nature of humanity this must be so, or the race would soon degenerate, and moral contagion eat out the heart of society. The purity of home is the safeguard to American manhood.

[31]
Personal Purity.
"Self-reverence, self-knowledge, self-control,
These three alone lead life to sovereign power."—TENNYSON.

1. **Words of the Great Teacher.**—Mark the words of the Great Teacher: "If thy right hand or foot cause thee to fall, cut it off and cast it from thee. If thy right eye cause thee to fall, pluck it out. It is better for thee to enter into life maimed and halt, than having two eyes to be cast into hell-fire, where the worm dieth not, and the fire is not quenched."

2. **A Melancholy Fact.**—It is a melancholy fact, in human experience, that the noblest gifts which men possess are constantly prostituted to other purposes than those for which they are designed. The most valuable and useful organs of the body are those which are capable of the greatest dishonor, abuse, and corruption. What a snare the wonderful organism of the eye may become, when used to read corrupt books, or to look upon licentious pictures, or vulgar theater scenes, or when used to meet the fascinating gaze of the harlot! What an instrument for depraving the whole man may be found in the matchless powers of the brain, the hand, the mouth, or the tongue! What potent instruments may these become in accomplishing the ruin of the whole being, for time and eternity![32]

3. **Abstinence.**—Some can testify with thankfulness that they never knew the sins of gambling, drunkenness, fornication, or adultery. In all these cases abstinence has been, and continues to be, liberty. Restraint is the noblest freedom. No man can affirm that self-denial ever injured him; on the contrary, self-restraint has been liberty, strength and blessing. Solemnly ask young men to remember this when temptation and passion strive as a floodtide to move them from the anchorage and peace of self-restraint. Beware of the deceitful stream of temporary gratification, whose eddying current drifts towards license, shame, disease and death. Remember how quickly moral power declines, how rapidly the edge of the fatal maelstrom is reached, how near the vortex, how terrible the penalty, how fearful the sentence of everlasting punishment!

4. **Frank Discussion.**—The time has arrived for a full and frank discussion of those things which affect the personal purity. Thousands are suffering to-day from various weaknesses, the causes of which they have never learned. Manly vigor is not increasing with that rapidity which a Christian age demands. Means of dissipation are on the increase. It is high time, therefore, that every lover of the race should call a halt, and inquire into the condition of things. Excessive modesty on this subject is not virtue. Timidity in presenting unpleasant but important truths has permitted untold damage in every age.

5. **Man Is a Careless Being.**—He is very much inclined to sinful things. He more often does that which is wrong than that which is right, because it is easier, and, for the moment, perhaps, more satisfying to the flesh. The Creator is often blamed for man's weaknesses and inconsistencies. This is wrong. God did not intend that we should be mere machines, but free moral agents. We are privileged to choose between good and evil. Hence,

if we perseveringly choose the latter, and make a miserable failure of life, we should blame only ourselves.

6. **The Pulpit.**—Would that every pulpit in the land might join hands with the medical profession and cry out with no uncertain sound against the mighty evils herein stigmatized! It would work a revolution for which coming society could never cease to be grateful.

7. **Strive to Attain a Higher Life.**—Strive to attain unto a higher and better life. Beware of all excesses, of whatever nature, and guard your personal purity with sacred determination. Let every aspiration be upward, and be strong in every good resolution. Seek the light, for in light there is life, while in darkness there is decay and death.[33]

CONFIDENCE THAT SOMETIMES MAKES TROUBLE.

[34]

How to Write All Kinds of Letters.

1. From the President in his cabinet to the laborer in the street; from the lady in her parlor to the servant in her kitchen; from the millionaire to the beggar; from the emigrant to the settler; from every country and under every combination of circumstances, letter writing in all its forms and varieties is most important to the advancement, welfare and happiness of the human family.

2. **Education.**—The art of conveying thought through the medium of written language is so valuable and so necessary, a thorough knowledge of the practice must be desirable to every one. For merely to write a good letter requires the exercise of much of the education and talent of any writer.

3. **A Good Letter.**—A good letter must be correct in every mechanical detail, finished in style, interesting in substance, and intelligible in construction. Few there are who do not need write them; yet a letter perfect in detail is rarer than any other specimen of composition.

4. **Penmanship.**—It is folly to suppose that the faculty for writing a good hand is confined to any particular persons. There is no one who can write at all, but what can write well, if only the necessary pains are practiced. Practice makes perfect. Secure a few copy books and write an hour each day. You will soon write a good hand.[35]

5. **Write Plainly.**—Every word of even the most trifling document should be written in such clear characters that it would be impossible to mistake it for another word, or the writer may find himself in the position of the Eastern merchant who, writing to the Indies for five thousand mangoes, received by the next vessel five hundred monkies, with a promise of more in the next cargo.

6. **Haste.**—Hurry is no excuse for bad writing, because any one of sense knows that everything hurried is liable to be ruined. Dispatch may be acquired, but hurry will ruin everything. If, however, you must write slowly to write well, then be careful not to hurry at all, for the few moments you will gain by rapid writing will never compensate you for the disgrace of sending an ill-written letter.

7. **Neatness.**—Neatness is also of great importance. A fair white sheet with handsomely written words will be more welcome to any reader than a blotted, bedaubed page covered with erasures and dirt, even if the matter in each be of equal value and interest. Erasures, blots, interlineations always spoil the beauty of any letter.

8. **Bad Spelling.**—When those who from faulty education, or forgetfulness are doubtful about the correct spelling of any word, it is best to keep a dictionary at hand, and refer to it upon such occasions. It is far better to spend a few moments in seeking for a doubtful word, than to dispatch an ill-spelled letter, and the search will probably impress the spelling upon the mind for a future occasion.

9. **Carelessness.**—Incorrect spelling will expose the most important or interesting letter to the severest sarcasm and ridicule. However perfect in all other respects, no epistle that is badly spelled will be regarded as the work of an educated gentleman or lady. Carelessness will never be considered, and to be ignorant of spelling is to expose an imperfect education at once.

10. **An Excellent Practice.**—After writing a letter, read it over carefully, correct all the errors and re-write it. If you desire to become a good letter writer, improve your penmanship, improve your language and grammar, re-writing once or twice every letter that you have occasion to write, whether on social or business subjects.

11. **Punctuation.**—A good rule for punctuation is to punctuate where the sense requires it, after writing a letter and reading it over carefully you will see where the punctuation marks are required, you can readily determine where the sense requires it, so that your letter will convey the desired meaning.[36]

12. **Correspondence.**—There is no better school or better source for self-improvement than a pleasant correspondence between friends. It is not at all difficult to secure a good list of correspondents if desired. The young people who take advantage of such opportunities for self-improvement will be much more popular in the community and in society. Letter writing cultivates the habit of study; it cultivates the mind, the heart, and stimulates self-improvement in general.

13. **Folding.**—Another bad practice with those unaccustomed to corresponding is to fold the sheet of writing in such a fantastic manner as to cause the receiver much annoyance in opening it. To the sender it may appear a very ingenious performance, but to the receiver it is only a source of vexation and annoyance, and may prevent the communication receiving the attention it would otherwise merit.

14. **Simple Style.**—The style of letter writing should be simple and unaffected, not raised on stilts and indulging in pedantic displays which are mostly regarded as cloaks of ignorance. Repeated literary quotations, involved sentences, long-sounding words and scraps of Latin, French and other languages are, generally speaking, out of place, and should not be indulged in.

15. **The Result.**—A well written letter has opened the way to prosperity for many a one, has led to many a happy marriage and constant friendship, and has secured many a good service in time of need; for it is in some measure a photograph of the writer, and may inspire love or hatred, regard or aversion in the reader, just as the glimpse of a portrait often determine us, in our estimate, of the worth of the person represented. Therefore, one of the roads to fortune runs through the ink bottle, and if we want to attain a certain end in love, friendship or business, we must trace out the route correctly with the pen in our hand.

[37]

HOW TO WRITE A LOVE LETTER.

1. **Love.**—There is no greater or more profound reality than love. Why that reality should be obscured by mere sentimentalism, with all its train of absurdities is incomprehensible. There is no nobler possession than the love of another. There is no higher gift from one human being to another than love. The gift and the possession are true sanctifiers of life, and should be worn as precious jewels without affectation and without bashfulness. For this reason there is nothing to be ashamed of in a love letter, provided it be sincere.

2. **Forfeits.**—No man need consider that he forfeits dignity if he speaks with his whole heart: no woman need fear she forfeits her womanly attributes if she responds as her heart bids her respond. "Perfect love casteth out fear" is as true now as when the maxim was first given to the world.

3. **Telling Their Love.**—The generality of the sex is love to be loved: how are they to know the fact that they [38]are loved unless they are told? To write a sensible love letter requires more talent than to solve, with your pen, a profound problem in philosophy. Lovers must not then expect much from each other's epistles.

4. **Confidential.**—Ladies and gentlemen who correspond with each other should never be guilty of exposing any of the contents of any letters written expressing confidence, attachment or love. The man who confides in a lady and honors her with his confidence should be treated with perfect security and respect, and those who delight in showing their confidential letters to others are unworthy, heartless and unsafe companions.

5. **Return of Letters.**—If letters were written under circumstances which no longer exist and all confidential relations are at an end, then all letters should be promptly returned.

6. **How to Begin a Love Letter.**—How to begin a love letter has been no doubt the problem of lovers and suitors of all ages and nations. Fancy the youth of Young America with lifted pen, thinking how he shall address his beloved. Much depends upon this letter. What shall he say, and how shall he say it, is the great question. Perseverance, however, will solve the problem and determine results.

7. **Forms of Beginning a Love Letter.**—Never say, "My Dearest Nellie," "My Adored Nellie," or "My Darling Nellie," until Nellie has first called you "My Dear," or has given you to understand that such familiar terms are permissible. As a rule a gentleman will never err if he says "Dear Miss Nellie," and if the letters are cordially reciprocated the "Miss" may in time be omitted, or other familiar terms used instead. In addressing a widow "Dear Madam," or, "My Dear Madam," will be a proper form until sufficient intimacy will justify the use of other terms.

8. **Respect.**—A lady must always be treated with respectful delicacy, and a gentleman should never use the term "Dear" or "My Dear" under any circumstances unless he knows it is perfectly acceptable or a long and friendly acquaintance justifies it.

9. **How to Finish a Letter.**—A letter will be suggested by the remarks on how to begin one. "Yours respectfully," "Yours truly," "Yours sincerely," "Yours affectionately," "Yours ever affectionately," "Yours most affectionately," "Ever yours," "Ever your own," or "Yours," are all appropriate, each depending upon the beginning of the letter. It is difficult to see any phrase which could be added to them which would carry more meaning than they [39]contain. People can sign themselves "adorers" and such like, but they do so at the peril of good taste. It is not good that men or women "worship" each other—if they succeed in preserving reciprocal love and esteem they will have cause for great contentment.

10. **Permission.**—No young man should ever write to a young lady any letter, formal or informal, unless he has first sought her permission to do so.

11. **Special Forms.**—We give various forms or models of love letters to be *studied, not copied*. We have given no replies to the forms given, as every letter written will naturally suggest an answer. A careful study will be a great help to many who have not enjoyed the advantages of a literary education.

FORMS OF SOCIAL LETTERS.

1.—From a Young Lady to a Clergyman Asking a Recommendation.

Nantwich, May 18th, 1894.

Reverend and Dear Sir:

Having seen an advertisement for a school mistress in the Daily Times, I have been recommended to offer myself as a candidate. Will you kindly favor me [40]with a testimonial as to my character, ability and conduct while at Boston Normal School? Should you consider that I am fitted for the position, you would confer a great favor on me if you would interest yourself in my behalf.

I remain, Reverend Sir,

Your most obedient and humble servant,

LAURA B. NICHOLS.

2.—Applying for a Position as a Teacher of Music.

Scotland, Conn., January 21st, 1894.

Madam:

Seeing your advertisement in The Clarion of to-day, I write to offer my services as a teacher of music in your family.

I am a graduate of the Peabody Institute, of Baltimore, where I was thoroughly instructed in instrumental and vocal music.

I refer by permission to Mrs. A. J. Davis, 1922 Walnut Street; Mrs. Franklin Hill, 2021 Spring Garden Street, and Mrs. William Murray, 1819 Spruce Street, in whose families I have given lessons.

Hoping that you may see fit to employ me, I am,

Very respectfully yours,
NELLIE REYNOLDS.

3.—*Applying for a Situation as a Cook.*

Charlton Place, September 8th, 1894.

Madam:

Having seen your advertisement for a cook in today's Times, I beg to offer myself for your place. I am a thorough cook. I can make clear soups, entrees, jellies, and all kinds of made dishes. I can bake, and am also used to a dairy. My wages are $4 per week, and I can give good reference from my last place, in which I lived for two years. I am thirty-three years of age.

I remain, Madam,
Yours very respectfully,
MARY MOONEY.

4.—*Recommending a School Teacher.*

Ottawa, Ill., February 10th, 1894.

Col.   Geo.   H.   Haight,
President Board of Trustees, etc.

Dear Sir: I take pleasure in recommending to your favorable consideration the application of Miss Hannah Alexander for the position of teacher in the public school at Weymouth.[41]

Miss Alexander is a graduate of the Davidson Seminary, and for the past year has taught a school in this place. My children have been among her pupils, and their progress has been entirely satisfactory to me.

Miss Alexander is a strict disciplinarian, an excellent teacher, and is thoroughly competent to conduct the school for which she applies.

Trusting that you may see fit to bestow upon her the appointment she seeks, I am,
Yours very respectfully,
ALICE MILLER.

5.—*A Business Introduction.*

Chicago., Ill., May 1st, 1894.

J.   W.   Brown,
Earlville, Ill.

My Dear Sir: This will introduce to you Mr. William Channing, of this city, who visits Earlville on a matter of business, which he will explain to you in person. You can rely upon his statements, as he is a gentleman of high character, and should you be able to render him any assistance, it would be greatly appreciated by
Yours truly,
HAIGHT LARABEE.

6.—*Introducing One Lady to Another.*

Dundee, Tenn., May 5th, 1894.

Dear Mary:

Allow me to introduce to you my ever dear friend, Miss Nellie Reynolds, the bearer of this letter. You have heard me speak of her so often that you will know at once who she is. As I am sure you will be mutually pleased with each other, I have asked her to inform you of her presence in your city. Any attention you may show her will be highly appreciated by
Yours affectionately,
LIZZIE EICHER.

7.—*To a Lady, Apologizing for a Broken Engagement.*

Albany, N. Y., May 10th, 1894.

My Dear Miss Lee:

Permit me to explain my failure to keep my appointment with you this evening. I was on my way to your house, with the assurance of a pleasant evening, when unfortunately I was very unexpectedly called from home on very important business.

I regret my disappointment, but hope that the future may afford us many pleasant meetings.

Sincerely your friend,

IRVING GOODRICH.

[42]

8.—*Form of an Excuse for a Pupil.*

Thursday Morning, April 4th.

Mr. Bunnel:

You will please excuse William for non-attendance at school yesterday, as I was compelled to keep him at home to attend to a matter of business.

MRS. A. SMITH.

9.—*Form of Letter Accompanying a Present.*

Louisville, July 6, 1894.

My Dearest Nelly:

Many happy returns of the day. So fearful was I that it would escape your memory, that I thought I would send you this little trinket by way of reminder. I beg you to accept it and wear it for the sake of the giver. With love and best wishes.

Believe me ever, your sincere friend,

CAROLINE COLLINS.

10.—*Returning Thanks for the Present.*

Louisville, July 6, 1894.

Dear Mrs. Collins:

I am very much obliged to you for the handsome bracelet you have sent me. How kind and thoughtful it was of you to remember me on my birthday. I am sure I have every cause to bless the day, and did I forget it, I have many kind friends to remind me of it. Again thanking you for your present, which is far too beautiful for me, and also for your kind wishes.

Believe me, your most grateful

BERTHA SMITH.

11.—*Congratulating a Friend Upon His Marriage.*

Menton, N.Y., May 24th, 1894.

My Dear Everett:

I have to-day received the invitation to your wedding, and as I cannot be present at that happy event to offer my congratulations in person, I write.

I am heartily glad you are going to be married, and congratulate you upon the wisdom of your choice. You have won a noble as well as a beautiful woman, and one whose love will make you a happy man to your life's end. May God grant that trouble may not come near you, but should it be your lot, you will have a wife to whom you can look with confidence for comfort, and whose good sense and devotion to you will be your sure and unfailing support.

That you may both be very happy, and that your happiness may increase with your years, is the prayer of

Your Friend,

FRANK HOWARD.

[43]

Declaration of Affection

Any extravagant flattery should be avoided, both as tending to disgust those to whom it is addressed, as well as to degrade the writers, and to create suspicion as to their sincerity. The sentiments should spring from the tenderness of the heart, and, when faithfully and delicately expressed, will never be read without exciting sympathy or emotion in all hearts not absolutely deadened by insensibility.

[44]

FORMS OF LOVE LETTERS.

12.—*An Ardent Declaration..*

Naperville, Ill., June 10th, 1894.

My Dearest Laura:

I can no longer restrain myself from writing to you, dearest and best of girls, what I have often been on the point of saying to you. I love you so much that I cannot find words in which to express my feelings. I have loved you from the very first day we met, and always shall. Do you blame me because I write so freely? I should be unworthy of you if I did not tell you the whole truth. Oh, Laura, can you love me in return? I am sure I shall not be able to bear it if your answer is unfavorable. I will study your every wish if you will give me the right to do so. May I hope? Send just one kind word to your sincere friend,

HARRY SMITH.

13.—*A Lover's Good-bye Before Starting on a Journey.*

Pearl St., New York, March 11th, 1894.

My Dearest Nellie: I am off to-morrow, and yet not altogether, for I leave my heart behind in your gentle keeping. You need not place a guard over it, however, for it is as impossible that it should stay away, as for a bit of steel [45]to rush from a magnet. The simile is eminently correct, for you, my dear girl, are a magnet, and my heart is as true to you as steel. I shall make my absence as brief as possible. Not a day, not an hour, not a minute, shall I waste either in going or returning. Oh, this business; but I won't complain, for we must have something for our hive besides honey—something that rhymes with it—and that we must have it, I must bestir myself. You will find me a faithful correspondent. Like the spider, I shall drop a line by (almost) every post; and mind, you must give me letter for letter. I can't give you credit. Your returns must be prompt and punctual.

Passionately yours,

LEWIS SHUMAN.

To   Miss   Nellie   Carter, No. —— Fifth Avenue, New York.

14.—*From an Absent Lover.*

Chicago, Ill., Sept. 10, 1894.

My Dearest Kate: This sheet of paper, though I should cover it with loving words, could never tell you truly how I long to see you again. Time does not run on with me now at the same pace as with other people; the hours seem days, the days weeks, while I am absent from you, and I have no faith in the accuracy of clocks and almanacs. Ah! if there were truth in clairvoyance, wouldn't I be with you at this moment! I wonder if you are as impatient to see me as I am to fly to you? Sometimes it seems as if I must leave business and everything else to the Fates, and take the first train to Dawson. However, the hours do move, though they don't appear to, and in a few more weeks we shall meet again. Let me hear from you as frequently as possible in the meantime. Tell me of your health, your amusements and your affections.

Remember that every word you write will be a comfort to me.

Unchangeably yours,

WILLIAM MILLER.

To   Miss   Kate   Martin, Dawson, N. D.

15.—*A Declaration of Love at First Sight.*

Waterford, Maine, May 8th, 1894.

Dear Miss Searles:

Although I have been in your society but once, the impression you have made upon me is so deep and powerful that I cannot forbear writing to you, in defiance of all rules of etiquette. Affection is sometimes of slow growth: [46]but sometimes it springs up in a moment. In half an hour after I was introduced to you my heart was no longer my own. I have not the assurance to suppose that I have been fortunate enough to create any interest in yours; but will you allow me to cultivate your acquaintance in the hope of being able to win your regard in the course of time? Petitioning for a few lines in reply,

I remain, dear Miss Searles,

Yours devotedly,

E. C. NICKS.

Miss   E.   Searles, Waterford, Maine.

16.—Proposing Marriage.

Wednesday, October 20th, 1894.

Dearest Etta:

The delightful hours I have passed in your society have left an impression on my mind that is altogether indelible, and cannot be effaced even by time itself. The frequent opportunities I have possessed, of observing the thousand acts of amiability and kindness which mark the daily tenor of your life, have ripened my feelings of affectionate regard into a passion at once ardent and sincere, until I have at length associated my hopes of future happiness with the idea of you as a life partner, in them. Believe me, dearest Etta, this is no puerile fancy, but the matured results of a long and warmly cherished admiration of your many charms of person and mind. It is love—pure, devoted love, and I feel confident that your knowledge of my character will lead you to ascribe my motives to their true source.

May I then implore you to consult your own heart, and should this avowal of my fervent and honorable passion for you be crowned with your acceptance and approval, to grant me permission to refer the matter to your parents. Anxiously awaiting your answer,

I am, dearest Etta,

Your sincere and faithful lover,

GEO. COURTRIGHT.

To   Miss   Etta   Jay,

Malden, Ill.

[47]

17.—From a Gentleman to a Widow.

Philadelphia, May 10th, 1894.

My Dear Mrs. Freeman:

I am sure you are too clear-sighted not to have observed the profound impression which your amiable qualities, intelligence and personal attractions have made upon my heart, and as you have not repelled my attentions nor manifested displeasure when I ventured to hint at the deep interest I felt in your welfare and happiness, I cannot help hoping that you will receive an explicit expression of my attachments, kindly and favorably. I wish it were in my power to clothe the feelings I entertain for you in such words as should make my pleadings irresistible; but, after all, what could I say, more than you are very dear to me, and that the most earnest desire of my soul is to have the privilege of calling you my wife? Do you, can you love me? You will not, I am certain, keep me in suspense, for you are too good and kind to trifle for a moment with sincerity like mine. Awaiting your answer,

I remain with respectful affection,

Ever yours,

HENRY MURRAY.

Mrs.   Julia   Freeman,

Philadelphia.

18.—From a Lady to an Inconstant Lover.

Dear Harry:

It is with great reluctance that I enter upon a subject which has given me great pain, and upon which silence has become impossible if I would preserve my self-respect. You cannot but be aware that I have just reason for saying that you have much displeased me. You have apparently forgotten what is due to me, circumstanced as we are, thus far at least. You cannot suppose that I can tamely see you disregard my feelings, by conduct toward other ladies from which I should naturally have the right to expect you to abstain. I am not so vulgar a person as to be jealous. When there is cause to infer changed feelings, or unfaithfulness to promises of constancy, jealousy is not the remedy. What the remedy is I need not say—we both of us have it in our hands. I am sure you will agree with me that we must come to some understanding by which the future shall be governed. Neither you nor I can bear a divided allegiance. Believe me that I write more in sorrow than in anger. You have made me very unhappy, and perhaps thoughtlessly. But it will take much to reassure me of your unaltered regard.

Yours truly,

EMMA.

MODESTY.
ACT NATURAL AND SPEAK WELL OF ALL PEOPLE.

Hints and Helps on Good Behavior at all Times and at all Places.
THE HUMAN FACE, LIKE A FLOWER, SPEAKS FOR ITSELF.

1. It takes acquaintance to found a noble esteem, but politeness prepares the way. Indeed, as Montaigne says, Courtesy begets esteem at sight. Urbanity·is half of affability, and affability is a charm worth possessing.

2. A pleasing demeanor is often the scales by which the pagan weighs the Christian. It is not virtue, but virtue inspires it. There are circumstances in which it takes a great and strong soul to pass under the little yoke of courtesy, but it is a passport to a greater soul standard.

3. Matthew Arnold says, "Conduct is three-fourths of character," and Christian benignity draws the line for conduct. A high sense of rectitude, a lowly soul, with a pure and kind [50]heart are elements of nobility which will work out in the life of a human being at home—everywhere. "Private refinement makes public gentility."

4. If you would conciliate the favor of men, rule your resentment. Remember that if you permit revenge or malice to occupy your soul, you are ruined.

5. Cultivate a happy temper; banish the blues; a cheerful saguine spirit begets cheer and hope.

6. Be trustworthy and be trustful.

7. Do not place a light estimate upon the arts of good reading and good expression; they will yield perpetual interest.

8. Study to keep versed in world events as well as in local occurrences, but abhor gossip, and above all scandal.

9. Banish a self-conscience spirit—the source of much awkwardness—with a constant aim to make others happy. Remember that it is incumbent upon gentlemen and ladies alike to be neat in habits.

10. The following is said to be a correct posture for walking. Head erect—not too rigid—chin in, shoulders back. Permit no unnecessary motion about the thighs. Do not lean over to one side in walking, standing or sitting; the practice is not only ungraceful, but it is deforming and therefore unhealthful.

11. Beware of affectation and of Beau Brummel airs.

12. If the hands are allowed to swing in walking, the arc should be limited, and the lady will manage them much more gracefully, if they almost touch the clothing.

13. A lady should not stand with her hands behind her. We could almost say, forget the hands except to keep them clean, including the nails, cordial and helpful. One hand may rest easily in the other. Study repose of attitude here as well as in the rest of the body.

14. Gestures are for emphasis in public speaking; do not point elsewhere, as a rule.

15. Greet your acquaintances as you meet them with a slight bow and smile, as you speak.

16. Look the person to whom you speak in the eye. Never under any circumstances wink at another or communicate by furtive looks.

17. Should you chance to be the rejected suitor of a lady, bear in mind your own self-respect, as well as the inexorable laws [51]of society, and bow politely when you meet her. Reflect that you do not stand before all woman-kind as you do at her bar. Do not resent the bitterness of flirtation. No lady or gentleman will flirt. Remember ever that painful prediscovery is better than later disappointment. Let such experience spur you to higher exertion.

18. Discretion should be exercised in introducing persons. Of two gentlemen who are introduced, if one is superior in rank or age, he is the one to whom the introduction should be made. Of two social equals, if one be a stranger in the place, his name should be mentioned first.

19. In general the simpler the introduction the better.

20. Before introducing a gentleman to a lady, remember that she is entitled to hold you responsible for the acquaintance. The lady is the one to whom the gentleman is presented, which may be done thus: "Miss A, permit me to introduce to you my friend, Mr. B."; or, "Miss A., allow me to introduce Mr. B." If mutual and near friends of yours, say simply, "Miss A., Mr. B."

21. Receive the introduction with a slight bow and the acknowledgment, "Miss A., I am happy to make your acquaintance"; or, "Mr. B., I am pleased to meet you." There is no reason why such stereotyped expressions should always be used, but something similar is expected. Do not extend the hand usually.

22. A true lady will avoid familiarity in her deportment towards gentlemen. A young lady should not permit her gentlemen friends to address her by her home name, and the reverse is true. Use the title Miss and Mr. respectively.

23. Ladies should be frank and cordial towards their lady friends, but never gushing.

24. Should you meet a friend twice or oftener, at short intervals, it is polite to bow slightly each time after the first.

25. A lady on meeting a gentleman with whom she has slight acquaintance will make a medium bow—neither too decided nor too slight or stiff.

26. For a gentleman to take a young lady's arm, is to intimate that she is feeble, and young ladies resent the mode.

27. If a young lady desires to visit any public place where she expects to meet a gentleman acquaintance, she should have a chaperon to accompany her, a person of mature years when possible, and never a giddy girl.

28. A lady should not ask a gentleman to walk with her.

[52]

A COMPLETE ETIQUETTE IN A FEW PRACTICAL RULES.

1. If you desire to be respected, keep clean. The finest attire and decorations will add nothing to the appearance or beauty of an untidy person.

2. Clean clothing, clean skin, clean hands, including the nails, and clean, white teeth, are a requisite passport for good society.

3. A bad breath should be carefully remedied, whether it proceeds from the stomach or from decayed teeth.

4. To pick the nose, finger about the ears, or scratch the head or any other part of the person, in company, is decidedly vulgar.

5. When you call at any private residence, do not neglect to clean your shoes thoroughly.

6. A gentleman should always remove his hat in the presence of ladies, except out of doors, and then he should lift or touch his hat in salutation. On meeting a lady a well-bred gentleman will always lift his hat.

7. An invitation to a lecture, concert, or other entertainment, may be either verbal or written, but should always be made at least twenty-four hours before the time.[53]

8. On entering a hall or church the gentleman should precede the lady in walking up the aisle, or walk by her side, if the aisle is broad enough.

9. A gentleman should always precede a lady upstairs, and follow her downstairs.

10. Visitors should always observe the customs of the church with reference to standing, sitting, or kneeling during the services.

11. On leaving a hall or church at the close of entertainment or services, the gentleman should precede the lady.

12. A gentleman walking with a lady should carry the parcels, and never allow the lady to be burdened with anything of the kind.

13. A gentleman meeting a lady on the street and wishing to speak to her, should never detain her, but may turn around and walk in the same direction she is going, until the conversation is completed.

14. If a lady is traveling with a gentleman, simply as a friend, she should place the amount of her expenses in his hands, or insist on paying the bills herself.

15. Never offer a lady costly gifts unless you are engaged to her, for it looks as if you were trying to purchase her goodwill; and when you make a present to a lady use no ceremony whatever.

21

Children should early be taught the lesson of Propriety and Good Manners.

16. Never carry on a private conversation in company. If secrecy is necessary, withdraw from the company.

17. Never sit with your back to another without asking to be excused.

18. It is as unbecoming for a gentleman to sit with legs crossed as it is for a lady.

19. Never thrum with your fingers, rub your hands, yawn, or sigh aloud in company.

20. Loud laughter, loud talking, or other boisterous manifestations should be checked in the society of others, especially on the street and in public places.[54]

21. When you are asked to sing or play in company, do so without being urged, or refuse in a way that shall be final; and when music is being rendered in company, show politeness to the musician by giving attention. It is very impolite to keep up a conversation. If you do not enjoy the music, keep silent.

22. Contentions, contradictions, etc., in society should be carefully avoided.

23. Pulling out your watch in company, unless asked the time of day, is a mark of the demi-bred. It looks as if you were tired of the company and the time dragged heavily.

24. You should never decline to be introduced to any one or all of the guests present at a party to which you have been invited.

25. A gentleman who escorts a lady to a party, or who has a lady placed under his care, is under particular obligations to attend to her wants and see that she has proper attention. He should introduce her to others, and endeavor to make the evening pleasant. He should escort her to the supper table and provide for her wants.

26. To take small children or dogs with you on a visit of ceremony is altogether vulgar, though in visiting familiar friends, children are not objectionable.

[55]

AN EGYPTIAN BRIDE'S WEDDING OUTFIT.

[56]

ETIQUETTE OF CALLS.

In the matter of making calls it is the correct thing:

For the caller who arrived first to leave first.

To return a first call within a week and in person.

To call promptly and in person after a first invitation.

For the mother or chaperon to invite a gentleman to call.

To call within a week after any entertainment to which one has been invited.

You should call upon an acquaintance who has recently returned from a prolonged absence.

It is proper to make the first call upon people in a higher social position, if one is asked to do so.

It is proper to call, after an engagement has been announced, or a marriage has taken place, in the family.

For the older residents in the city or street to call upon the newcomers to their neighborhood is a long recognized custom.

It is proper, after a removal from one part of the city to another, to send out cards with one's new address upon them.

To ascertain what are the prescribed hours for calling in the place where one is living, or making a visit, and to adhere to those hours is a duty that must not be overlooked.

A gentleman should ask for the lady of the house as well as the young ladies, and leave cards for her as well as for the head of the family.[57]

Improve Your Speech by Reading.

ETIQUETTE IN YOUR SPEECH.

Don't say Miss or Mister without the person's name.

Don't say pants for trousers.

Don't say gents for gentlemen.

Don't say female for woman.

Don't say elegant to mean everything that pleases you.

Don't say genteel for well-bred.

Don't say ain't for isn't.

Don't say I done it for I did it.

Don't say he is older than me; say older than I.

Don't say she does not see any; say she does not see at all.

Don't say not as I know; say not that I know.

Don't say he calculates to get off; say he expects to get off.

Don't say he don't; say he doesn't.

Don't say she is some better; say she is somewhat better.

Don't say where are you stopping? say where are you staying?

Don't say you was; say you were.

Don't say I say, says I, but simply say I said.

Don't sign your letters yours etc., but yours truly.

Don't say lay for lie; lay expresses action; lie expresses rest.

Don't say them bonnets; say those bonnets.

Don't say party for person.

Don't say it looks beautifully, but say it looks beautiful.[58]

Don't say feller, winder, to-morrer, for fellow, window, tomorrow.

Don't use slangy words; they are vulgar.

Don't use profane words; they are sinful and foolish.

Don't say it was her, when you mean it was she.

Don't say not at once for at once.

Don't say he gave me a recommend, but say he gave me a recommendation.

Don't say the two first for the first two.

Don't say he learnt me French; say he taught me French.

Don't say lit the fire; say lighted the fire.

Don't say the man which you saw; say the man whom you saw.

Don't say who done it; say who did it.

Don't say if I was rich I would buy a carriage; say if I were rich.

Don't say if I am not mistaken you are in the wrong; say if I mistake not.

Don't say who may you be; say who are you?

Don't say go lay down; say go lie down.

Don't say he is taller than me; say taller than I.

Don't say I shall call upon him; say I shall call on him.

Don't say I bought a new pair of shoes; say I bought a pair of new shoes.

Don't say I had rather not; say I would rather not.

Don't say two spoonsful; say two spoonfuls.

ETIQUETTE OF DRESS AND HABITS.

Don't let one day pass without a thorough cleansing of your person.

Don't sit down to your evening meal before a complete toilet if you have company.

Don't cleanse your nails, your nose or your ears in public.

Don't use hair dye, hair oil or pomades.

Don't wear evening dress in daytime.

Don't wear jewelry of a gaudy character; genuine jewelry modestly worn is not out of place.

Don't overdress yourself or walk affectedly.

Don't wear slippers or dressing-gown or smoking-jacket out of your own house.

Don't sink your hands in your trousers' pockets.

Don't whistle in public places, nor inside of houses either.

Don't use your fingers or fists to beat a tattoo upon floor, desk or window panes.

Don't examine other people's papers or letters scattered on their desk.[59]

Don't bring a smell of spirits or tobacco into the presence of ladies.

Never use either in the presence of ladies.

Don't drink spirits; millions have tried it to their sorrow.

ETIQUETTE ON THE STREET.

1. Your conduct on the street should always be modest and dignified. Ladies should carefully avoid all loud and boisterous conversation or laughter and all undue liveliness in public.

2. When walking on the street do not permit yourself to be absent-minded, as to fail to recognize a friend; do not go along reading a book or newspaper.

3. In walking with a lady on the street give her the inner side of the walk, unless the outside is the safer part; in which case she is entitled to it.

4. Your arm should not be given to any lady except your wife or a near relative, or a very old lady, during the day, unless her comfort or safety requires it. At night the arm should always be offered; also in ascending the steps of a public building.

5. In crossing the street a lady should gracefully raise her dress a little above her ankle with one hand. To raise the dress with both hands is vulgar, except in places where the mud is very deep.

6. A gentleman meeting a lady acquaintance on the street should not presume to join her in her walk without first asking her permission.

7. If you have anything to say to a lady whom you may happen to meet in the street, however intimate you may be, do not stop her, but turn round and walk in company with her; you can take leave at the end of the street.

8. A lady should not venture out upon the street alone after dark. By so doing she compromises her dignity, and exposes herself to indignity at the hands of the rougher class.

9. Never offer to shake hands with a lady in the street if you have on dark or soiled gloves, as you may soil hers.

10. A lady does not form acquaintances upon the street, or seek to attract the attention of the other sex or of persons of her own sex. Her conduct is always modest and unassuming. Neither does a lady demand services or favors from a gentleman. She accepts them graciously, always [60]expressing her thanks. A gentleman will not stand on the street corners, or in hotel doorways, or store windows and gaze impertinently at ladies as they pass by. This is the exclusive business of loafers.

11. In walking with a lady who has your arm, should you have to cross the street, do not disengage your arm and go around upon the outside, unless the lady's comfort renders it necessary. In walking with a lady, where it is necessary for you to proceed singly, always go before her.

ETIQUETTE BETWEEN SEXES.

1. A lady should be a lady, and a gentleman a gentleman under any and all circumstances.

2. **Female Indifference to Man.**—There is nothing that affects the nature and pleasure of man so much as a proper and friendly recognition from a lady, and as women are more or less dependent upon man's good-will, either for gain or pleasure, it surely stands to their interest to be reasonably pleasant and courteous in his presence or society. Indifference is always a poor investment, whether in society or business.

3. **Gallantry and Ladyism** should be a prominent feature in the education of young people. Politeness to ladies cultivates the intellect and refines the soul, and he who can be easy and entertaining in the society of ladies has mastered one of the greatest accomplishments. There is nothing taught in school, academy or college, that contributes so much to the happiness of man as a full development of his social and moral qualities.

4. **Ladylike Etiquette.**—No woman can afford to treat men rudely. A lady must have a high intellectual and moral ideal and hold herself above reproach. She must remember that the art of pleasing and entertaining gentlemen is infinitely more ornamental than laces, ribbons or diamonds. Dress and glitter may please man, but it will never benefit him.

5. **Cultivate Deficiencies.**—Men and women poorly sexed treat each other with more or less indifference, whereas a hearty sexuality inspires both to a right estimation of the faculties and qualities of each other. Those who are deficient should seek society and

overcome their deficiencies. While some naturally inherit faculties as entertainers, others are compelled to acquire them by cultivation.[61]

6. Ladies' Society.—He who seeks ladies' society should seek an education and should have a pure heart and a pure mind. Read good, pure and wholesome literature and study human nature, and you will always be a favorite in the society circle.

7. Woman Haters.—Some men with little refinement and strong sensual feelings virtually insult and thereby disgust and repel every female they meet. They look upon woman with an inherent vulgarity, and doubt the virtue and integrity of all alike. But it is because they are generally [62]insincere and impure themselves, and with such a nature culture and refinement are out of the question, there must be a revolution.

8. Men Haters.—Women who look upon all men as odious, corrupt or hateful, are no doubt so themselves, though they may be clad in silk and sparkle with diamonds and be as pretty as a lily; but their hypocrisy will out, and they can never win the heart of a faithful, conscientious and well balanced man. A good woman has broad ideas and great sympathy. She respects all men until they are proven unworthy.

9. Fond of Children.—The man who is naturally fond of children will make a good husband and a good father. So it behooves the young man, to notice children and cultivate the art of pleasing them. It will be a source of interest, education and permanent benefit to all.

10. Excessive Luxury.—Although the association with ladies is an expensive luxury, yet it is not an expensive education. It elevates, refines, sanctifies and purifies, and improves the whole man. A young man who has a pure and genuine respect for ladies, will not only make a good husband, but a good citizen as well.

11. Masculine Attention.—No woman is entitled to any more attention than her loveliness and ladylike conduct will command. Those who are most pleasing will receive the most attention, and those who desire more should aspire to acquire more by cultivating those graces and virtues which ennoble woman, but no lady should lower or distort her own true ideal, or smother and crucify her conscience, in order to please any living man. A good man will admire a good woman, and deceptions cannot long be concealed. Her show of dry goods or glitter of jewels cannot long cover up her imperfections or deceptions.

12. Purity.—Purity of purpose will solve all social problems. Let all stand on this exalted sexual platform, and teach every man just how to treat the female sex, and every woman how to behave towards the masculine; and it will incomparably adorn the manners of both, make both happy in each other, and mutually develop each other's sexuality and humanity.

[63]

Practical Rules on Table Manners.

1. Help ladies with a due appreciation; do not overload the plate of any person you serve. Never pour gravy on a plate without permission. It spoils the meat for some persons.

2. Never put anything by force upon any one's plate. It is extremely ill-bred, though extremely common, to press one to eat of anything.

3. If at dinner you are requested to help any one to sauce or gravy, do not pour it over the meat or vegetables, but on one side of them. Never load down a person's plate with anything.

4. As soon as you are helped, begin to eat, or at least begin to occupy yourself with what you have before you. Do not wait till your neighbors are served—a custom that was long ago abandoned.

5. Should you, however, find yourself at a table where they have the old-fashioned steel forks, eat with your knife, as the others do, and do not let it be seen that you have any objection to doing so.

6. Bread should be broken. To butter a large piece of bread and then bite it, as children do, is something the knowing never do.[64]

7. In eating game or poultry do not touch the bones with your fingers. To take a bone in the fingers for the purpose of picking it, is looked upon as being very inelegant.

8. Never use your own knife or fork to help another. Use rather the knife or fork of the person you help.

9. Never send your knife or fork, or either of them, on your plate when you send for second supply.

10. Never turn your elbows out when you use your knife and fork. Keep them close to your sides.

11. Whenever you use your fingers to convey anything to your mouth or to remove anything from the mouth, let it be the fingers of the left hand.

12. Tea, coffee, chocolate and the like are drank from the cup and never from the saucer.

13. In masticating your food, keep your mouth shut; otherwise you will make a noise that will be very offensive to those around you.

14. Don't attempt to talk with a full mouth. One thing at a time is as much as any man can do well.

15. Should you find a worm or insect in your food, say nothing about it.

16. If a dish is distasteful to you, decline it, and without comment.

17. Never put bones or bits of fruit on the table cloth. Put them on the side of your plate.

18. Do not hesitate to take the last piece on the dish, simply because it is the last. To do so is to directly express the fear that you would exhaust the supply.

19. If you would be what you would like to be—abroad, take care that you *are* what you would like to be—at home.

20. Avoid picking your teeth at the table if possible; but if you must, do it, if you can, where you are not observed.

21. If an accident of any kind soever should occur during dinner, the cause being who or what it may, you should not seem to note it.

22. Should you be so unfortunate as to overturn or to break anything, you should make no apology. You might let your regret appear in your face, but it would not be proper to put it in words.

[65]

Social Duties.

Man in Society is like a flower,
Blown in its native bed. 'Tis there alone
His faculties expanded in full bloom
Shine out, there only reach their proper use.—COWPER.
The primal duties shine aloft like stars;
The charities that soothe, and heal, and bless,
Are scatter'd at the feet of man like flowers.—WORDSWORTH.

[66]

GIVING A PARLOR RECITATION.

1. **Membership in Society.**—Many fail to get hold of the idea that they are members of society. They seem to suppose that the social machinery of the world is self-operating. They cast their first ballot with an emotion of pride, perhaps, but are sure to pay their first tax with a groan. They see political organizations in active existence; the parish, and the church, and other important bodies that embrace in some form of society all men, are successfully operated; and yet these young men have no part or lot in the matter. They do not think of giving a day's time to society.

2. **Begin Early.**—One of the first things a young man should do is to see that he is acting his part in society. The earlier this is begun the better. I think that the opponents of secret societies in colleges have failed to estimate the benefit which it must be to every member to be obliged to contribute to the support of his particular organization, and to

assume personal care and responsibility as a member. If these societies have a tendency to teach the lessons of which I speak, they are a blessed thing.

3. **Do Your Part.**—Do your part, and be a man among men. Assume your portion of social responsibility, and see that you discharge it well. If you do not do this, then you are mean, and society has the right to despise you just as much as it chooses to do so. You are, to use a word more emphatic than agreeable, a sneak, and have not a claim upon your neighbors for a single polite word.

4. **A Whining Complainer.**—Society, as it is called, is far more apt to pay its dues to the individual than the individual to society. Have you, young man, who are at home whining over the fact that you cannot get into society, done anything to give you a claim to social recognition? Are you able to make any return for social recognition and social privileges? Do you know anything? What kind of coin do you propose to pay in the discharge of the obligation which comes upon you with social recognition? In other words, as a return for what you wish to have society do for you, what can you do for society? This is a very important question—more important to you than to society. The question is, whether you will be a member of society by right, or by courtesy. If you have so mean a spirit as to be content to be a beneficiary of society—to receive favors and to confer none—you have no business in the society to which you aspire. You are an exacting, conceited fellow.

5. **What Are You Good For?**—Are you a good beau, and are you willing to make yourself useful in waiting on the [67]ladies on all occasions? Have you a good set of teeth, which you are willing to show whenever the wit of the company gets off a good thing? Are you a true, straightforward, manly fellow, with whose healthful and uncorrupted nature it is good for society to come in contact? In short, do you possess anything of any social value? If you do, and are willing to impart it, society will yield itself to your touch. If you have nothing, then society, as such, owes you nothing. Christian philanthropy may put its arm around you, as a lonely young man, about to spoil for want of something, but it is very sad and humiliating for a young man to be brought to that. There are people who devote themselves to nursing young men, and doing them good. If they invite you to tea, go by all means, and try your hand. If, in the course of the evening, you can prove to them that your society is desirable, you have won a point. Don't be patronized.

6. **The Morbid Condition.**—Young men, you are apt to get into a morbid state of mind, which declines them to social intercourse. They become devoted to business with such exclusiveness, that all social intercourse is irksome. They go out to tea as if they were going to jail, and drag themselves to a party as to an execution. This disposition is thoroughly morbid, and to be overcome by going where you are invited, always, and with a sacrifice of feeling.

7. **The Common Blunder.**—Don't shrink from contact with anything but bad morals. Men who affect your unhealthy minds with antipathy, will prove themselves very frequently to be your best friends and most delightful companions. Because a man seems uncongenial to you, who are squeamish and foolish, you have no right to shun him. We become charitable by knowing men. We learn to love those whom we have despised by rubbing against them. Do you not remember some instance of meeting a man or woman whom you had never previously known or cared to know—an individual, perhaps, against whom you have entertained the strongest prejudices—but to whom you became bound by a lifelong friendship through the influence of a three days' intercourse? Yet, if you had not thus met, you would have carried through life the idea that it would be impossible for you to give your fellowship to such an individual.

8. **The Foolishness of Man.**—God has introduced into human character infinite variety, and for you to say that you do not love and will not associate with a man because he is unlike you, is not only foolish but wrong. You are to remember that in the precise manner and decree in which [68]a man differs from you, do you differ from him; and that from his standpoint you are naturally as repulsive to him, as he, from your standpoint, is to you. So, leave all this talk of congeniality to silly girls and transcendental dreamers.

GATHERING ORANGES IN THE SUNNY SOUTH.

9. **Do Business in Your Way and Be Honest.**—Do your business in your own way, and concede to every man the privilege which you claim for yourself. The more you

27

mix with men, the less you will be disposed to quarrel, and the more charitable and liberal will you become. The fact that you do not understand a man, is quite as likely to be your fault as his. There are a good many chances in favor of the conclusion that, if you fail to like an individual whose acquaintance you make it is through your own ignorance and illiberality. So I say, meet every man honestly; seek to know him; and you will find that in those points in which he differs from you rests his power to instruct you, enlarge you, and do you good. Keep your heart open for everybody, and be sure that you shall have your reward. You shall find a jewel under the most uncouth exterior; and associated with homeliest manners and oddest ways and ugliest faces, you will find rare virtues, fragrant little humanities, and inspiring heroisms.

10. **Without Society, Without Influence.**—Again: you can have no influence unless you are social. An unsocial man is as devoid of influence as an ice-peak is of verdure. It is through social contact and absolute social value alone that you can accomplish any great social good. It is through the invisible lines which you are able to attach to the minds with which you are brought into association alone that you can tow society, with its deeply freighted interests, to the great haven of your hope.

11. **The Revenge of Society.**—The revenge which society takes upon the man who isolates himself, is as terrible as it is inevitable. The pride which sits alone will have the privilege of sitting alone in its sublime disgust till it drops into the grave. The world sweeps by the man, carelessly, remorselessly, contemptuously. He has no hold upon society, because he is no part of it.

12. **The Conclusion of the Whole Matter.**—You cannot move men until you are one of them. They will not follow you until they have heard your voice, shaken your hand, and fully learned your principles and your sympathies. It makes no difference how much you know, or how much you are capable of doing. You may pile accomplishment upon acquisition mountain high; but if you fail to be a social man, demonstrating to society that your lot is with the rest, a [69]little child with a song in its mouth, and a kiss for all and a pair of innocent hands to lay upon the knees, shall lead more hearts and change the direction of more lives than you.

[70]
Politeness.

1. **Beautiful Behavior.**—Politeness has been described as the art of showing, by external signs, the internal regard we have for others. But one may be perfectly polite to another without necessarily paying a special regard for him. Good manners are neither more nor less than beautiful behavior. It has been well said that "a beautiful form is better than a beautiful face, and a beautiful behavior is better than a beautiful form; it gives a higher pleasure than statues or pictures—it is the finest of the fine arts."

2. **True Politeness.**—The truest politeness comes of sincerity. It must be the outcome of the heart, or it will make no lasting impression; for no amount of polish can dispense with truthfulness. The natural character must be allowed to appear, freed of its angularities and asperities. Though politeness, in its best form, should resemble water—"best when clearest, most simple, and without taste"—yet genius in a man will always cover many defects of manner, and much will be excused to the strong and the original. Without genuineness and individuality, human life would lose much of its interest and variety, as well as its manliness and robustness of character.

3. **Personality of Others.**—True politeness especially exhibits itself in regard for the personality of others. A man will respect the individuality of another if he wishes to be respected himself. He will have due regard for his views and opinions, even though they differ from his own. The well-mannered man pays a compliment to another, and sometimes even secures his respect by patiently listening to him. He is simply tolerant and forbearant, and refrains from judging harshly; and harsh judgments of others will almost invariably provoke harsh judgments of ourselves.

4. **The Impolite.**—The impolite, impulsive man will, however, sometimes rather lose his friend than his joke. He may surely be pronounced a very foolish person who secures another's hatred at the price of a moment's gratification. It was a saying of Burnel, the

engineer—himself one of the kindest-natured of men—that "spite and ill-nature are among the most expensive luxuries in life." Dr. Johnson once said: "Sir, a man has no more right to say a rude thing to another than to knock him down."

5. **Feelings of Others.**—Want of respect for the feelings of others usually originates in selfishness, and issues in [71]hardness and repulsiveness of manner. It may not proceed from malignity so much, as from want of sympathy, and want of delicacy—a want of that perception of, and attention to, those little and apparently trifling things, by which pleasure is given or pain occasioned to others. Indeed, it may be said that in self-sacrifice in the ordinary intercourse of life, mainly consists the difference between being well and ill bred. Without some degree of self-restraint in society a man may be found almost insufferable. No one has pleasure in holding intercourse with such a person, and he is a constant source of annoyance to those about him.

6. **Disregard of Others.**—Men may show their disregard to others in various impolite ways, as, for instance, by neglect of propriety in dress, by the absence of cleanliness, or by indulging in repulsive habits. The slovenly, dirty person, by rendering himself physically disagreeable, sets the tastes and feelings of others at defiance, and is rude and uncivil, only under another form.

7. **The Best School of Politeness.**—The first and best school of politeness, as of character, is always the home, where woman is the teacher. The manners of society at large are but the reflex of the manners of our collective homes, neither better nor worse. Yet, with all the disadvantages of ungenial homes, men may practice self-culture of manner as of intellect, and learn by good examples to cultivate a graceful and agreeable behavior towards others. Most men are like so many gems in the rough, which need polishing by contact with other and better natures, to bring out their full beauty and lustre. Some have but one side polished, sufficient only to show the delicate graining of the interior; but to bring out the full qualities of the gem, needs the discipline of experience, and contact with the best examples of character in the intercourse of daily life.

8. **Captiousness of Manner.**—While captiousness of manner, and the habit of disputing and contradicting every thing said, is chilling and repulsive, the opposite habit of assenting to, and sympathizing with, every statement made, or emotion expressed, is almost equally disagreeable. It is unmanly, and is felt to be dishonest. "It may seem difficult," says Richard Sharp, "to steer always between bluntness and plain dealing, between merited praises and lavishing indiscriminate flattery; but it is very easy—good humor, kindheartedness, and perfect simplicity, being all that are requisite to do what is right in the right way." At the same time many are impolite, not because they mean to be so, but because they are awkward, and perhaps know no better.[72]

9. **Shy People.**—Again many persons are thought to be stiff, reserved, and proud, when they are only shy. Shyness is characteristic of most people of the Teutonic race. From all that can be learned of Shakespeare, it is to be inferred that he was an exceedingly shy man. The manner in which his plays were sent into the world—for it is not known that he edited or authorized the publication of a single one of them,—and the dates at which they respectively appeared, are mere matters of conjecture.

10. **Self-Forgetfulness.**—True politeness is best evinced by self-forgetfulness, or self-denial in the interest of others. Mr. Garfield, our martyred president, was a gentleman of royal type. His friend, Col. Rockwell, says of him: "In the midst of his suffering he never forgets others. For instance, to-day he said to me, 'Rockwell, there is a poor soldier's widow who came to me before this thing occurred, and I promised her, she should be provided for. I want you to see that the matter is attended to at once.' He is the most docile patient I ever saw."

11. **Its Bright Side.**—We have thus far spoken of shyness as a defect. But there is another way of looking at it; for even shyness has its bright side, and contains an element of good. Shy men and shy races are ungraceful and undemonstrative, because, as regards society at large, they are comparatively unsociable. They do not possess those elegancies of manner acquired by free intercourse, which distinguish the social races, because their tendency is to shun society rather than to seek it. They are shy in the presence of strangers, and shy even in their own families. They hide their affections under a robe of reserve, and

when they do give way to their feelings, it is only in some very hidden inner chamber. And yet, the feelings are there, and not the less healthy and genuine, though they are not made the subject of exhibition to others.

12. **Worthy of Cultivation.**—While, therefore, grace of manner, politeness of behavior, elegance of demeanor, and all the arts that contribute to make life pleasant and beautiful, are worthy of cultivation, it must not be at the expense of the more solid and enduring qualities of honesty, sincerity, and truthfulness. The fountain of beauty must be in the heart more than in the eye, and if it does not tend to produce beautiful life and noble practice, it will prove of comparatively little avail. Politeness of manner is not worth much, unless it is accompanied by polite actions.

[73]
Influence of Good Character.
"Unless above himself he can
Erect himself, how poor a thing is man!"—DANIEL.

"Character is moral order seen through the medium of an individual nature—Men of character are the conscience of the society to which they belong."—EMERSON.

The purest treasure mortal times afford,
Is—spotless reputation; that away,
Men are but gilded loam, or painted clay.
A jewel in a ten-times-barr'd-up chest
Is—a bold Spirit in a loyal breast.—SHAKSPEARE.

1. **Reputation.**—The two most precious things this side the grave are our reputation and our life. But it is to be lamented that the most contemptible whisper may deprive us of the one, and the weakest weapon of the other. A wise man, therefore, will be more anxious to deserve a fair name than to possess it, and this will teach him so to live, as not to be afraid to die.

2. **Character.**—Character is one of the greatest motive powers in the world. In its noblest embodiments, it exemplifies human nature in its highest forms, for it exhibits man at his best.

3. **The Heart That Rules in Life.**—Although genius always commands admiration, character most secures respect. The former is more the product of brain power, the latter of heart power; and in the long run it is the heart that rules in life. Men of genius stand to society in the relation of its intellect as men of character of its conscience: and while the former are admired, the latter are followed.

4. **The Highest Ideal of Life and Character.**—Commonplace though it may appear, this doing of one's duty embodies the highest ideal of life and character. There may be nothing heroic about it; but the common lot of men is not heroic. And though the abiding sense of duty upholds man in his highest attitudes, it also equally sustains him in the transaction of the ordinary affairs of every-day existence. Man's life is "centered in the sphere of common duties." The most influential of all the virtues are those which are the most in request for daily use. They wear the best, and last the longest.

5. **Wealth.**—Wealth in the hands of men of weak purpose, or deficient self-control, or of ill regulated passions, is [74]only a temptation and a snare—the source, it may be, of infinite mischief to themselves, and often to others.

On the contrary, a condition of comparative poverty is compatible with character in its highest form. A man may possess only his industry, his frugality, his integrity, and yet stand high in the rank of true manhood. The advice which Burns' father gave him was the best:

"He bade me act a manly part, though I had ne'er a farthing,
For without an honest, manly heart no man was worth regarding."

6. **Character is Property.**—It is the noblest of possessions. It is an estate in the general good-will and respect of men; they who invest in it—though they may not become rich in this world's goods—will find their reward in esteem and reputation fairly and honorably won. And it is right that in life good qualities should tell—that industry, virtue, and goodness should rank the highest—and that the really best men should be foremost.

7. **Simple Honesty of Purpose.**—This in a man goes a long way in life, if founded on a just estimate of himself and a steady obedience to the rule he knows and feels to be right. It holds a man straight, gives him strength and sustenance, and forms a mainspring of vigorous action. No man is bound to be rich or great—no, nor to be wise—but every man is bound to be honest and virtuous.

[76]

Family Government.
HEAVENLY MUSIC.

1. **Gentleness Must Characterize Every Act of Authority.**—The storm of excitement that may make the child start, bears no relation to actual obedience. The inner firmness, that sees and feels a moral conviction and expects obedience, is only disguised and defeated by bluster. The more calm and direct it is, the greater certainty it has of dominion.

2. **For the Government of Small Children.**—For the government of small children speak only in the authority of love, yet authority, loving and to be obeyed. The most important lesson to impart is obedience to authority as authority. The question of salvation with most children will be settled as soon as they learn to obey parental authority. It establishes a habit and order of mind that is ready to accept divine authority. This precludes skepticism and disobedience, and induces that childlike trust and spirit set forth as a necessary state of salvation. Children that are never made to obey are left to drift into the sea of passion where the pressure for surrender only tends to drive them at greater speed from the haven of safety.

3. **Habits of Self-Denial.**—Form in the child habits of self-denial. Pampering never matures good character.

4. **Emphasize Integrity.**—Keep the moral tissues tough in integrity; then it will hold a hook of obligations when once set in a sure place. There is nothing more vital. Shape all your experiments to preserve the integrity. Do not so reward it that it becomes mercenary. Turning State's evidence is a dangerous experiment in morals. Prevent deceit from succeeding.

5. **Guard Modesty.**—To be brazen is to imperil some of the best elements of character. Modesty may be strengthened into a becoming confidence, but brazen facedness can seldom be toned down into decency. It requires the miracle of grace.

6. **Protect Purity.**—Teach your children to loathe impurity. Study the character of their playmates. Watch their books. Keep them from corruption at all cost. The groups of youth in the school and in society, and in business places, seed with improprieties of word and thought. Never relax your vigilance along this exposed border.
BOTH PUZZLED.

7. **Threaten the Least Possible.**—In family government threaten the least possible. Some parents rattle off their commands with penalties so profusely that there is a steady [78]roar of hostilities about the child's head. These threats are forgotten by the parent and unheeded by the child. All government is at an end.

8. **Do Not Enforce Too Many Commands.**—Leave a few things within the range of the child's knowledge that are not forbidden. Keep your word good, but do not have too much of it out to be redeemed.

9. **Punish as Little as Possible.**—Sometimes punishment is necessary, but the less it is resorted to the better.

10. **Never Punish in a Passion.**—Wrath only becomes cruelty. There is no moral power in it. When you seem to be angry you can do no good.

11. **Brutish Violence Only Multiplies Offenders.**—Striking and beating the body seldom reaches the soul. Fear and hatred beget rebellion.

12. **Punish Privately.**—Avoid punishments that break down self-respect. Striking the body produces shame and indignation. It is enough for the other children to know that discipline is being administered.

13. **Never Stop Short of Success.**—When the child is not conquered the punishment has been worse than wasted. Reach the point where neither wrath nor sullenness remain. By firm persistency and persuasion require an open look of recognition

and peace. It is only evil to stir up the devil unless he is cast out. Ordinarily one complete victory will last a child for a lifetime. But if the child relapses, repeat the dose with proper accompaniments.

14. **Do Not Require Children to Complain of Themselves for Pardon.**—It begets either sycophants or liars. It is the part of the government to detect offences. It reverses the order of matters to shirk this duty.

15. **Grade Authority Up to Liberty.**—The growing child must have experiments of freedom. Lead him gently into the family. Counsel with him. Let him plan as he can. By and by he has the confidence of courage without the danger of exposures.

16. **Respect.**—Parents must respect each other. Undermining either undermines both. Always govern in the spirit of love.

[79]

CONVERSATION.

Some men are very entertaining for a first interview, but after that they are exhausted, and run out; on a second meeting we shall find them very flat and monotonous; like hand-organs, we have heard all their tunes.—COULTON.

He who sedulously attends, pointedly asks, calmly speaks, coolly answers, and ceases when he has no more to say, is in possession of some of the best requisites of man.—LAVATER.

Beauty is never so lovely as when adorned with the smile, and conversation never sits easier upon us than when we know and then discharge ourselves in a symphony of Laughter, which may not improperly be called the Chorus of Conversation.—STEELE.

The first ingredient in Conversation is Truth, the next Good Sense, the third Good Humor, and the fourth Wit.—SIR WILLIAM TEMPLE.

[80]

Home Lessons in Conversation.

Say nothing unpleasant when it can be avoided.

Avoid satire and sarcasm.

Never repeat a word that was not intended for repetition.

Cultivate the supreme wisdom, which consists less in saying what ought to be said than in not saying what ought not to be said.

Often cultivate "flashes of silence."

It is the larger half of the conversation to listen well.

Listen to others patiently, especially the poor.

Sharp sayings are an evidence of low breeding.

Shun faultfindings and faultfinders.

Never utter an uncomplimentary word against anyone.

Compliments delicately hinted and sincerely intended are a grace in conversation.

Commendation of gifts and cleverness properly put are in good taste, but praise of beauty is offensive.

Repeating kind expressions is proper.

Compliments given in a joke may be gratefully received in earnest.

The manner and tone are important parts of a compliment.

Avoid egotism.

Don't talk of yourself, or of your friends or your deeds.

Give no sign that you appreciate your own merits.

Do not become a distributer of the small talk of a community. The smiles of your auditors do not mean respect.

Avoid giving the impression of one filled with "suppressed egotism."

Never mention your own peculiarities; for culture destroys vanity.

Avoid exaggeration.

Do not be too positive.

Do not talk of display oratory.

Do not try to lead in conversation, looking around to enforce silence.

Lay aside affected silly etiquette for the natural dictates of the heart.

Direct the conversation where others can join with you and impart to you useful information.

Avoid oddity. Eccentricity is shallow vanity.

Be modest.

Be what you wish to seem.

Avoid repeating a brilliant or clever saying.

[82]

THINKING ONLY OF DRESS.

If you find bashfulness or embarrassment coming upon you, do or say something at once. The commonest matter gently stated is better than an embarrassing silence. Sometimes changing your position, or looking into a book for a moment may relieve your embarrassment, and dispel any settling stiffness.

Avoid telling many stories, or repeating a story more than once in the same company.

Never treat any one as if you simply wanted him to tell stories. People laugh and despise such a one.

Never tell a coarse story. No wit or preface can make it excusable.

Tell a story, if at all, only as an illustration, and not for itself. Tell it accurately.

Be careful in asking questions for the purpose of starting conversation or drawing out a person, not to be rude or intrusive.

Never take liberties by staring, or by any rudeness.

Never infringe upon any established regulations among strangers.

Do not always prove yourself to be the one in the right. The right will appear. You need only give it a chance.

Avoid argument in conversation. It is discourteous to your host.

Cultivate paradoxes in conversation with your peers. They add interest to commonplace matters. To strike the harmless faith of ordinary people in any public idol is waste, but such a movement with those able to reply is better.

Never discourse upon your ailments.

Never use words of the meaning or pronunciation of which you are uncertain.

Avoid discussing your own or other people's domestic concerns.

Never prompt a slow speaker, as if you had all the ability. In conversing with a foreigner who may be learning our language, it is excusable to help him in some delicate way.

Never give advice unasked.

Do not manifest impatience.

Do not interrupt another when speaking.

Do not find fault, though you may gently criticise.

Do not appear to notice inaccuracies of speech in others.

Do not always commence a conversation by allusion to the weather.

Do not, when narrating an incident, continually say, "you see," "you know."[83]

Do not allow yourself to lose temper or speak excitedly.

Do not introduce professional or other topics that the company generally cannot take an interest in.

Do not talk very loud. A firm, clear, distinct, yet mild, gentle, and musical voice has great power.

Do not be absent-minded, requiring the speaker to repeat what has been said that you may understand.

Do not try to force yourself into the confidence of others.

Do not use profanity, vulgar terms, words of double meaning, or language that will bring the blush to anyone.

Do not allow yourself to speak ill of the absent one if it can be avoided. The day may come when some friend will be needed to defend you in your absence.

Do not speak with contempt and ridicule of a locality which you may be visiting. Find something to truthfully praise and commend; thus make yourself agreeable.

Do not make a pretense of gentility, nor parade the fact that you are a descendant of any notable family. You must pass for just what you are, and must stand on your own merit.

Do not contradict. In making a correction say, "I beg your pardon, but I had the impression that it was so and so." Be careful in contradicting, as you may be wrong yourself.

Do not be unduly familiar; you will merit contempt if you are. Neither should you be dogmatic in your assertions, arrogating to yourself such consequences in your opinions.

Do not be too lavish in your praise of various members of your own family when speaking to strangers; the person to whom you are speaking may know some faults that you do not.

Do not feel it incumbent upon yourself to carry your point in conversation. Should the person with whom you are conversing feel the same, your talk may lead into violent argument.

Do not try to pry into the private affairs of others by asking what their profits are, what things cost, whether Melissa ever had a beau, and why Amarette never got married? All such questions are extremely impertinent and are likely to meet with rebuke.

Do not whisper in company; do not engage in private conversation; do not speak a foreign language which the general company present may not understand, unless it is understood that the foreigner is unable to speak your own language.

[84]

OR
The Care of the Person.

IMPORTANT RULES.
Widower Jones and Widow Smith.

1. **Good Appearance.**—The first care of all persons should be for their personal appearance. Those who are slovenly or careless in their habits are unfit for refined society, and cannot possibly make a good appearance in it. A well-bred person will always cultivate habits of the most scrupulous neatness. A gentleman or lady is always well dressed. The garment may be plain or of coarse material, or even worn "thin and shiny," but if it is carefully brushed and neat it can be worn with dignity.[85]

2. **Personal Cleanliness.**—Personal appearance depends greatly on the careful toilet and scrupulous attention to dress. The first point which marks the gentleman or lady in appearance is rigid cleanliness. This remark supplies to the body and everything which covers it. A clean skin—only to be secured by frequent baths—is indispensable.

3. **The Teeth.**—The teeth should receive the utmost attention. Many a young man has been disgusted with a lady by seeing her unclean and discolored teeth. It takes but a few moments, and if necessary secure some simple tooth powder or rub the teeth thoroughly every day with a linen handkerchief, and it will give the teeth and mouth a beautiful and clean appearance.

4. **The Hair and Beard.**—The hair should be thoroughly brushed and well kept, and the beard of men properly trimmed. Men should not let their hair grow long and shaggy.

5. **Underclothing.**—The matter of cleanliness extends to all articles of clothing, underwear as well as the outer clothing. Cleanliness is a mark of true utility. The clothes need not necessarily be of a rich and expensive quality, but they can all be kept clean. Some persons have an odor about them that is very offensive, simply on account of their underclothing being worn too long without washing. This odor of course cannot be detected by the person who wears the soiled garments, but other persons easily detect it and are offended by it.

6. **The Bath.**—No person should think for a moment that they can be popular in society without regular bathing. A bath should be taken at least once a week, and if the feet perspire they should be washed several times a week, as the case may require. It is not unfrequent that young men are seen with dirty ears and neck. This is unpardonable and boorish, and shows gross neglect. Occasionally a young lady will be called upon unexpectedly when her neck and smiling face are not emblems of cleanliness. Every lady owes it to herself to be fascinating; every gentleman is bound, for his own sake, to be

presentable; but beyond this there is the obligation to society, to one's friends, and to those with whom we may be brought in contact.

7. **Soiled Garments.**—A young man's garments may not be expensive, yet there is no excuse for wearing a soiled collar and a soiled shirt, or carrying a soiled handkerchief. No one should appear as though he had slept in a stable, shaggy hair, soiled clothing or garments indifferently put on and carelessly buttoned. A young man's vest should always be kept buttoned in the presence of ladies.[86]

8. **The Breath.**—Care should be taken to remedy an offensive breath without delay. Nothing renders one so unpleasant to one's acquaintance, or is such a source of misery to one's self. The evil may be from some derangement of the stomach or some defective condition of the teeth, or catarrhal affection of the throat and nose. See remedies in other portions of the book.

A YOUNG MAN'S PERSONAL APPEARANCE.

Dress changes the manners.—VOLTAIRE.

Whose garments wither, shall receive faded smiles.—SHERIDAN KNOWLES.

Men of sense follow fashion so far that they are neither conspicuous for their excess nor peculiar by their opposition to it.—ANONYMOUS.

1. A well-dressed man does not require so much an extensive as a varied wardrobe. He does not need a different suit for every season and every occasion, but if he is careful to select clothes that are simple and not striking or conspicuous, he may use the garment over and over again without their being noticed, provided they are suitable to the season and the occasion.

2. A clean shirt, collar and cuffs always make a young man look neat and tidy, even if his clothes are not of the latest pattern and are somewhat threadbare.

3. Propriety is outraged when a man of sixty dresses like a youth of sixteen. It is bad manners for a gentleman to use perfumes to a noticeable extent. Avoid affecting singularity in dress. Expensive clothes are no sign of a gentleman.

The Dude of the 17th Century.

4. When dressed for company, strive to appear easy and natural. Nothing is more distressing to a sensitive person, or more ridiculous to one gifted with refinement, than to see a lady laboring under the consciousness of a fine gown; or a gentleman who is stiff, awkward and ungainly in a brand-new coat.

5. Avoid what is called the "ruffianly style of dress" or the slouchy appearance of a half-unbottoned vest, and suspenderless pantaloons. That sort of affectation is, if possible, even more disgusting than the painfully elaborate frippery of the dandy or dude. Keep your clothes well brushed and keep them cleaned. Slight spots can be removed with a little sponge and soap and water.

6. A gentleman should never wear a high hat unless he has on a frock coat or a dress suit.

7. A man's jewelry should be good and simple. Brass or false jewelry, like other forms of falsehood, is vulgar. Wearing many cheap decorations is a serious fault.[87]

8. If a man wears a ring it should be on the third finger of the left hand. This is the only piece of jewelry a man is allowed to wear that does not serve a purpose.

9. Wearing imitations of diamonds is always in very bad taste.

10. Every man looks better in a full beard if he keeps it well trimmed. If a man shaves he should shave at least every other day, unless he is in the country.

11. The finger-nails should be kept cut, and the teeth should be cleaned every morning, and kept clear from tartar. A man who does not keep his teeth clean does not look like a gentleman when he shows them.

[88]

Dress.

We sacrifice to dress, till household joys
And comforts cease. Dress drains our cellar dry,
And keeps our larder lean. Puts out our fires,

And introduces hunger, frost and woe,
Where peace and hospitality might reign.—COWPER.

1. **God is a Lover of Dress.**—We cannot but feel that God is a lover of dress. He has put on robes of beauty and glory upon all his works. Every flower is dressed in richness; every field blushes beneath a mantle of beauty; every star is veiled in brightness; every bird is clothed in the [89]habiliments of the most exquisite taste. The cattle upon the thousand hills are dressed by the hand divine. Who, studying God in his works, can doubt, that he will smile upon the evidence of correct taste manifested by his children in clothing the forms he has made them?

2. **Love of Dress.**—To love dress is not to be a slave of fashion; to love dress only is the test of such homage. To transact the business of charity in a silken dress, and to go in a carriage to the work, injures neither the work nor the worker. The slave of fashion is one who assumes the livery of a princess, and then omits the errand of the good human soul; dresses in elegance, and goes upon no good errand, and thinks and does nothing of value to mankind.

3. **Beauty in Dress.**—Beauty in dress is a good thing, rail at it who may. But it is a lower beauty, for which a higher beauty should not be sacrificed. They love dresses too much who give it their first thought, their best time, or all their money; who for it neglect the culture of their mind or heart, or the claims of others on their service; who care more for their dress than their disposition; who are troubled more by an unfashionable bonnet than a neglected duty.

4. **Simplicity of Dress.**—Female lovliness never appears to so good advantage as when set off by simplicity of dress. No artist ever decks his angels with towering feathers and gaudy jewelry; and our dear human angels—if they would make good their title to that name—should carefully avoid ornaments, which properly belong to Indian squaws and African princesses. These tinselries may serve to give effect on the stage, or upon the ball room floor, but in daily life there is no substitute for the charm of simplicity. A vulgar taste is not to be disguised by gold or diamonds. The absence of a true taste and refinement of delicacy cannot be compensated for by the possession of the most princely fortune. Mind measures gold, but gold cannot measure mind. Through dress the mind may be read, as through the delicate tissue the lettered page. A modest woman will dress modestly; a really refined and intelligent woman will bear the marks of careful selection and faultless taste.

5. **People of Sense.**—A coat that has the mark of use upon it, is a recommendation to the people of sense, and a hat with too much nap, and too high lustre, a derogatory circumstance. The best coats in our streets are worn on the backs of penniless fops, broken down merchants, clerks with pitiful salaries, and men that do not pay up. The heaviest gold chains dangle from the fobs of gamblers and gentlemen of very limited means; costly ornaments on [90]ladies, indicate to the eyes that are well opened, the fact of a silly lover or husband cramped for funds.

6. **Plain and Neat.**—When a pretty woman goes by in plain and neat apparel, it is the presumption that she has fair expectations, and a husband that can show a balance in his favor. For women are like books,—too much gilding makes men suspicious, that the binding is the most important part. The body is the shell of the soul, and the dress is the husk of the body; but the husk generally tells what the kernel is. As a fashionably dressed young lady passed some gentlemen, one of them raised his hat, whereupon another, struck by the fine appearance of the lady, made some inquiries concerning her, and was answered thus: "She makes a pretty ornament in her father's house, but otherwise is of no use."

7. **The Richest Dress.**—The richest dress is always worn on the soul. The adornments that will not perish, and that all men most admire, shine from the heart through this life. God has made it our highest, holiest duty, to dress the soul he has given us. It is wicked to waste it in frivolity. It is a beautiful, undying, precious thing. If every young woman would think of her soul when she looks in the glass, would hear the cry of her naked mind when she dallies away her precious hours at her toilet, would listen to the sad moaning

of her hollow heart, as it wails through her idle, useless life, something would be done for the elevation of womanhood.

8. **Dressing Up.**—Compare a well-dressed body with a well-dressed mind. Compare a taste for dress with a taste for knowledge, culture, virtue, and piety. Dress up an ignorant young woman in the "height of fashion"; put on plumes and flowers, diamonds and gewgaws; paint her face, girt up her waist, and I ask you, if this side of a painted and feathered savage you can find anything more unpleasant to behold. And yet such young women we meet by the hundred every day on the street and in all our public places. It is awful to think of.

9. **Dress Affects our Manners.**—A man who is badly dressed, feels chilly, sweaty, and prickly. He stammers, and does not always tell the truth. He means to, perhaps, but he can't. He is half distracted about his pantaloons, which are much to short, and are constantly hitching up; or his frayed jacket and crumpled linen harrow his soul, and quite unman him. He treads on the train of a lady's dress, and says, "Thank you", sits down on his hat, and wishes the "desert were his dwelling place."

[91]

Beauty.

"She walks in beauty, like the night
Of cloudless climes and starry skies:
And all that's best of dark and bright
Meet her in aspect and in her eyes;
Thus mellowed to that tender light
Which heaven to gaudy day denies."—BYRON.

1. **The Highest Style of Beauty.**—The highest style of beauty to be found in nature pertains to the human form, as animated and lighted up by the intelligence within. It is the expression of the soul that constitutes this superior beauty. It is that which looks out of the eye, which sits in calm majesty on the brow, lurks on the lip, smiles on the cheek, is set forth in the chiselled lines and features of the countenance, in the general contour of figure and form, in the movement, and gesture, and tone; it is this looking out of the invisible spirit that dwells within, this manifestation of the higher nature, that we admire and love; this constitutes to us the beauty of our species.[92]

2. **Beauty Which Perishes Not.**—There is a beauty which perishes not. It is such as the angels wear. It forms the washed white robes of the saints. It wreathes the countenance of every doer of good. It adorns every honest face. It shines in the virtuous life. It molds the hands of charity. It sweetens the voice of sympathy. It sparkles on the brow of wisdom. It flashes in the eye of love. It breathes in the spirit of piety. It is the beauty of the heaven of heavens. It is that which may grow by the hand of culture in every human soul. It is the flower of the spirit which blossoms on the tree of life. Every soul may plant and nurture it in its own garden, in its own Eden.

3. **We May All Be Beautiful.**—This is the capacity of beauty that God has given to the human soul, and this the beauty placed within the reach of all. We may all be beautiful. Though our forms may be uncomely and our features not the prettiest, our spirits may be beautiful. And this inward beauty always shines through. A beautiful heart will flash out in the eye. A lovely soul will glow in the face. A sweet spirit will tune the voice, wreathe the countenance in charms. Oh, there is a power in interior beauty that melts the hardest heart!

4. **Woman the Most Perfect Type of Beauty.**—Woman, by common consent, we regard as the most perfect type of beauty on earth. To her we ascribe the highest charms belonging to this wonderful element so profusely mingled in all God's works. Her form is molded and finished in exquisite delicacy of perfection. The earth gives us no form more perfect, no features more symmetrical, no style more chaste, no movements more graceful, no finish more complete; so that our artists ever have and ever will regard the woman-form of humanity as the most perfect earthly type of beauty. This form is most perfect and symmetrical in the youth of womanhood; so that the youthful woman is earth's queen of

beauty. This is true, not only by the common consent of mankind, but also by the strictest rules of scientific criticism.

A REJECTED LOVER.

5. **Fadeless Beauty.**—There cannot be a picture without its bright spots; and the steady contemplation of what is bright in others, has a reflex influence upon the beholder. It reproduces what it reflects. Nay, it seems to leave an impress even upon the countenance. The feature, from having a dark, sinister aspect, becomes open, serene, and sunny. A countenance so impressed, has neither the vacant stare of the idiot, nor the crafty, penetrating look of the basilisk, but the clear, placid aspect of truth and goodness. The woman [94]who has such a face is beautiful. She has a beauty which changes not with the features, which fades not with years. It is beauty of expression. It is the only kind of beauty which can be relied upon for a permanent influence with the other sex. The violet will soon cease to smile. Flowers must fade. The love that has nothing but beauty to sustain it, soon withers away.

6. **A Pretty Woman Pleases the Eye**, a good woman, the heart. The one is a jewel, the other a treasure. Invincible fidelity, good humor, and complacency of temper, outlive all the charms of a fine face, and make the decay of it invisible. That is true beauty which has not only a substance, but a spirit; a beauty that we must intimately know to justly appreciate.

7. **The Woman You Love Best.**—Beauty, dear reader, is probably the woman you love best, but we trust it is the beauty of soul and character, which sits in calm majesty on the brow, lurks on the lip, and will outlive what is called a fine face.

8. **The Wearing of Ornaments.**—Beauty needs not the foreign aid of ornament, but is when unadorned adorned the most, is a trite observation; but with a little qualification it is worthy of general acceptance. Aside from the dress itself, ornaments should be very sparingly used—at any rate, the danger lies in over-loading oneself, and not in using too few. A young girl, and especially one of a light and airy style of beauty, should never wear gems. A simple flower in her hair or on her bosom is all that good taste will permit. When jewels or other ornaments are worn, they should be placed where you desire the eye of the spectator to rest, leaving the parts to which you do not want attention called as plain and negative as possible. There is no surer sign of vulgarity than a profusion of heavy jewelry carried about upon the person.

[95]

Sensible Helps to Beauty.

1. FOR SCRAWNY NECK.—Take off your tight collars, feather boas and such heating things. Wash neck and chest with hot water, then rub in sweet oil all that you can work in. Apply this every night before you retire and leave the skin damp with it while you sleep.

2. FOR RED HANDS.—Keep your feet warm by soaking them often in hot water, and keep your hands out of the water as much as possible. Rub your hands with the skin of a lemon and it will whiten them. If your skin will bear glycerine after you have washed, pour into the palm a little glycerine and lemon juice mixed, and rub over the hands and wipe off.

3. NECK AND FACE.—Do not bathe the neck and face just before or after being out of doors. It tends to wrinkle the skin.

4. SCOWLS.—Never allow yourself to scowl, even if the sun be in your eyes. That scowl will soon leave its trace and no beauty will outlive it.[96]

5. WRINKLED FOREHEAD.—If you wrinkle your forehead when you talk or read, visit an oculist and have your eyes tested, and then wear glasses to fit them.

6. OLD LOOKS.—Sometimes your face looks old because it is tired. Then apply the following wash and it will make you look younger: Put three drops of ammonia, a little borax, a tablespoonful of bay rum, and a few drops of camphor into warm water and apply to your face. Avoid getting it into your eyes.

7. THE BEST COSMETIC.—Squeeze the juice of a lemon into a pint of sweet milk. Wash the face with it every night and in the morning wash off with warm rain water. This will produce a very beautiful effect upon the skin.

8. SPOTS ON THE FACE.—Moles and many other discolorations may be removed from the face by a preparation composed of one part chemically pure carbolic acid and two parts pure glycerine. Touch the spots with a camel's-hair pencil, being careful that the preparation does not come in contact with the adjacent skin. Five minutes after touching, bathe with soft water and apply a little vaseline. It may be necessary to repeat the operation, but if persisted in, the blemishes will be entirely removed.

9. WRINKLES.—This prescription is said to cure wrinkles: Take one ounce of white wax and melt it to a gentle heat. Add two ounces of the juice of lily bulbs, two ounces of honey, two drams of rose water, and a drop or two of ottar of roses. Apply twice a day, rubbing the wrinkles the wrong way. Always use tepid water for washing the face.

10. THE HAIR.—The hair must be kept free from dust or it will fall out. One of the best things for cleaning it, is a raw egg rubbed into the roots and then washed out in several waters. The egg furnishes material for the hair to grow on, while keeping the scalp perfectly clean. Apply once a month.

11. LOSS OF HAIR.—When through sickness or headache the hair falls out, the following tonic may be applied with good effect: Use one ounce of glycerine, one ounce of bay rum, one pint of strong sage tea, and apply every other night, rubbing well into the scalp.

[97]

How to Keep the Bloom and Grace of Youth.
THE SECRET OF ITS PRESERVATION.
MRS. WM. MCKINLEY.

1. The question most often asked by women is regarding the art of retaining, with advancing years, the bloom and grace of youth. This secret is not learned through the analysis of chemical compounds, but by a thorough study of nature's laws peculiar to their sex. It is useless for women with wrinkled faces, dimmed eyes and blemished skins to seek for external applications of beautifying balms and lotions to bring the glow of life and health into the face, and yet there are truths, simple yet wonderful, whereby the bloom of early life can be restored and retained, as should be the heritage of all God's children, sending the light of beauty into every woman's face. The secret:

2. Do not bathe in hard water; soften it with a few drops of ammonia, or a little borax.

3. Do not bathe the face while it is very warm, and never use very cold water.

4. Do not attempt to remove dust with cold water; give your face a hot bath, using plenty of good soap, then give it a thorough rinsing with warm water.

5. Do not rub your face with a coarse towel.

6. Do not believe you can remove wrinkles by filling in the crevices with powder. Give your face a Russian bath every night; that is, bathe it with water so hot that you wonder how you can bear it, and then, a minute after, with moderately cold water, that will make your face glow with warmth; dry it with a soft towel.

[98]

Form and Deformity.
MALE. FEMALE.
Showing the Difference in Form and Proportion.

1. **Physical Deformities.**—Masquerading is a modern accomplishment. Girls wear tight shoes, burdensome skirts, corsets, etc., all of which prove so fatal to their health. At the age of seventeen or eighteen, our "young ladies" are sorry specimens of feminality; and palpitators, cosmetics and all the modern paraphernalia are required to make them appear fresh and blooming. Man is equally at fault. A devotee to all the absurd devices of fashion, he practically asserts that "dress makes the man." But physical deformities are of far less importance than moral imperfections.

2. **Development of the Individual.**—It is not possible for human beings to attain their full stature of humanity, except by loving long and perfectly. Behold that venerable man! he is mature in judgment, perfect in every action and expression, and saintly in goodness. You almost worship as you behold. What rendered him thus perfect?

39

What [99]rounded off his natural asperities, and moulded up his virtues? Love, mainly. It permeated every pore, and seasoned every fibre of his being, as could nothing else. Mark that matronly woman. In the bosom of her family she is more than a queen and goddess combined. All her looks and actions express the outflowing of some or all of the human virtues. To know her is to love her. She became thus perfect, not in a day or year, but by a long series of appropriate means. Then by what? Chiefly in and by love, which is specially adapted thus to develop this maturity.

3. **Physical Stature.**—Men and women generally increase in stature until the twenty-fifth year, and it is safe to assume, that perfection of function is not established until maturity of bodily development is completed. The physical contour of these representations plainly exhibits the difference in structure, and also implies difference of function. Solidity and strength are represented by the organization of the male, grace and beauty by that of the female. His broad shoulders represent physical power and the right of dominion, while her bosom is the symbol of love and nutrition.

HOW TO DETERMINE A PERFECT HUMAN FIGURE.

Lady's Dress in the days of Greece.

The proportions of the perfect human figure are strictly mathematical. The whole figure is six times the length of the foot. Whether the form be slender or plump, this rule holds good. Any deviation from it is a departure from the highest beauty of proportion. The Greeks made all their statues according to this rule. The face, from the highest point of the forehead, where the hair begins, to the end of the chin, is one-tenth of the whole stature. The hand, from the wrist to the end of the middle finger, is the same. The chest is a fourth, and from the nipples to the top of the head is the same. From the top of the chest to the highest point of the forehead is a seventh. If the length of the face, from the roots of the hair to the chin, be divided into three equal parts, the first division determines the point where the eyebrows meet, and the second the place of the nostrils. The navel is the central point of the human body, and if a man should lie on his back with his arms and legs extended, the periphery of the circle which might be described around him, with the navel for its center, would touch the extremities of his hands and feet. The height from the feet to the top of the head is the same as the [100]distance from the extremity of one hand to the extremity of the other when the arms are extended.

The Venus de Medici is considered the most perfect model of the female forms, and has been the admiration of the world for ages. Alexander Walker, after minutely describing this celebrated statue, says: "All these admirable characteristics of the female form, the mere existence of which in woman must, one is temped to imagine, be, even to herself, a source of ineffable pleasure, these constitute a being worthy, as the personification of beauty, of occupying the temples of Greece; present an object finer, alas, than Nature even seems capable of producing; and offer to all nations and ages a theme of admiration and delight." Well might Thomson say:

So stands the statue that enchants the world,
So, bending, tries to vail the matchless boast—
The mingled beauties of exulting Greece.

We beg our readers to observe the form of the waist (evidently innocent of corsets and tight dresses) of this model woman, and also that of the Greek Slave in the accompanying outlines. These forms are such as unperverted nature and the highest art alike require. To compress the waist, and thereby change its form, pushing the ribs inward, displacing the vital organs, and preventing the due expansion of the lungs, is as destructive to beauty as it is to health.[101]

THE HISTORY, MYSTERY, BENEFITS AND INJURIES OF THE CORSET.

The Corset in the 18th Century.

1. The origin of the corset is lost in remote antiquity. The figures of the early Egyptian women show clearly an artificial shape of the waist produced by some style of corset. A similar style of dress must also have prevailed among the ancient Jewish maidens; for Isaiah, in calling upon the women to put away their personal adornments, says: "Instead of a girdle there shall be a rent, and instead of a stomacher (corset) a girdle of sackcloth."

2. Homer also tells us of the cestus or girdle of Venus, which was borrowed by the haughty Juno with a view to increasing her personal attractions, that Jupiter might be a more tractable and orderly husband.

3. Coming down to the later times, we find the corset was used in France and England as early as the 12th century.

4. The most extensive and extreme use of the corset occurred in the 16th century, during the reign of Catherine de Medici of France and Queen Elizabeth of England. With Catherine de Medici a thirteen-inch waist measurement was considered the standard of fashion, while a thick waist was an abomination. No lady could consider her figure of proper shape unless she could span her waist with her two hands. To produce this result a strong rigid corset was worn night and day until the waist was laced down to the required size. Then over this corset was placed the steel apparatus shown in the illustration on next page. This corset-cover reached from the hip to the throat, and [102]produced a rigid figure over which the dress would fit with perfect smoothness.

5. During the 18th century corsets were largely made from a species of leather known as "Bend," which was not unlike that used for shoe soles, and measured nearly a quarter of an inch in thickness. One of the most popular corsets of the time was the corset and stomacher shown in the accompanying illustration.

Steel Corset worn in Catherine's time.

6. About the time of the French Revolution a reaction set in against tight lacing, and for a time there was a return to the early classical Greek costume. This style of dress prevailed, with various modifications, until about 1810, when corsets and tight lacing again returned with threefold fury. Buchan, a prominent writer of this period, says that it was by no means uncommon to see "a mother lay her daughter down upon the carpet, and, placing her foot upon her back, break half a dozen laces in tightening her stays."

7. It is reserved to our own time to demonstrate that corsets and tight lacing do not necessarily go hand in hand. Distortion and feebleness are not beauty. A proper proportion should exist between the size of the waist and the breadth of the shoulders and hips, and if the waist is diminished below this proportion, it suggests disproportion and invalidism rather than grace and beauty.

8. The perfect corset is one which possesses just that degree of rigidity which will prevent it from wrinkling, but will at the same time allow freedom in the bending and twisting of the body. Corsets boned with whalebone, horn or steel are necessarily stiff, rigid and uncomfortable. After a few days' wear the bones or steels become bent and set in position, or, as more frequently happens, they break and cause injury or discomfort to the wearer.

9. About seven years ago an article was discovered for the stiffening of corsets, which has revolutionized the corset industry of the world. This article is manufactured from [103]the natural fibers of the Mexican Ixtle plant, and is known as Coraline. It consists of straight, stiff fibers like bristles bound together into a cord by being wound with two strands of thread passing in opposite directions. This produces an elastic fiber intermediate in stiffness between twine and whalebone. It cannot break, but it possesses all the stiffness and flexibility necessary to hold the corset in shape and prevent its wrinkling.

We congratulate the ladies of to-day upon the advantages they enjoy over their sisters of two centuries ago, in the forms and the graceful and easy curves of the corsets now made as compared with those of former times.

Forms of Corsets in the time of Elizabeth of England.

[104]

TIGHT-LACING.
EGYPTIAN CORSET.
THE NATURAL WAIST.
THE EFFECTS OF LACING.

It destroys natural beauty and creates an unpleasant and irritable temper. A tight-laced chest and a good disposition cannot go together. The human form has been molded by nature, the best shape is undoubtedly that which she has given it. To endeavor to render it more elegant by artificial means is to change it; to make it much smaller below and much larger above is to destroy its beauty; to keep it cased up in a kind of domestic cuirass is not only to deform it, but to expose the internal parts to serious injury. Under such compression as is commonly practiced by ladies, the [105]development of the bones, which are still tender, does not take place conformably to the intention of nature, because nutrition is necessarily stopped, and they consequently become twisted and deformed.

Those who wear these appliances of tight-lacing often complain that they cannot sit upright without them—are sometimes, indeed, compelled to wear them during all the twenty-four hours; a fact which proves to what extent such articles weaken the muscles of the trunk. The injury does not fall merely on the internal structure of the body, but also on its beauty, and on the temper and feelings with which that beauty is associated. Beauty is in reality but another name for expression of countenance, which is the index of sound health, intelligence, good feelings and peace of mind. All are aware that uneasy feelings, existing habitually in the breast speedily exhibit their signature on the countenance, and that bitter thoughts or a bad temper spoil the human expression of its comeliness and grace.

[107]
The Care of the Hair.
NATURAL HAIR.
1. **The Color of the Hair.**—The color of the hair corresponds with that of the skin—being dark or black, with a dark complexion, and red or yellow with a fair skin. When a white skin is seen in conjunction with black hair, as among the women of Syria and Barbary, the apparent exception arises from protection from the sun's rays, and opposite colors are often found among people of one prevailing feature. Thus red-haired Jews are not uncommon, though the nation in general have dark complexion and hair.

2. **The Imperishable Nature of Hair.**—The imperishable nature of hair arises from the combination of salt and metals in its composition. In old tombs and on mummies it has been found in a perfect state, after a lapse of over two thousand years. There are many curious accounts proving the indestructibility of the human hair.

3. **Tubular.**—In the human family the hairs are tubular, the tubes being intersected by partitions, resembling in some degree the cellular tissue of plants. Their hollowness prevents incumbrance from weight, while their power of resistance is increased by having their traverse sections rounded in form.

4. **Cautions.**—It is ascertained that a full head of hair, beard and whiskers, are a prevention against colds and consumptions. Occasionally, however, it is found necessary to remove the hair from the head, in cases of fever or disease, to stay the inflammatory symptoms, and to relieve the brain. The head should invariably be kept cool. Close night-caps are unhealthy, and smoking-caps and coverings for the head within doors are alike detrimental to the free growth of the hair, weakening it, and causing it to fall out.

HOW TO BEAUTIFY AND PRESERVE THE HAIR.
1. **To Beautify the Hair.**—Keep the head clean, the pores of the skin open, and the whole circulatory system in a healthy condition, and you will have no need of bear's grease (alias hog's lard). Where there is a tendency in the hair to fall off on account of the weakness or sluggishness of the circulation, or an unhealthy state of the skin, cold water and friction with a tolerably stiff brush are probably the best remedial agents.

2. **Barber's Shampoos.**—Are very beneficial if properly prepared. They should not be made too strong. Avoid strong shampoos of any kind. Great caution should be exercised in this matter.[108]

3. **Care of the Hair.**—To keep the hair healthy, keep the head clean. Brush the scalp well with a stiff brush, while dry. Then wash with castile soap, and rub into the roots, bay rum, brandy or camphor water. This done twice a month will prove beneficial. Brush the scalp thoroughly twice a week. Dampen the hair with soft water at the toilet, and do not use oil.

4. **Hair Wash.**—Take one ounce of borax, half an ounce of camphor powder—these ingredients fine—and dissolve them in one quart of boiling water. When cool, the solution

will be ready for use. Dampen the hair frequently. This wash is said not only to cleanse and beautify, but to strengthen the hair, preserve the color and prevent baldness.

Another Excellent Wash.—The best wash we know for cleansing and softening the hair is an egg beaten up and rubbed well into the hair, and afterwards washed out with several washes of warm water.

5. **The Only Sensible and Safe Hair Oil.**—The following is considered a most valuable preparation: Take of extract of yellow Peruvian bark, fifteen grains; extract of rhatany root, eight grains; extract of burdoch root and oil of nutmegs (fixed), of each two drachms; camphor (dissolve with spirits of wine), fifteen grains; beef marrow, two ounces; best olive oil, one ounce; citron juice, half a drachm; aromatic essential oil, as much as sufficient to render it fragrant; mix and make into an ointment. Two drachms of bergamot, and a few drops of attar of roses would suffice.

6. **Hair Wash.**—A good hair wash is soap and water, and the oftener it is applied the freer the surface of the head will be from scurf. The hair-brush should also be kept in requisition morning and evening.

7. **To Remove Superfluous Hair.**—With those who dislike the use of arsenic, the following is used for removing superfluous hair from the skin: Lime, one ounce; carbonate of potash, two ounces; charcoal powder, one drachm. For use, make it into a paste with a little warm water, and apply it to the part, previously shaved close. As soon as it has become thoroughly dry, it may be washed off with a little warm water.

8. **Coloring for Eyelashes and Eyebrows.**—In eyelashes the chief element of beauty consists in their being long and glossy; the eyebrows should be finely arched and clearly divided from each other. The most innocent darkener of the brow is the expressed juice of the elderberry, or a burnt clove.[109]

DISCUSSING THE FASHIONS.

9. **Crimping Hair.**—To make the hair stay in crimps, take five cents worth of gum arabic and add to it just enough boiling water to dissolve it. When dissolved, add enough alcohol to make it rather thin. Let this stand all night and then bottle it to prevent the alcohol from evaporating. This put on the hair at night, after it is done up in papers or pins, will make it stay in crimp the hottest day, and is perfectly harmless.

10. **To Curl the Hair.**—There is no preparation that will make naturally straight hair assume a permanent curl. The following will keep the hair in curl for a short time: Take borax, two ounces; gum arabic, one drachm; and hot [110]water, not boiling, one quart; stir, and, as soon as the ingredients are dissolved, add three tablespoonfuls of strong spirits of camphor. On retiring to rest, wet the hair with the above liquid, and roll in twists of paper as usual. Do not disturb the hair until morning, when untwist and form into ringlets.

11. **For Falling or Loosening of the Hair.**—Take:

Alcohol, a half pint.

Salt, as much as will dissolve.

Glycerine, a tablespoonful.

Flour of sulphur, teaspoonful. Mix.

Rub on the scalp every morning.

12. **To Darken the Hair without Bad Effects.**—Take:

Blue vitriol (powdered), one drachm.

Alcohol, one ounce.

Essence of roses, ten drops.

Rain-water, a half-pint.

Shake together until they are thoroughly dissolved.

13. **Gray Hair.**—There are no known means by which the hair can be prevented from turning gray, and none which can restore it to its original hue, except through the process of dyeing. The numerous "hair color restorers" which are advertised are chemical preparations which act in the manner of a dye or as a paint, and are nearly always dependent for their power on the presence of lead. This mineral, applied to the skin, for a long time, will lead to the most disastrous maladies—lead-palsy, lead colic, and other symptoms of poisoning. It should, therefore, never be used for this purpose.

How to Cure Pimples or Other Facial Eruptions.

1. It requires self-denial to get rid of pimples, for persons troubled with them will persist in eating fat meats and other articles of food calculated to produce them. Avoid the use of rich gravies, or pastry, or anything of the kind in excess. Take all the out-door exercise yon can and never indulge in a late supper. Retire at a reasonable hour, and rise early in the morning. Sulphur to purify the blood may be taken three times a week—a thimbleful in a glass of milk before breakfast. It takes some time for the sulphur to do its work, therefore persevere in its use till the humors, or pimples, or blotches, disappear. Avoid getting wet while taking the sulphur.

2. **Try This Recipe**: Wash the face twice a day in warm water, and rub dry with a coarse towel. Then with a soft towel rub in a lotion made of two ounces of white brandy, one ounce of cologne, and one-half ounce of liquor potassa. [112]Persons subject to skin eruptions should avoid very salty or fat food. A dose of Epsom salts occasionally might prove beneficial.

3. Wash the face in a dilution of carbolic acid, allowing one teaspoonful to a pint of water. This is an excellent and purifying lotion, and may be used on the most delicate skins. Be careful about letting this wash get into the eyes.

4. Oil of sweet almonds, one ounce; fluid potash, one drachm. Shake well together, and then add rose water, one ounce; pure water, six ounces. Mix. Rub the pimples or blotches for some minutes with a rough towel, and then dab them with the lotion.

5. Dissolve one ounce of borax, and sponge the face with it every night. When there are insects, rub on flower of sulphur dry after washing, rub well and wipe dry; use plenty of castile soap.

6. Dilute corrosive sublimate with oil of almonds. A few days' application will remove them.

BLACK-HEADS AND FLESH WORMS.
A Regular Flesh Worm Greatly Magnified.

A HEALTHY COMPLEXION.
This is a minute little creature, scientifically called *Demodex folliculorum*, hardly visible to the naked eye, with comparatively large fore body, a more slender hind body and eight little stumpy processes that do duty as legs. No specialized head is visible, although of course there is a mouth orifice. These creatures live on the sweat glands or pores of the human face, and owing to the appearance that they give to the infested pores, they are usually known as "black-heads." It is not at all uncommon to see an otherwise pretty face disfigured by these ugly creatures, although the insects themselves are nearly transparent white. The black appearance is really due the accumulation of dirt which gets under the edges of the skin of the enlarged sweat glands and cannot be removed in the ordinary way by washing, because the abnormal, hardened secretion of the gland itself becomes stained. These insects are so lowly organized that it is almost impossible to satisfactorily deal with them. [113]and they sometimes cause the continual festering of the skin which they inhabit.

Remedy.—Press them out with a hollow key or with the thumb and fingers, and apply a mixture of sulphur and cream every evening. Wash every morning with the best toilet soap, or wash the face with hot water with a soft flannel at bedtime.

Love.

But there's nothing half so sweet in life
As love's young dream.—MOORE.
All love is sweet,

Given or returned. Common as light is love,
And its familiar voice wearies not ever.—SHELLEY.
Doubt thou the stars are fire,
Doubt that the sun doth move;
Doubt truth to be a liar,
But never doubt I love.—SHAKESPEARE.
Let those love now who never loved before,
Let those that always loved now love the more.—PARNELL.

LOVE'S YOUNG DREAM.

1. **Love Blends Young Hearts.**—Love blends young hearts in blissful unity, and, for the time, so ignores past ties and affections, as to make willing separation of the son from his father's house, and the daughter from all the sweet endearments of her childhood's home, to go out together, and rear for themselves an altar, around which shall cluster all the cares and delights, the anxieties and sympathies, of the family relationship; this love, if pure, unselfish, and discreet, constitutes the chief usefulness and happiness of human life.

2. **Without Love.**—Without love there would be no organized households, and, consequently, none of that earnest endeavor for competence and respectability, which is the mainspring to human effort; none of those sweet, softening, restraining and elevating influences of domestic life, which can alone fill the earth with the glory of the Lord and make glad the city of Zion. This love is indeed heaven upon earth; but above would not be heaven without it; where there is not love, there is fear; but, "love casteth out fear." And yet we naturally do offend what we most love.

3. **Love Is the Sun of Life.**—Most beautiful in morning and evening, but warmest and steadiest at noon. It is the sun of the soul. Life without love is worse than death; a world without a sun. The love which does not lead to labor will soon die out, and the thankfulness which does not embody itself in sacrifices is already changing to gratitude. Love is not ripened in one day, nor in many, nor even in a human lifetime. It is the oneness of soul with soul in appreciation and perfect trust. To be blessed it must rest in that faith in the Divine which underlies every other motion. To be true, it must be eternal as God himself.

4. **Love Is Dependent.**—Remember that love is dependent upon forms; courtesy of etiquette guards and protects courtesy of heart. How many hearts have been lost irrevocably, and how many averted eyes and cold looks have been gained from what seemed, perhaps, but a trifling negligence of forms?

[116]

LOVE MAKING IN THE EARLY COLONIAL DAYS.

5. **Radical Differences.**—Men and women should not be judged by the same rules. There are many radical differences in their affectional natures. Man is the creature of interest and ambition. His nature leads him forth into the struggle and bustle of the world. Love is but the embellishment of his early life, or a song piped in the intervals of the acts. He seeks for fame, for fortune, for space in the world's thoughts, and dominion over his fellow-men. But a woman's whole life is a history of the affections. The heart is her world; it is there her ambition strives for empire; it is there her ambition seeks for hidden treasures. She sends forth her sympathies on adventure; she embarks her whole soul in the traffic of affection; and if shipwrecked her case is hopeless, for it is bankruptcy of the heart.

6. **Woman's Love.**—Woman's love is stronger than death; it rises superior to adversity, and towers in sublime beauty above the niggardly selfishness of the world. Misfortune cannot suppress it; enmity cannot alienate it; temptation cannot enslave it. It is the guardian angel of the nursery and the sick bed; it gives an affectionate concord to the partnership of life and interest, circumstances cannot modify it; it ever remains the same to sweeten existence, to purify the cup of life, on the rugged pathway to the grave, and melt to moral pliability the brittle nature of man. It is the ministering spirit of home, hovering in soothing caresses over the cradle, and the death-bed of the household, and filling up the urn of all its sacred memories.

7. **A Lady's Complexion.**—He who loves a lady's complexion, form and features, loves not her true self, but her soul's old clothes. The love that has nothing but beauty to sustain it, soon withers and dies. The love that is fed with presents always requires feeding.

Love, and love only, is the loan for love. Love is of the nature of a burning glass, which, kept still in one place, fireth; changed often, it doth nothing. The purest joy we can experience in one we love, is to see that person a source of happiness to others. When you are with the person loved, you have no sense of being bored. This humble and trivial circumstance is the great test—the only sure and abiding test of love.

8. **Two Souls Come Together.**—When two souls come together, each seeking to magnify the other, each in subordinate sense worshiping the other, each help the other; the two flying together so that each wing-beat of the one helps each wing-beat of the other—when two souls come together thus, they are lovers. They who unitedly move themselves away from grossness and from earth, toward the throne of crystaline and the pavement golden, are, indeed, true lovers.

[118]

CUPID'S CAPTURED VICTIM.
The Power and Peculiarities of Love.

LOVE IS A TONIC AND A REMEDY FOR DISEASE, MAKES PEOPLE LOOK YOUNGER, CREATES INDUSTRY, ETC.

"All thoughts, all passions, all desires,
Whatever stirs this mortal frame,
Are ministers of Love,
And feed his sacred flame."

1. It is a physiological fact long demonstrated that persons possessing a loving disposition borrow less of the cares of life, and also live much longer than persons with a strong, narrow and selfish nature. Persons who love scenery, love domestic animals, show great attachment for all friends; love their home dearly and find interest and enchantment in almost everything have qualities of mind and heart which indicate good health and a happy disposition.

2. Persons who love music and are constantly humming or whistling a tune, are persons that need not be feared, they are kind-hearted and with few exceptions possess a loving disposition. Very few good musicians become criminals.

3. Parents that cultivate a love among then children will find that the same feeling will soon be manifested in their children's disposition. Sunshine in the hearts of the parents will blossom in the lives of the children. The parent who continually cherishes a feeling of dislike and rebellion in his soul, cultivating moral hatred against his fellow-man, will soon find the same things manifested by his son. As the son resembles his father in looks so he will to a certain extent resemble him in character. Love in the heart of the parent will beget kindness and affection in the heart of a child. Continuous scolding and fretting in the home will soon make love a stranger.[119]

THE TURKISH WAY OF MAKING LOVE

4. If you desire to cultivate love, create harmony in all your feelings and faculties. Remember that all that is pure, holy and virtuous in love flows from the deepest fountain of the human soul. Poison the fountain and you change virtue to vice, and happiness to misery.

5. Love strengthens health, and disappointment cultivates disease. A person in love will invariably enjoy the best of health. Ninety-nine per cent. of our strong constitutioned men, now in physical ruin, have wrecked themselves on the breakers of an unnatural love. Nothing but right love and a right marriage will restore them to health.

6. All men feel much better for going a courting, providing they court purely. Nothing tears the life out of man more than lust, vulgar thoughts and immoral conduct. The libertine or harlot has changed love, God's purest gift to man, into lust. They cannot acquire love in its purity again, the sacred flame has vanished forever. Love is pure, and cannot be found in the heart of a seducer.

7. A woman is never so bright and full of health as when deeply in love. Many sickly and frail women are snatched from the clutches of some deadly disease and restored to health by falling in love.

46

8. It is a long established fact that married persons are healthier than unmarried persons; thus it proves that health and happiness belong to the home. Health depends upon mind. Love places the mind into a delightful state and quickens every human function, makes the blood circulate and weaves threads of joy into cables of domestic love.

PREPARING TO ENTERTAIN HER LOVER.

9. An old but true proverb: "A true man loving one woman will speak well of all women. A true woman loving one man will speak well of all men. A good wife praises all men, but praises her husband most. A good man praises all women, but praises his wife most."

10. Persons deeply in love become peculiarly pleasant, winning and tender. It is said that a musician can never excel or an artist do his best until he has been deeply in love. A good orator, a great statesman or great men in general are greater and better for having once been thoroughly in love. A man who truly loves his wife and home is always a safe man to trust.

11. Love makes people look younger in years. People in unhappy homes look older and more worn and fatigued. A woman at thirty, well courted and well married, looks five or ten years younger than a woman of the same age unhappily married. Old maids and bachelors always look older [120]than they are. A flirting widow always looks younger than an old maid of like age.

12. Love renders women industrious and frugal, and a loving husband spends lavishly on a loved wife and children, though miserly towards others.

13. Love cultivates self-respect and produces beauty. Beauty in walk and beauty in looks; a girl in love is at her best; it brings out the finest traits of her character, she walks more erect and is more generous and forgiving; her voice is sweeter and she makes happy all about her. She works better, sings better and is better.

14. Now in conclusion, a love marriage is the best life insurance policy; it pays dividends every day, while every other insurance policy merely promises to pay after death. Remember that statistics demonstrate that married people outlive old maids and old bachelors by a goodly number of years and enjoy healthier and happier lives.

[122]
Amativeness or Connubial Love.
CONFIDENCE.

1. **Multiplying the Race.**—Some means for multiplying our race is necessary to prevent its extinction by death. Propagation and death appertain to man's earthly existence. If the Deity had seen fit to bring every member of the human family into being by a direct act of creative power, without the agency of parents, the present wise and benevolent arrangements of husbands and wives, parents and children, friends and neighbors, would have been superseded, and all opportunities for exercising parental and connubial love, in which so much enjoyment is taken, cut off. But the domestic feelings and relations, as now arranged, must strike every philosophical observer as inimitably beautiful and perfect—as the offspring of infinite Wisdom and Goodness combined.

2. **Amativeness and its Combinations** constitute their origin, counterpart, and main medium of manifestation. Its primary function is connubial love. From it, mainly, spring those feelings which exist between the sexes as such and [123]result in marriage and offspring. Combined with the higher sentiments, it gives rise to all those reciprocal kind feelings and nameless courtesies which each sex manifests towards the other; refining and elevating both, promoting gentility and politeness, and greatly increasing social and general happiness.

3. **Renders Men More Polite to Women.**—So far from being in the least gross or indelicate, its proper exercise is pure, chaste, virtuous, and even an ingredient in good manners. It is this which renders men always more polite towards women than to one another, and more refined in their society, and which makes women more kind, grateful, genteel and tender towards men than women. It makes mothers love their sons more than their daughters, and fathers more attached to their daughters. Man's endearing recollections of his mother or wife form his most powerful incentives to virtue, study, and good deeds, as

47

well as restraints upon his vicious inclinations; and, in proportion as a young man is dutiful and affectionate to his mother, will he be fond of his wife; for, this faculty is the parent of both.

4. **All Should Cultivate the Faculty of Amativeness or Connubial Lore.**—Study the personal charms and mental accomplishments of the other sex by ardent admirers of beautiful forms, and study graceful movements and elegant manners, and remember, much depends upon the tones and accents of the voice. Never be gruff if you desire to be winning. Seek and enjoy and reciprocate fond looks and feelings. Before you can create favorable impressions you must first be honest and sincere and natural, and your conquest will be sure and certain.

Love and Common-Sense.

1. Do you love her because she goes to the altar with her head full of book learning, her hands of no earthly use, save for the piano and brush; because she has no conception of the duties and responsibilities of a wife; because she hates housework, hates its everlasting routine and ever recurring duties; because she hates children and will adopt every means to evade motherhood; because she loves her ease, loves to have her will supreme, loves, oh how well, to be free to go and come, to let the days slip idly by, to be absolved from all responsibility, to live without labor, without care? Will you love her selfish, shirking, calculating nature after twenty years of close companionship?

2. Do you love him because he is a man, and therefore, no matter how weak mentally, morally or physically he may [124]be, he has vested in him the power to save you from the ignominy of an old maid's existence? Because you would rather be Mrs. Nobody, than make the effort to be Miss Somebody? because you have a great empty place in your head and heart that nothing but a man can fill? because you feel you cannot live without him? God grant the time may never come when you cannot live with him.

AN EARNEST CALLER.

3. Do you love her because she is a thoroughly womanly woman; for her tender sympathetic nature; for the jewels of her life, which are absolute purity of mind and heart; for the sweet sincerity of her disposition; for her loving, charitable thought; for her strength of character? because she is pitiful to the sinful, tender to the sorrowful, capable, self-reliant, modest, true-hearted? in brief, because she is the embodiment of all womanly virtues?

4. Do you love him because he is a manly man; because the living and operating principle of his life is a tender reverence for all women; because his love is the overflow of the best part of his nature; because he has never soiled his soul with an unholy act or his lips with an oath; because mentally he is a man among men; because physically he stands head and shoulders above the masses; because morally he is far beyond suspicion, in his thought, word or deed; because his earnest manly consecrated life is a mighty power on God's side?

5. But there always has been and always will be unhappy marriages until men learn what husbandhood means; how to care for that tenderly matured, delicately constituted being, that he takes into his care and keeping. That if her wonderful adjusted organism is overtaxed and overburdened, her happiness, which is largely dependent upon her health, is destroyed.

6. Until men give the women they marry the undivided love of their heart; until constancy is the key-note of a life which speaks eloquently of clean thoughts and clean hearts.

7. Until men and women recognize that self-control in a man, and modesty in a woman, will bring a mutual respect that years of wedded life will only strengthen. Until they recognize that love is the purest and holiest of all things known to humanity, will marriage continue to bring unhappiness and discontent, instead of that comfort and restful peace which all loyal souls have a right to expect and enjoy.

8. Be sensible and marry a sensible, honest and industrious companion, and happiness through life will be your reward.

[126]

What Women Love in Men.

1. Women naturally love courage, force and firmness in men. The ideal man in a woman's eye must be heroic and brave. Woman naturally despises a coward, and she has little or no respect for a bashful man.

2. Woman naturally loves her lord and master. Women who desperately object to be overruled, nevertheless admire men who overrule them, and few women would have any respect for a man whom they could completely rule and control.

3. Man is naturally the protector of woman; as the male wild animal of the forest protects the female, so it is natural for man to protect his wife and children, and therefore woman admires those qualities in a man which make him a protector.

4. Large Men.—Women naturally love men of strength, size and fine physique, a tall, large and strong man rather than a short, small and weak man. A woman always pities a weakly man, but rarely ever has any love for him.

5. Small and Weakly Men.—All men would be of good size in frame and flesh, were it not for the infirmities visited upon them by the indiscretion of parents and ancestors of generations before.

6. Youthful Sexual Excitement.—There are many children born healthy and vigorous who destroy the full vigor of their generative organs in youth by self-abuse, and if they survive and marry, their children will have small bones, small frames and sickly constitutions. It is therefore not strange that instinct should lead women to admire men not touched with these symptoms of physical debility.

7. Generosity.—Woman generally loves a generous man. Religion absorbs a great amount of money in temples, churches, ministerial salaries, etc., and ambition and appetite absorb countless millions, yet woman receives more gifts from man than all these combined: she [127]loves a generous giver. *Generosity and Gallantry* are the jewels which she most admires. A woman receiving presents from a man implies that she will pay him back in love, and the woman who accepts a man's presents, and does not respect him, commits a wrong which is rarely ever forgiven.

8. Intelligence.—Above all other qualities in man, woman admires his intelligence. Intelligence is man's woman-captivating card. This character in woman is illustrated by an English army officer, as told by O. S. Fowler, betrothed in marriage to a beautiful, loving heiress, summoned to India, who wrote back to her:

"I have lost an eye, a leg, an arm, and been so badly marred and begrimmed besides, that you never could love this poor, maimed soldier. Yet, I love you too well to make your life wretched by requiring you to keep your marriage-vow with me, from which I hereby release you. Find among English peers one physically more perfect, whom you can love better."

She answered, as all genuine women must answer:

"Your noble mind, your splendid talents, your martial prowess which maimed you, are what I love. As long as you retain sufficient body to contain the casket of your soul, which alone is what I admire, I love you all the same, and long to make you mine forever."

9. Soft Men.—All women despise soft and silly men more than all other defects in their character. Woman never can love a man whose conversation is flat and insipid. Every man seeking woman's appreciation or love should always endeavor to show his intelligence and manifest an interest in books and daily papers. He should read books and inform himself so that he can talk intelligently upon the various topics of the day. Even an ignorant woman always loves superior intelligence.

10. Sexual Vigor.—Women love sexual vigor in men. This is human nature. Weakly and delicate fathers have weak and puny children, though the mother may be strong and robust. A weak mother often bears strong children, if the father is physically and sexually vigorous. Consumption is often inherited from fathers, because they furnish the body, yet more women die with it because of female obstructions. Hence women love passion in men, because it endows their offspring with strong functional vigor.

11. Passionate Men.—The less passion any woman possesses, the more she prizes a strong passionate man. This is a natural consequence, for if she married one equally[128]passionless, their children would be poorly endowed or they would have none;

49

she therefore admires him who makes up the deficiency. Hence very amorous men prefer quiet, modest and reserved women.

12. Homely Men are admired by women if they are large, strong and vigorous and possess a good degree of intelligence. Looks are trifles compared with the other qualities which man may possess.

13. Young Man, If you desire to win the love and admiration of young ladies, first, be intelligent; read books and papers; remember what you read, so you can talk about it. Second, be generous and do not show a stingy and penurious disposition when in the company of ladies. Third, be sensible, original, and have opinions of your own and do not agree with everything that someone else says, or agree with everything that a lady may say. Ladies naturally admire genteel and intelligent discussions and conversations when there is someone to talk with who has an opinion of his own. Woman despises a man who has no opinion of his own; she hates a trifling disposition and admires leadership, original ideas, and looks up to man as a leader. Women despise all men whom they can manage, overrule, cow-down and subdue.

14. Be Self-Supporting.—The young man who gives evidence of thrift is always in demand. Be enthusiastic and drive with success all that you undertake. A young man, sober, honest and industrious, holding a responsible position or having a business of his own, is a prize that some bright and beautiful young lady would like to draw. Woman admires a certainty.

15. Uniformed Men.—It is a well known fact that women love uniformed men. The soldier figures as a hero in about every tale of fiction and it is said by good authority that a man in uniform has three more chances to marry than the man without uniform. The correct reason is, the soldier's profession is bravery, and he is dressed and trained for that purpose, and it is that which makes him admired by ladies rather than the uniform which he wears. His profession is also that of a protector.

[129]

KATE SHELLEY
The Heroine of Honey Creek, who July 6, 1881, crept across the
trembling bridge in the darkness of a terrific storm, and
stopped the approaching Passenger Train.

What Men Love in Women.

1. Female Beauty.—Men love beautiful women, for woman's beauty is the highest type of all beauty. A handsome woman needs no diamonds, no silks or satins; her brilliant face outshines diamonds and her form is beautiful in calico.

2. False Beautifiers.—Man's love of female beauty surpasses all other love, and whatever artificial means are used to beautify, to a certain extent are falsehoods which lead to distrust or dislike. Artificial beauty is always an imitation, and never can come into competition with the genuine. No art can successfully imitate nature.

3. True Kind of Beauty.—Facial beauty is only skin-deep. A beautiful form, a graceful figure, graceful movements and a kind heart are the strongest charms in the perfection of female beauty. A brilliant face always outshines what may be called a pretty face, for intelligence is that queenly grace which crowns woman's influence over men. Good looks and good and pure conduct awaken a man's love for women. A girl must therefore be charming as well [130]as beautiful, for a charming girl will never become a charmless wife.

4. A Good Female Body.—No weakly, poor-bodied woman can draw a man's love like a strong, well developed body. A round, plump figure with an overflow of animal life is the woman most commonly sought, for nature in man craves for the strong qualities in women, as the health and life of offspring depend upon the physical qualities of wife and mother. A good body and vigorous health, therefore, become indispensable to female beauty.

5. Broad Hips.—A woman with a large pelvis gives her a superior and significant appearance, while a narrow pelvis always indicate weak sexuality. The other portions of the body however must be in harmony with the size and breadth of the hips.

6. Full Busts.—In the female beauty of physical development there is nothing that can equal full breasts. It is an indication of good health and good maternal qualities. As a face looks bad without a nose, so the female breast, when narrow and flat, produces a bad effect. The female breasts are the means on which a new-born child depends for its life and growth, hence it is an essential human instinct for men to admire those physical proportions in women which indicate perfect motherhood. Cotton and all other false forms simply show the value of natural ones. All false forms are easily detected, because large natural ones will generally quiver and move at every step, while the artificial ones will manifest no expression of life. As woman looks so much better with artificial paddings and puffings than she does without, therefore modern society should waive all objections to their use. A full breast has been man's admiration through all climes and ages, and whether this breast-loving instinct is right or wrong, sensible or sensual, it is a fact well known to all, that it is a great disappointment to a husband and father to see his child brought up on a bottle. Men love full breasts, because it promotes maternity. If, however, the breasts are abnormally large, it indicates maternal deficiency the same as any disproportion or extreme.

7. Small Feet.—Small feet and small ankles are very attractive, because they are in harmony with a perfect female form, and men admire perfection. Small feet and ankles indicate modesty and reserve, while large feet and ankles indicate coarseness, physical power, authority, predominance. Feet and ankles however must be in harmony with the body, as small feet and small ankles on a large woman would be out of proportion and consequently not beautiful.[131]

8. Beautiful Arms.—As the arm is always in proportion with the other portions of the body, consequently a well-shaped arm, small hands and small wrists, with full muscular development, is a charm and beauty not inferior to the face itself, and those who have well-shaped arms may be proud of them, because they generally keep company with a fine bust and a fine figure.

9. Intelligence.—A mother must naturally possess intelligence, in order to rear her children intelligently, consequently it is natural for man to chiefly admire mental qualities in women, for utility and practicability depend upon intelligence. Therefore a man generally loves those charms in women which prepare her for the duties of companionship. If a woman desires to be loved, she must cultivate her intellectual gifts, be interesting and entertaining in society, and practical and helpful in the home, for these are some of the qualifications which make up the highest type of beauty.

10. Piety and Religion in Women.—Men who love home and the companionship of their wives, love truth, honor and honesty. It is this higher moral development that naturally leads them to admire women of moral and religious natures. It is therefore not strange that immoral men love moral and church-loving wives. Man naturally admires the qualities which tend to the correct government of the home. Men want good and pure children, and it is natural to select women who insure domestic contentment and happiness. A bad man, of course, does not deserve a good wife, yet he will do his utmost to get one.

11. False Appearance.—Men love reserved, coy and discreet women much more than blunt, shrewd and boisterous. Falsehood, false hair, false curls, false forms, false bosoms, false colors, false cheeks, and all that is false, men naturally dislike, for in themselves they are a poor foundation on which to form family ties, consequently duplicity and hypocrisy in women is very much disliked by men, but a frank, honest, conscientious soul is always lovable and lovely and will not become an old maid, except as a matter of choice and not of necessity.

[132]

History of Marriage.

1. "It is not good for man to be alone," was the Divine judgment, and so God created for him an helpmate; therefore sex is as Divine as the soul.[133]

2. Polygamy.—Polygamy has existed in all ages. It is and always has been the result of moral degradation and wantonness.

3. The Garden of Eden.—The Garden of Eden was no harem. Primeval nature knew no community of love; there was only the union of two souls, and the twain were made one flesh. If God had intended man to be a polygamist he would have created for him two or more wives; but he only created one wife for the first man. He also directed Noah to take into the ark two of each sort—a male and female—another evidence that God believed in pairs only.

4. Abraham no doubt was a polygamist, and the general history of patriarchal life shows that the plurality of wives and concubinage were national customs, and not the institutions authorized by God.

5. Egyptian History.—Egyptian history, in the first ostensible form we have, shows that concubinage and polygamy were in common practice.

6. Solomon.—It is not strange that Solomon, with his thousand wives, exclaimed: "All is vanity and vexation of spirit." Polygamy is not the natural state of man.

7. Concubinage and Polygamy continued till the fifth century, when the degraded condition of woman became to some extent matters of some concern and recognition. Before this woman was regarded simply as an instrument of procreation, or a mistress of the household, to gratify the passions of man.

8. The Chinese marriage system was, and is, practically polygamous, for from their earliest traditions we learn, although a man could have but one wife, he was permitted to have as many concubines as he desired.

9. Mohammedanism.—Of the 150,000,000 Mohammedans all are polygamists. Their religion appeals to the luxury of animal propensities, and the voluptuous character of the Orientals has penetrated western Europe and Africa.

10. Mormonism.—The Mormon Church, founded by Joseph Smith, practiced polygamy until the beginning of 1893, when the church formally declared and resigned polygamy as a part or present doctrine of their religious institution. Yet all Mormons are polygamists at heart. It is a part of their religion; national law alone restrains them.

11. Free Lovers.—There is located at Lenox, Madison County, New York, an organization popularly known as Free Lovers. The members advocate a system of complex marriage, a sort of promiscuity, with a freedom of love for [134]any and all. Man offers woman support and love, woman enjoying freedom, self-respect, health, personal and mental competency, gives herself to man in the boundless sincerity of an unselfish union. In their system, love is made synonymous with sexuality, and there is no doubt but what woman is only a plaything to gratify animal caprice.

12. Monogamy (Single Wife), is a law of nature evident from the fact that it fulfills the three essential conditions of man, viz.: the development of the individual, the welfare of society and reproduction. In no nation with a system of polygamy do we find a code of political and moral rights, and the condition of woman is that of a slave. In polygamous countries nothing is added to the education and civilization. The natural tendency is sensualism, and sensualism tends to mental starvation.

13. Christian Civilization has lifted woman from slavery to liberty. Wherever Christian civilization prevails there are legal marriages, pure homes and education. May God bless the purity of the home.

Marriage.

"Thus grief still treads upon the heel of pleasure,
Married in haste we may repent at leisure."—SHAKSPEARE.

The parties are wedded. The priest or clergyman has pronounced as one those hearts that before beat in unison with each other. The assembled guests congratulate the happy pair. The fair bride has left her dear mother bedewed with tears and sobbing just as if her heart would break, and as if the happy bridegroom was leading her away captive against her will. They enter the carriage. It drives off on the wedding tour, and his arms encircles the yielding waist of her now all his own, while her head reclines on the breast of the man of her choice. If she be young and has married an old man, she will be sad. If she has married for a home, or position, or wealth, a pang will shoot across her fair bosom. If she has married without due consideration or on too light an acquaintance, it will be her sorrow before long. But, if loving and beloved, she has united her destiny with a worthy man, she will rejoice, and on her journey feel a glow of satisfaction and delight unfelt before and which will be often renewed, and daily prove as the living waters from some perennial spring.

[135]
The Advantages of Wedlock.
'Tis sweet to hear the watch-dog's honest bark,
Bay deep-mouthed welcome as we draw near home;
'Tis sweet to know there is an eye will mark
Our coming, and look brighter when we come.—BYRON, DON JUAN.

1. Marriage is the natural state of man and woman. Matrimony greatly contributes to the wealth and health of man.

2. Circumstances may compel a man not to select a companion until late in life. Many may have parents or relatives, dependent brothers and sisters to care for, yet family [136]ties are cultivated, notwithstanding the home is without a wife.

3. In Christian countries the laws of marriage have greatly added to the health of man. Marriage in barbarous countries, where little or no marriage ceremonies are required, benefits man but little. There can be no true domestic blessedness without loyalty and love for the select and married companion. All the licentiousness and lust of a libertine, whether civilized or uncivilized, bring him only unrest and premature decay.

4. A man, however, may be married and not mated, and consequently reap trouble and unhappiness. A young couple should first carefully learn each other by making the courtship a matter of business, and sufficiently long that the disposition and temper of each may be thoroughly exposed and understood.

5. First see that there is love; secondly, that there is adaptation; thirdly, see that there are no physical defects; and if these conditions are properly considered, cupid will go with you.

6. The happiest place on all earth is home. A loving wife and lovely children are jewels without price, as Payne says:

"'Mid pleasures and palaces though we may roam,
Be it ever so humble, there's no place like home."

7. Reciprocated love produces a general exhilaration of the system. The elasticity of the muscles is increased, the circulation is quickened, and every bodily function is stimulated to renewed activity by a happy marriage.

8. The consummation desired by all who experience this affection, is the union of souls in a true marriage. Whatever of beauty or romance there may have been in the lover's dream, is enhanced and spiritualized in the intimate communion of married life. The crown of wifehood and maternity is purer, more divine than that of the maiden. Passion is lost— emotions predominate.

AN ALGERIAN BRIDE.

9. **Too Early Marriages.**—Too early marriage is always bad for the female. If a young girl marries, her system is weakened and a full development of her body is prevented, and the dangers of confinement are considerably increased.

10. Boys who marry young derive but little enjoyment from the connubial state. They are liable to excesses and thereby lose much of the vitality and power of strength and physical endurance.

11. **Long Life.**—Statistics show that married men live longer than bachelors. Child-bearing for women is conducive to longevity.

[137]
12. **Complexion.**—Marriage purifies the complexion, removes blotches from the skin, invigorates the body, fills up the tones of the voice, gives elasticity and firmness to the step, and brings health and contentment to old age.

13. **Temptations Removed.**—Marriage sanctifies a home, while adultery and libertinism produce unrest, distrust and misery. It must be remembered that a married man can practice the most absolute continence and enjoy a far better state of health than the licentious man. The comforts of companionship develop purity and give rest to the soul.

14. **Total Abstention.**—It is no doubt difficult for some men to fully abstain from sexual intercourse and be entirely chaste in mind. The great majority of men experience frequent strong sexual desire. Abstention is very apt to produce in their minds voluptuous images and untamable desires which require an iron will to banish or control. The hermit in his seclusion, or the monk in his retreat, are often flushed with these passions and trials. It is, however, natural; for remove these passions and man would be no longer a man. It is evident that the natural state of man is that of marriage; and he who avoids that state is not in harmony with the laws of his being.

15. **Prostitution.**—Men who inherit strong passions easily argue themselves into the belief, either to practice [138]masturbation or visit places of prostitution, on the ground that their health demands it. Though medical investigation has proven it repeatedly to be false, yet many believe it. The consummation of marriage involves the mightiest issues of life and is the most holy and sacred right recognized by man, and it is the Balm of Gilead for many ills. Masturbation or prostitution soon blight the brightest prospects a young man may have. Manhood is morality and purity of purpose, not sensuality.

Disadvantages of Celibacy.
Disadvantages of Celibacy.
Keeping Bachelor's Hall.
The Old Bachelor Sewing on His Buttons.

1. To live the life of a bachelor has many advantages and many disadvantages. The man who commits neither fornication, adultery nor secret vice, and is pure in mind, surely has all the moral virtues that make a good man and a good citizen, whether married or unmarried.

2. If a good pure-minded man does not marry, he will suffer no serious loss of vital power; there will be no tendency to spermatorrhœa or congestion, nor will he be afflicted with any one of those ills which certain vicious writers and quacks would lead many people to believe. Celibacy is perfectly consistent with mental vigor and physical strength. Regularity in the habits of life will always have its good effects on the human body.

3. The average life of a married man is much longer than that of a bachelor. There is quite an alarming odds in the United States in favor of a man with a family. It is claimed that the married man lives on an average from five to twenty years longer than a bachelor. The married man lives a more regular life. He has his meals more regularly and is better nursed in sickness, and in every way a happier and more contented man. The happiness of wife and children will always add comfort and length of days to the man who is happily married.

4. It is a fact well answered by statistics that there is more crime committed, more vices practiced, and more immorality among single men than among married men. Let the young man be pure in heart like Bunyan's Pilgrim, and he can pass the deadly dens, the roaring lions, and overcome the ravenous fires of passion, unscathed. The vices of single men support the most flagrant of evils of modern society, hence let every young man beware and keep his body clean and pure. His future happiness largely depends upon his chastity while a single man.

[140]

Old Maids.
"WE SHALL NEVER MARRY."

1. **Modern Origin.**—The prejudice which certainly still exists in the average mind against unmarried women must be of comparatively modern origin. From the earliest ages, in ancient Greece, and Rome particularly, the highest [141]honors were paid them. They were the ministers of the old religions, and regarded with superstitious awe.

2. **Matrimony.**—Since the reformation, especially during the last century, and in our own land, matrimony has been so much esteemed, notably by women, that it has come to be

regarded as in some sort discreditable for them to remain single. Old maids are mentioned on every hand with mingled pity and disdain, arising no doubt from the belief, conscious or unconscious, that they would not be what they are if they could help it. Few persons have a good word for them as a class. We are constantly hearing of lovely maidens, charming wives, buxom widows, but almost never of attractive old maids.

3. **Discarding Prejudice.**—The real old maid is like any other woman. She has faults necessarily, though not those commonly conceived of. She is often plump, pretty, amiable, interesting, intellectual, cultured, warm-hearted, benevolent, and has ardent friends of both sexes. These constantly wonder why she has not married, for they feel that she must have had many opportunities. Some of them may know why; she may have made them her confidantes. She usually has a sentimental, romantic, frequently a sad and pathetic past, of which she does not speak unless in the sacredness of intimacy.

4. **Not Quarrelsome.**—She is not dissatisfied, querulous nor envious. On the contrary, she is, for the most part, singularly content, patient and serene,—more so than many wives who have household duties and domestic cares to tire and trouble them.

5. **Remain Single from Necessity.**—It is a stupid, as well as a heinous mistake, that women who remain single do so from necessity. Almost any woman can get a husband if she is so minded, as daily observation attests. When we see the multitudes of wives who have no visible signs of matrimonial recommendation, why should we think that old maids have been totally neglected? We may meet those who do not look inviting. But we meet any number of wives who are even less inviting.

"WE HAVE CHANGED OUR MINDS."

6. **First Offer.**—The appearance and outgiving of many wives denote that they have accepted the first offer; the appearance and outgiving of many old maids that they have declined repeated offers. It is undeniable, that wives, in the mass, have no more charm than old maids have, in the mass. But, as the majority of women are married, they are no more criticised nor commented on, in the bulk, than the whole sex are. They are spoken of individually as pretty or[143]plain, bright or dull, pleasant or unpleasant; while old maids are judged as a species, and almost always unfavorable.

7. **Becomes a Wife.**—Many an old maid, so-called, unexpectedly to her associates becomes a wife, some man of taste, discernment and sympathy having induced her to change her state. Probably no other man of his kind has proposed before, which accounts for her singleness. After her marriage hundreds of persons who had sneered at her condition find her charming, thus showing the extent of their prejudice against feminine celibacy. Old maids in general, it is fair to presume, do not wait for opportunities, but for proposers of an acceptable sort. They may have, indeed they are likely to have, those, but not to meet these.

8. **No Longer Marry for Support.**—The time has changed and women have changed with it. They have grown more sensible, more independent in disposition as well as circumstances. They no longer marry for support; they have proved their capacity to support themselves, and self-support has developed them in every way. Assured that they can get on comfortably and contentedly alone they are better adapted by the assurance for consortship. They have rapidly increased from this and cognate causes, and have so improved in person, mind and character that an old maid of to-day is wholly different from an old maid of forty years ago.

CONVINCING HIS WIFE.

[144]

When and Whom to Marry.

1. **Early Marriages.**—Women too early married always remain small in stature, weak, pale, emaciated, and more or less miserable. We have no natural nor moral right to perpetuate unhealthy constitutions, therefore women should not marry too young and take upon themselves the responsibility, by producing a weak and feeble generation of children. It is better not to consummate a marriage until a full development of body and mind has taken place. A young woman of twenty-one to twenty-five, and a young man of twenty-three to twenty-eight, are considered the right age in order to produce an intelligent and healthy offspring. "First make the tree good, then shall the fruit be good also."

2. If marriage is delayed too long in either sex, say from thirty to forty-five, the offspring will often be puny and more liable to insanity, idiocy, and other maladies.

3. **Puberty.**—This is the period when childhood passes from immaturity of the sexual functions to maturity. Woman attains this state a year or two sooner than man. In the hotter climates the period of puberty is from twelve to fifteen years of age, while in cold climates, such as Russia, the United States, and Canada, puberty is frequently delayed until the seventeenth year.

4. **Diseased Parents.**—We do the race a serious wrong in multiplying the number of hereditary invalids. Whole families of children have fallen heir to lives of misery and suffering by the indiscretion and poor judgment of parents. No young man in the vigor of health should think for a moment of marrying a girl who has the impress of consumption or other disease already stamped upon her feeble constitution. It only multiplies his own suffering, and brings no material happiness to his invalid wife. On the other hand, no healthy, vigorous young woman ought to unite her destiny with a man, no matter how much she adored him, who is not healthy and able to brave the hardships of life. If a young man or young woman with feeble body cannot find permanent relief either by medicine or change of climate, no thoughts of marriage should be entertained. Courting a patient may be pleasant, but a hard thing in married life to enjoy. The young lady who supposes that any young man wishes to marry her for the sake of nursing her through life makes a very grave mistake.

THE BASHFUL YOUNG COUPLE.
"A faint heart never won a fair lady."

5. **Whom to Choose for a Husband.**—The choice of a husband requires the coolest judgment and the most [146]vigilant sagacity. A true union based on organic law is happiness, but let all remember that oil and water will not mix; the lion will not lie down with the lamb, nor can ill-assorted marriages be productive of aught but discord.

"Let the woman take
An elder than herself, so wears she to him—
So sways she, rules in her husband's heart."

Look carefully at the disposition.—See that your intended spouse is kind-hearted, generous, and willing to respect the opinions of others, though not in sympathy with them. Don't marry a selfish tyrant who thinks only of himself.

6. **Be Careful.**—Don't marry an intemperate man with a view of reforming him. Thousands have tried it and failed. Misery, sorrow and a very hell on earth have been the consequences of too many such generous undertakings.

7. **The True and Only Test** which any man should look for in woman is modesty in demeanor before marriage, absence both of assumed ignorance and disagreeable familiarity, and a pure and religious frame of mind. Where these are present, he need not doubt that he has a faithful and a chaste wife.

8. **Marrying First Cousins** is dangerous to offspring. The observation is universal, the children of married first cousins are too often idiots, insane, clump-footed, crippled, blind, or variously diseased. First cousins are always sure to impart all the hereditary disease in both families to their children. If both are healthy there is less danger.

9. **Do Not Choose One Too Good**, or too far above you, lest the inferior dissatisfying the superior, breed those discords which are worse than the trials of a single life. Don't be too particular; for you might go farther and fare worse. As far as you yourself are faulty, you should put up with faults. Don't cheat a consort by getting one much better than you can give. We are not in heaven yet, and must put up with their imperfections, and instead of grumbling at them, be glad they are no worse; remembering that a faulty one is a great deal better than none, if he loves you.

10. **Marrying for Money.**—Those who seek only the society of those who can boast of wealth will nine times out of ten suffer disappointment. Wealth cannot manufacture true love nor money buy domestic happiness. Marry because you love each other, and God will bless your home. A cottage with a loving wife is worth more than a royal palace with a discontented and unloving queen.[147]

56

11. **Difference in Age.**—It is generally admitted that the husband should be a few years older than the wife. The question seems to be how much difference. Up to twenty-two those who propose marriage should be about the same age; however, other things being equal, a difference of fifteen years after the younger is twenty-five, need not prevent a marriage. A man of forty-five may marry a woman of twenty-five much more safely than one of thirty a girl below nineteen, because her mental sexuality is not as mature as his, and again her natural coyness requires more delicate and affectionate treatment than he is likely to bestow. A girl of twenty or under should seldom if ever marry a man of thirty or over, because the love of an elderly man for a girl is more parental than conjugal; while hers for him is like that of a daughter to a father. He may pet, flatter and indulge her as he would a grown-up daughter, yet all this is not genuine masculine and feminine love, nor can she exert over him the influence every man requires from his wife.

12. **The Best Time.**—All things considered, we advise the male reader to keep his desires in check till he is at least twenty-five, and the female not to enter the pale of wedlock until she has attained the age of twenty. After those periods, marriage is the proper sphere of action, and one in which nearly every individual is called by nature to play his proper part.

13. **Select Carefully.**—While character, health, accomplishments and social position should be considered, yet one must not overlook mental construction and physical conformation. The rule always to be followed in choosing a life partner is *identity of taste and diversity of temperament*. Another essential is that they be physically adapted to each other. For example: The pelvis—that part of the anatomy containing all the internal organs of gestation—is not only essential to beauty and symmetry, but is a matter of vital importance to her who contemplates matrimony, and its usual consequences. Therefore, the woman with a very narrow and contracted pelvis should never choose a man of giant physical development lest they cannot duly realize the most important of the enjoyments of the marriage state, while the birth of large infants will impose upon her intense labor pains, or even cost her her life.[148]

CHOOSE INTELLECTUALLY—LOVE AFTERWARD.
Explaining the Necessity for a New Bonnet.

1. **Love.**—Let it ever be remembered that love is one of the most sacred elements of our nature, and the most dangerous with which to tamper. It is a very beautiful and delicately contrived faculty, producing the most delightful results, but easily thrown out of repair—like a tender plant, the delicate fibers of which incline gradually to entwine themselves around its beloved one, uniting two willing hearts by a thousand endearing ties, and making of "twain one flesh"; but they are easily torn asunder, and then adieu to the joys of connubial bliss![149]

2. **Courting by the Quarter.**—This courting by the quarter, "here a little and there a little," is one of the greatest evils of the day. This getting a little in love with Julia, and then a little with Eliza, and a little more with Mary,—this fashionable flirtation and coquetry of both sexes—is ruinous to the domestic affections; besides, effectually preventing the formation of true connubial love. I consider this dissipation of the affections one of the greatest sins against Heaven, ourselves, and the one trifled with, that can be committed.

3. **Frittering Away Affections.**—Young men commence courting long before they think of marrying, and where they entertain no thoughts of marriage. They fritter away their own affections, and pride themselves on their conquests over the female heart; triumphing in having so nicely fooled them. They pursue this sinful course so far as to drive their pitiable victims, one after another, from respectable society, who, becoming disgraced, retaliate by heaping upon them all the indignities and impositions which the fertile imagination of woman can invent or execute.

4. **Courting Without Intending to Marry.**—Nearly all this wide-spread crime and suffering connected with public and private licentiousness and prostitution, has its origin in these unmeaning courtships—this premature love—this blighting of the affections, and every young man who courts without intending to marry, is throwing himself or his sweetheart into *this hell upon earth*. And most of the blame rests on young men, because they

take the liberty of paying their addresses to the ladies and discontinuing them, at pleasure, and thereby mainly cause this vice.

5. **Setting Their Caps.**—True, young ladies sometimes "set their caps," sometimes court very hard by their bewitching smiles and affectionate manners; by the natural language of love, or that backward reclining and affectionate roll of the head which expresses it; by their soft and persuasive accents; by their low dresses, artificial forms, and many other unnatural and affected ways and means of attracting attention and exciting love; but women never court till they have been in love and experienced its interruption, till their first and most tender fibres of love have been frostbitten by disappointment. It is surely a sad condition of society.

"HASTY FAMILIARITY IS FRAUGHT WITH MANY DANGERS."

6. **Trampling the Affections of Women.**—But man is a self-privileged character. He may not only violate the laws of his own social nature with impunity, but he may even trample upon the affections of woman. He may even carry [151]this sinful indulgence to almost any length, and yet be caressed and smiled tenderly upon by woman; aye, even by virtuous woman. He may call out, only to blast the glowing affections of one young lady after another, and yet his addresses be cordially welcomed by others. Surely a gentleman is at perfect liberty to pay his addresses, not only to a lady, but even to the ladies, although he does not entertain the thought of marrying his sweet-heart, or, rather his victim. O, man, how depraved! O, woman, how strangely blind to your own rights and interests!

7. **An Infallible Sign.**—An infallible sign that a young man's intentions are improper, is his trying to excite your passions. If he loves you, he will never appeal to that feeling, because he respects you too much for that. And the woman who allows a man to take advantage of her just to compel him to marry her, is lost and heartless in the last degree, and utterly destitute of moral principle as well as virtue. A woman's riches is her virtue, that gone she has lost all.

8. **The Beginning of Licentiousness.**—Man it seldom drives from society. Do what he may, woman, aye, virtuous and even pious woman rarely excludes him from her list of visitors. But where is the point of propriety?—immoral transgression should exclude either sex from respectable society. Is it that one false step which now constitutes the boundary between virtue and vice? Or rather, the discovery of that false step? Certainly not! but it is all that leads to, and precedes and induces it. It is this courting without marrying. This is the beginning of licentiousness, as well as its main, procuring cause, and therefore infinitely worse than its consummation merely.

9. **Searing the Social Affections.**—He has seared his social affections so deeply, so thoroughly, so effectually, that when, at last, he wishes to marry, he is incapable of loving. He marries, but is necessarily cold-hearted towards his wife, which of course renders her wretched, if not jealous, and reverses the faculties of both towards each other; making both most miserable for life. This induces contention and mutual recrimination, if not unfaithfulness, and imbitters the marriage relations through life; and well it may.

10. **Unhappy Marriages.**—This very cause, besides inducing most of that unblushing public and private prostitution already alluded to, renders a large proportion of the marriages of the present day unhappy. Good people mourn over the result, but do not once dream of its cause. They even pray for moral reform, yet do the very things that increase the evil.[152]

AFTER THE ENGAGEMENT.

11. **Weeping Over Her Fallen Son.**—Do you see yonder godly mother, weeping over her fallen son, and remonstrating with him in tones of a mother's tenderness and importunity? That very mother prevented that very son marrying the girl he dearly loved, because she was poor, and this interruption of his love was the direct and procuring cause of his ruin; for, if she had allowed him to marry this beloved one, he never would have thought of giving his "strength unto strange women." True, the mother ruined her son ignorantly, but none the less effectually.

12. **Seduction and Ruin.**—That son next courts another virtuous fair one, engages her affections, and ruins her, or else leaves her broken-hearted, so that she is the more easily

58

ruined by others, and thus prepares the way for her becoming an inmate of a house "whose steps take hold on hell." His heart is now indifferent, he is ready for anything.

13. **The Right Principle.**—I say then, with emphasis, that no man should ever pay his addresses to any woman, until he has made his selection, not even to aid him in making that choice. He should first make his selection intellectually, and love afterward. He should go about the matter coolly and with judgment, just as he would undertake any other important matter. No man or woman, when blinded by love, is in a fit state to judge advantageously as to what he or she requires, or who is adapted to his or her wants.

14. **Choosing First and Loving Afterwards.**—I know, indeed, that this doctrine of choosing first and loving afterward, of excluding love from the councils, and of choosing by and with the consent of the intellect and moral sentiments, is entirely at variance with the feelings of the young and the customs of society; but, for its correctness, I appeal to the common-sense—not to the experience, for so few try this plan. Is not this the only proper method, and the one most likely to result happily? Try it.

15. **The Young Woman's Caution.**—And, especially, let no young lady ever once think of bestowing her affections till she is certain they will not be broken off—that is, until the match is fully agreed upon; but rather let her keep her heart whole till she bestows it for life. This requisition is as much more important, and its violation as much more disastrous to woman than to man, as her social faculties are stronger than his.

16. **A Burnt Child Dreads the Fire.**—As a "burnt child dreads the fire," and the more it is burnt, the greater the dread: so your affections, once interrupted, will recoil from a second love, and distrust all mankind. No! you cannot be too choice of your love—that pivot on which turn your destinies for life and future happiness.

[154]
Love-Spats.

For aught that ever I could read,
Could ever hear by tale or history,
The course of true love never did ran smooth."—SHAKESPEARE.

"Heaven has no rage like love to hatred turned,
Nor hell a fury like a woman scorned."—CONGREVE.

"Thunderstorms clear the atmosphere and promote vegetation; then why not Love-spats promote love, as they certainly often do?

They are almost universal, and in the nature of our differences cannot be helped. The more two love, the more they are aggrieved by each other's faults; of which these spats are but the correction.

Love-spats instead of being universal, they are consequent on imperfect love, and only aggravate, never correct errors. Sexual storms never improve, whereas love obviates faults by praising the opposite virtues. Every view of them, practical and philosophical, condemns them as being to love what poison is to health, both before and after marriage. They are nothing but married discords. Every law of mind and love condemns them. Shun them as you would deadly vipers, and prevent them by forestallment."—O. S. Fowler.

1. **The True Facts.**—Notwithstanding some of the above quotations, to the contrary, trouble and disagreement between lovers embitters both love and life. Contention is always dangerous, and will beget alienation if not final separation.

2. **Confirmed Affections.**—Where affections are once thoroughly confirmed, each one should be very careful in taking offense, and avoid all disagreements as far as possible, but if disagreements continually develop with more or less friction and irritation, it is better for the crisis to come and a final separation take place. For peace is better than disunited love.

CUPID'S REBELLION

3. **Hate-Spats.**—Hate-spats, though experienced by most lovers, yet, few realize how fatal they are to subsequent affections. Love-spats develop into hate-spats, and their effects upon the affections are blighting and should not under any circumstances be tolerated. Either agree, or agree to disagree. If there cannot be harmony before the ties of marriage are

assumed, then there cannot be harmony [156]after. Married life will be continually marred by a series of "hate-spats" that sooner or later will destroy all happiness, unless the couple are reasonably well mated.

4. More Fatal the Oftener They Occur.—As O. S. Fowler says: "'The poison of asps is under their lips.' The first spat is like a deep gash cut into a beautiful face, rendering it ghastly, and leaving a fearful scar, which neither time nor cosmetics can ever efface; including that pain so fatal to love, and blotting that sacred love-page with memory's most hideous and imperishable visages. Cannot many now unhappy remember them as the beginning of that alienation which embittered your subsequent affectional cup, and spoiled your lives? With what inherent repulsion do you look back upon them? Their memory is horrid, and effect on love most destructive."

5. Fatal Conditions.—What are all lovers' "spats" but disappointment in its very worst form? They necessarily and always produce all its terrible consequences. The finer feelings and sensibilities will soon become destroyed and nothing but hatred will remain.

6. Extreme Sorrow.—After a serious "spat" there generally follows a period of tender sorrow, and a feeling of humiliation and submission. Mutual promises are consequently made that such a condition of things shall never happen again, etc. But be sure and remember, that every subsequent difficulty will require stronger efforts to repair the breach. Let it be understood that these compromises are dangerous, and every new difficulty increases their fatality. Even the strongest will endure but few, nor survive many.

7. Distrust and Want of Confidence.—Most difficulties arise from distrust or lack of confidence or common-sense. When two lovers eye each other like two curs, each watching, lest the other should gain some new advantage, then this shows a lack of common-sense, and the young couple should get sensible or separate.

8. Jealousy.—When one of the lovers, once so tender, now all at once so cold and hardened; once so coy and familiar, now suddenly so reserved, distant, hard and austere, is always a sure case of jealousy. A jealous person is first talkative, very affectionate, and then all at once changes and becomes cold, reserved and repulsive, apparently without cause. If a person is jealous before marriage, this characteristic will be increased rather than diminished by marriage.[157]

9. Confession.—If you make up by confession, the confessor feels mean and disgraced; or if both confess and forgive, both feel humbled; since forgiveness implies inferiority and pity; from which whatever is manly and womanly shrinks. Still even this is better than continued "spats."

10. Prevention.—If you can get along well in your courtship you will invariably make a happy couple if you should unite your destinies in marriage. Learn not to give nor take offence. You must remember that all humanity is imperfect at best. We all have our faults, and must keep them in subordination. Those who truly love each other will have but few difficulties in their courtship or in married life.

11. Remedies.—Establishing a perfect love in the beginning constitutes a preventive. Fear that they are not truly loved usually paves the way for "spats." Let all who make any pretension guard against all beginnings of this reversal, and strangle these "hate-spats" the moment they arise. "Let not the sun go down upon thy wrath," not even an hour, but let the next sentence after they begin quench them forever. And let those who cannot court without "spats," stop; for those who spat before marriage, must quarrel after.

"Let not the sun go down upon thy wrath."

[159]

A Broken Heart.
A BROKEN HEART

1. Wounded Love.—'Tis true that love wields a magic, sovereign, absolute, and tyrannical power over both the body and the mind when it is given control. It often, in case of disappointment, works havoc and deals death blows to its victims, and leaves many in that morbid mental condition which no life-tonics simply can restore. Wounded love may be the result of hasty and indiscreet conduct of young people; or the outgrowth of lust, or the result of domestic infidelity and discord.

2. **Fatal Effects.**—Our cemeteries receive within the cold shadows of the grave thousands and thousands of victims that annually die from the results of "broken hearts." It is no doubt a fact that love troubles cause more disorders of the heart than everything else combined.

3. **Disrupted Love.**—It has long been known that dogs, birds, and even horses, when separated from their companions or friends, have pined away and died; so it is not strange that man with his higher intuitive ideas of affection should suffer from love when suddenly disrupted.

4. **Crucifying Love.**—Painful love feelings strike right to the heart, and the breaking up of love that cannot be consummated in marriage is sometimes allowed to crucify the affections. There is no doubt that the suffering from disappointed love is often deeper and more intense than meeting death itself.

5. **Healing.**—The paralyzing and agonizing consequences of ruptured love can only be remedied by diversion and society. Bring the mind into a state of patriotic independence with a full determination to blot out the past. Those who cannot bring into subordination the pangs of disappointment in love are not strong characters, and invariably will suffer disappointments in almost every department of life. Disappointment in love means rising above it, and conquering it, or demoralization, mental, physical and sexual.

6. **Love Runs Mad.**—Love comes unbidden. A blind ungovernable impulse seems to hold sway in the passions of the affections. Love is blind and seems to completely subdue and conquer. It often comes like a clap of thunder from a clear sky, and when it falls it falls flat, leaving only the ruins of a tornado behind.

7. **Bad, Dismal, and Blue Feelings.**—Despondency breathes disease, and those who yield to it can neither work, eat nor sleep; they only suffer. The spell-bound, fascinated, magnetized affections seem to deaden self-control and no [160]doubt many suffering from love-sickness are totally helpless; they are beside themselves, irrational and wild. Men and women of genius, influence and education, all seem to suffer alike, but they do not yield alike to the subduing influence; some pine away and die; others rise above it, and are the stronger and better for having been afflicted.

8. **Rise above It.**—Cheer up! If you cannot think pleasurably over your misfortune, forget it. You must do this or perish. Your power and influence is too much to blight by foolish and melancholy pining. Your own sense, your self-respect, your self-love, your love for others, command you not to spoil yourself by crying over "spilt milk."

MARRIAGE ON A DEATHBED.

9. **Retrieve Your Past Loss.**—Do sun, moon, and stars indeed rise and set in your loved one? Are there not "as good fish in the sea as ever were caught?" and can you not catch them? Are there not other hearts on earth just as loving and lovely, and in every way as congenial? If circumstances had first turned you upon another, you would have felt about that one as now about this. Love depends far less on the party loved than on the loving one. Or is this the way either to retrieve your past loss, or provide for the future? Is it not both unwise and self-destructive; and in every way calculated to render your case, present and prospective, still more hopeless?

10. **Find Something to Do.**—Idle hands are Satan's workshop. Employ your mind; find something to do; something in which you can find self-improvement; something that will fit you better to be admired by someone else, read, and improve your mind; get into society, throw your whole soul into some new enterprise, and you will conquer with glory and come out of the fire purified and made more worthy.

11. **Love Again.**—As love was the cause of your suffering, so love again will restore you, and you will love better and more consistently. Do not allow yourself to become soured and detest and shun association. Rebuild your dilapidated sexuality by cultivating a general appreciation of the excellence, especially of the mental and moral qualities of the opposite sex. Conquer your prejudices, and vow not to allow anyone to annoy or disturb your calmness.

61

12. **Love for the Dead.**—A most affectionate woman, who continues to love her affianced though long dead, instead of becoming soured or deadened, manifests all the richness and sweetness of the fully-developed woman thoroughly in love, along with a softened, mellow, twilight sadness which touches every heart, yet throws a peculiar lustre and beauty over her manners and entire character. She must mourn, [161]but not forever. It is not her duty to herself or to her Creator.

13. **A Sure Remedy.**—Come in contact with the other sex. You are infused with your lover's magnetism, which must remain till displaced by another's. Go to parties and picnics; be free, familiar, offhand, even forward; try your knack at fascinating another, and yield to fascinations yourself. But be honest, command respect, and make yourself attractive and worthy.

[162]

Former Customs and Peculiarities Among Men.

1. **Polygamy.**—There is a wide difference as regards the relations of the sexes in different parts of the world. In some parts polygamy has prevailed from time immemorial.

Most savage people are polygamists, and the Turks, though slowly departing from the practice, still allow themselves a plurality of wives.

2. **Rule Reversed.**—In Thibet the rule is reversed, and the females are provided with two or more husbands. It is said that in many instances a whole family of brothers have but one wife. The custom has at least one advantageous feature, viz.: the possibility of leaving an unprotected widow and a number of fatherless children is entirely obviated.

3. **The Morganatic Marriage** is a modification of polygamy. It sometimes occurs among the royalty of Europe, and is regarded as perfectly legitimate, but the morganatic wife is of lower rank than her royal husband, and her children do not inherit his rank or fortune. The Queen only is the consort of the sovereign, and entitled to share his rank.

4. **Different Manners of Obtaining Wives.**—Among the uncivilized almost any envied possession is taken by brute force or superior strength. The same is true in obtaining a wife. The strong take precedence of the weak. It is said that among the North American Indians it was the custom for men to wrestle for the choice of women. A weak man could seldom retain a wife that a strong man coveted.

The law of contest was not confined to individuals alone. Women were frequently the cause of whole tribes arraying themselves against each other in battle. The effort to excel in physical power was a great incentive to bodily development, and since the best of the men were preferred by the most superior women, the custom was a good one in this, that the race was improved.

5. **The Aboriginal Australian** employed low cunning and heartless cruelty in obtaining his wife. Laying in ambush, with club in hand, he would watch for the coveted woman,[163]and, unawares, spring upon her. If simply disabled he carried her off as his possession, but if the blow had been hard enough to kill, he abandoned her to watch for another victim. There is here no effort to attract or please, no contest of strength; his courtship, if courtship it can be called, would compare very unfavorably with any among the brute creation.

6. **The Kalmuck Tartar** races for his bride on horseback, she having a certain start previously agreed upon. The *nuptial knot* consists in catching her, but we are told that the result of the race all depends upon whether the girl wants to be caught or not.

7. **Sandwich Islanders.**—Marriage among the early natives of these islands was merely a matter of mutual inclination. There was no ceremony at all, the men and women united and separated as they felt disposed.

8. **The Feudal Lord**, in various parts of Europe, when any of his dependents or followers married, exercised the right of assuming the bridegroom's proper place in the marriage couch for the first night. Seldom was there any escape from this abominable practice. Sometimes the husband, if wealthy, succeeded in buying off the petty sovereign from exercising his privilege.

9. **The Spartans** had the custom of encouraging intercourse between their best men and women for the sake of a superior progeny, without any reference to a marriage

ceremony. Records show that the ancient Roman husband has been known to invite a friend, in whom he may have admired some physical or mental trait, to share the favors of his wife, that the peculiar qualities that he admired might be repeated in the offspring.

[164]
The Peasant Father Blessing His Daughter at Her Engagement.

[165]

Hasty marriage seldom proveth well.—*Shakespere, Henry VI.*

The reason why so few marriages are happy is, because young ladies spend their time in making nets, not in making cages.—*Swift, Thoughts on Various Subjects.*

Sensible Hints in Choosing a Partner.

1. There are many fatal errors and many love-making failures in courtship. Natural laws govern all nature and reduce all they govern to eternal right; therefore love naturally, not artificially. Don't love a somebody or a nobody simply because they have money.

2. **Court Scientifically.**—If you court at all, court scientifically. Bungle whatever else you will, but do not bungle courtship. A failure in this may mean more than a loss of wealth or public honors; it may mean ruin, or a life often worse than death. The world is full of wretched and mismated people.

Begin right and all will be right; begin wrong and all will end wrong. When you court, make a business of it and study your interest the same as you would study any other business proposition.

3. **Divorces.**—There is not a divorce on our court records that is not the result of some fundamental error in courtship. The purity or the power of love may be corrupted the same as any other faculty, and when a man makes up his mind to marry and shuts his eyes and grabs in the dark for a companion, he dishonors the woman he captures and commits a crime against God and society. In this enlightened age there should be comparatively few mistakes made in the selection of a suitable partner. Sufficient time should be taken to study each other's character and disposition. Association will soon reveal adaptability.

4. **False Love.**—Many a poor, blind and infatuated novice thinks he is desperately in love, when there is not the least genuine affection in his nature. It is all a momentary[166]passion, a sort of puppy love; his vows and pledges are soon violated, and in wedlock he will become indifferent and cold to his wife and children, and he will go through life without ambition, encouragement or success. He will be a failure. True love speaks for itself, and the casual observer can read its proclamations. True love does not speak in a whisper. It always makes itself heard. The follies of flirting develop into many unhappy marriages, and blight many a life. A man happily married has superior advantages both socially and financially.

5. **Flirting just for Fun.**—Who is the flirt, what is his reputation, motive, or character? Every young man and woman must have a reputation; if it is not good it is bad, there is no middle ground. Young people who are running in the streets after dark, boisterous and noisy in their conversation, gossiping and giggling, flirting with first one and then another, will soon settle their matrimonial prospects among good society. Modesty is a priceless jewel. No sensible young man with a future will marry a flirt.

6. **The Arch-Deceiver.**—They who win the affection simply for their own amusement are committing a great sin for which there is no adequate punishment. How can you shipwreck the innocent life of that confiding maiden, how can you forget her happy looks as she drank in your expressions of love, how can you forget her melting eyes and glowing cheeks, her tender tone reciprocating your pretended love? Remember that God is infinitely just, and "the soul that sinneth shall surely die." You may dash into business, seek pleasure in the club room, and visit gambling hells, but "Thou art the man" will ever stare you in the face. Her pale, sad cheeks, her hollow eyes will never cease to haunt you. Men should promote happiness, and not cause misery. Let the savage Indians torture captives to death by the slow flaming fagot, but let civilized man respect the tenderness and love of

confiding women. Torturing the opposite sex is double-distilled barbarity. Young men agonizing young ladies, is the cold-blooded cruelty of devils, not men.

7. **The Rule to Follow.**—Do not continually pay your attentions to the same lady if you have no desire to win her affections. Occasionally escorting her to church, concert, picnic, party, etc., is perfectly proper; but to give her your special attention, and extend invitations to her for all places of amusements where you care to attend, is an implied promise that you prefer her company above all others, and she has a right to believe that your attentions are serious.[167]

THE WEDDING RING.

8. **Every Girl Should Seal Her Heart** against all manifested affections, unless they are accompanied by a proposal. Woman's love is her all, and her heart should be as flint until she finds one who is worthy of her confidence. Young woman, never bestow your affections until by some word or deed at least you are fully justified in recognizing sincerity and faith in him who is paying you special attention. You are [168]then more competent to judge the honesty and falsity of man. Nature has thrown a wall of maidenly modesty around you. Preserve that and not let your affections be trifled with while too young by any youthful flirt who is in search of hearts to conquer.

9. **Female Flirtation.**—The young man who loves a young woman has paid her the highest compliment in the possession of man. Perpetrate almost any sin, inflict any other torture, but spare him the agony of disappointment. It is a crime that can never be forgiven, and a debt that never can be paid.

10. **Loyalty.**—Young persons with serious intentions, or those who are engaged should be thoroughly loyal to each other. If they seek freedom with others the flame of jealousy is likely to be kindled and love is often turned to hatred, and the severest anger of the soul is aroused. Loyalty, faithfulness, confidence, are the three jewels to be cherished in courtship. Don't be a flirt.

11. **Kissing, Fondling, and Caressing Between Lovers.**—This should never be tolerated under any circumstances, unless there is an engagement to justify it, and then only in a sensible and limited way. The girl who allows a young man the privilege of kissing her or putting his arms around her waist before engagement will at once fall in the estimation of the man she has thus gratified and desired to please. Privileges always injure, but never benefit.

SAYING "NO" WHEN MEANING "YES."

12. **Improper Liberties During Courtship Kill Love.**—Any improper liberties which are permitted by young ladies, whether engaged or not, will change love into sensuality, and her affections will become obnoxious, if not repellent. Men by nature love virtue, and for a life companion naturally shun an amorous woman. Young folks, as you love moral purity and virtue, never reciprocate love until you have required the right of betrothal. Remember that those who are thoroughly in love will respect the honor and virtue of each other. The purity of woman is doubly attractive, and sensuality in her becomes doubly offensive and repellent. It is contrary to the laws of nature for a man to love a harlot.

13. **A Seducer.**—The punishment of the seducer is best given by O. S. Fowler, in his "Creative Science." The sin and punishment rest on all you who call out only to blight a trusting, innocent, loving virgin's affections, and then discard her. You deserve to be horsewhipped by her father, cowhided by her brothers, branded villain by her mother, cursed by herself, and sent to the whipping-post and dungeon.[169]

14. **Caution.**—A young lady should never encourage the attentions of a young man, who shows no interest in his sisters. If a young man is indifferent to his sisters he will become indifferent to his wife as soon as the honey moon is over. There are few if any exceptions to this rule. The brother who will not be kind and loving in his mother's home will make a very poor husband.

15. **The Old Rule:** "Never marry a man that does not make his mother a Christmas present every Christmas," is a good one. The young lady makes no mistake in uniting her destinies with the man that loves his mother and respects his sisters and brothers.

[170]

SAFE HINTS.

A CHINESE BRIDE AND GROOM.

1. Marry in your own position in life. If there is any difference in social position, it is better that the husband should be the superior. A woman does not like to look down upon her husband, and to be obliged to do so is a poor guarantee for their happiness.

2. It is best to marry persons of your own faith and religious convictions, unless one is willing to adopt those of the other. Difference of faith is apt to divide families, and to produce great trouble in after life. A pious woman should beware of marrying an irreligious man.[171]

3. Don't be afraid of marrying a poor man or woman. Good health, cheerful disposition, stout hearts and industrious hands will bring happiness and comfort.

4. Bright red hair should marry jet black, and jet black auburn or bright red, etc. And the more red-faced and bearded or impulsive a man, the more dark, calm, cool and quiet should his wife be; and vice versa. The florid should not marry the florid, but those who are dark, in proportion as they themselves are light.

5. Red-whiskered men should marry brunettes, but no blondes; the color of the whiskers being more determinate of the temperament than that of the hair.

6. The color of the eyes is still more important. Gray eyes must marry some other color, almost any other except gray; and so of blue, dark, hazel, etc.

7. Those very fleshy should not marry those equally so, but those too spare and slim; and this is doubly true of females. A spare man is much better adapted to a fleshy woman than a round-favored man. Two who are short, thick-set and stocky, should not unite in marriage, but should choose those differently constituted; but on no account one of their own make. And, in general, those predisposed to corpulence are therefore less inclined to marriage.

8. Those with little hair or beard should marry those whose hair is naturally abundant; still those who once had plenty, but who have lost it, may marry those who are either bald or have but little; for in this, as in all other cases, all depends on what one is by nature, little on present states.

9. Those whose motive-temperament decidedly predominates, who are bony, only moderately fleshy, quite prominent-featured, Roman-nosed and muscular, should not marry those similarly formed.

10. Small, nervous men must not marry little, nervous or sanguine women, lest both they and their children have quite too much of the hot-headed and impulsive, and die suddenly.

Light, Life, Health and Beauty.

11. Two very beautiful persons rarely do or should marry; nor two extra homely. The fact is a little singular that very handsome women, who of course can have their pick, rarely marry good-looking men, but generally give preference to those who are homely; because that [173]exquisiteness in which beauty originates naturally blends with that power which accompanies huge noses and disproportionate features.

12. Rapid movers, speakers, laughers, etc., should marry those who are calm and deliberate, and impulsives those who are stoical; while those who are medium may marry those who are either or neither, as they prefer.

13. Noses indicate characters by indicating the organisms and temperaments. Accordingly, those noses especially marked either way should marry those having opposite nasal characteristics. Roman noses are adapted to those which turn up, and pug noses to those turning down; while straight noses may marry either.

14. Men who love to command must be especially careful not to marry imperious, women's-rights woman; while those who willingly "obey order;" need just such. Some men require a wife who shall take their part; yet all who do not need strong-willed women, should be careful how they marry them.

15. A sensible woman should not marry an obstinate but injudicious, unintelligent man; because she cannot long endure to see and help him blindly follow his poor, but spurn her good, plans.

16. The reserved or secretive should marry the frank. A cunning man cannot endure the least artifice in a wife. Those who are non-committal must marry those who are

demonstrative; else, however much they may love, neither will feel sure as to the other's affections, and each will distrust the other, while their children will be deceitful.

17. A timid woman should never marry a hesitating man, lest, like frightened children, each keep perpetually re-alarming the other by imaginary fears.

18. An industrious, thrifty, hard-working man should marry a woman tolerably saving and industrious. As the "almighty dollar" is now the great motor-wheel of humanity, and that to which most husbands devote their entire lives, to delve alone is uphill work.

[174]

Marriage Securities.
WE MUST PART.

1. **Seek Each Other's Happiness.**—A selfish marriage that seeks only its own happiness defeats itself. Happiness is a fire that will not burn long on one stick.[175]

2. **Do Not Marry Suddenly.**—It can always be done till it is done, if it is a proper thing to do.

3. **Marry in Your Own Grade in Society.**—It is painful to be always apologizing for any one. It is more painful to be apologized for.

4. **Do Not Marry Downward.**—It is hard enough to advance in the quality of life without being loaded with clay heavier than your own. It will be sufficiently difficult to keep your children up to your best level without having to correct a bias in their blood.

5. **Do Not Sell Yourself.**—It matters not whether the price be money or position.

6. **Do Not Throw Yourself Away.**—You will not receive too much, even if you are paid full price.

7. **Seek the Advice of Your Parents.**—Your parents are your best friends. They will make more sacrifice for you than any other mortals. They are elevated above selfishness concerning you. If they differ from you concerning your choice, it is because they must.

8. **Do Not Marry to Please Any Third Party.**—You must do the living and enduring.

9. **Do Not Marry to Spite Anybody.**—It would add wretchedness to folly.

10. **Do Not Marry Because Someone Else May Seek the Same Hand.**—One glove may not fit all hands equally well.

11. **Do Not Marry to Get Rid of Anybody.**—The coward who shot himself to escape from being drafted was insane.

12. **Do Not Marry Merely for the Impulse of Love.**—Love is a principle as well as an emotion. So far as it is a sentiment it is a blind guide. It does not wait to test the presence of exalted character in its object before breaking out into a flame. Shavings make a hot fire, but hard coal is better for the Winter.

13. **Do Not Marry Without Love.**—A body without a soul soon becomes offensive.

14. **Test Carefully the Effect of Protracted Association.**—If familiarity breeds contempt before marriage it will afterward.

15. **Test Carefully the Effect of Protracted Separation.**—True love will defy both time and space.

16. **Consider Carefully** the right of your children under the laws of heredity. It is doubtful whether you have a right to increase the number of invalids and cripples.

17. **Do Not Marry Simply Because You Have Promised to Do So.**—If a seam opens between you now it will widen into [176]a gulf. It is less offensive to retract a mistaken promise than to perjure your soul before the altar. Your intended spouse has a right to absolute integrity.

GOING TO BE MARRIED.

18. **Marry Character.**—It is not so much what one has as what one is.

19. **Do Not Marry the Wrong Object.**—Themistocles said he would rather marry his daughter to a man without [177]money than to money without a man. It is well to have both. It is fatal to have neither.

20. **Demand a Just Return.**—You give virtue and purity, and gentleness and integrity. You have a right to demand the same in return. Duty requires it.

66

21. **Require Brains.**—Culture is good, but will not be transmitted. Brain power may be.

22. **Study Past Relationship.**—The good daughter and sister makes a good wife. The good son and brother makes a good husband.

23. **Never Marry as a Missionary Deed.**—If one needs saving from bad habits he is not suitable for you.

24. **Marriage is a Sure and Specific Remedy** for all the ills known as seminal losses. As right eating cures a sick stomach and right breathing diseased lungs, so the right use of the sexual organs will bring relief and restoration. Many men who have been sufferers from indiscretions of youth, have married, and were soon cured of spermatorrhœa and other complications which accompanied it.

25. **A Good, Long Courtship** will often cure many difficulties or ills of the sexual organs. O. S. Fowler says: "See each other often spend many pleasant hours together," have many walks and talks, think of each other while absent, write many love letters, be inspired to many love feelings and acts towards each other, and exercise your sexuality in a thousand forms ten thousand times, every one of which tones up and thereby recuperates this very element now dilapidated. When you have courted long enough to marry, you will be sufficiently restored to be reimproved by it. Come,

Up and at it.—Dress up, spruce up, and be on the alert. Don't wait too long to get one much more perfect than you are; but settle on some one soon. Remember that your unsexed state renders you over-dainty, and easily disgusted. So contemplate only their lovable qualities.

26. **Purity of Purpose.**—Court with a pure and loyal purpose, and when thoroughly convinced that the disposition of other difficulties are in the way of a happy marriage life, then *honorably* discuss it and honorably treat each other in the settlement.

27. **Do not trifle** with the feelings or affections of each other. It is a sin that will curse you all the days of your life.

[178]
Women Who Make the Best Wives.

1. **Conscious of the Duties of Her Sex.**—A woman conscious of the duties of her sex, one who unflinchingly discharges the duties allotted to her by nature, would no doubt make a good wife.

2. **Good Wives and Mothers.**—The good wives and mothers are the women who believe in the sisterhood of women as well as in the brotherhood of men. The highest exponent of this type seeks to make her home something more than an abode where children are fed, clothed and taught the catechism. The State has taken her children into politics by making their education a function of politicians. The good wife and homemaker says to her children, "Where thou goest, I will go." She puts off her own inclinations to ease and selfishness. She studies the men who propose to educate her children; she exhorts mothers to sit beside fathers on the school-board; she will even herself accept such thankless office in the interests of the helpless youth of the schools who need a mother's as well as a father's and a teacher's care in this field of politics.

3. **A Busy Woman.**—As to whether a busy woman, that is, a woman who labors for mankind in the world outside her home,—whether such an one can also be a good housekeeper, and care for her children, and make a real "Home, Sweet Home!" with all the comforts by way of variation, why! I am ready, as the result of years practical experience as a busy woman, to assert that women of affairs can also be women of true domestic tastes and habits.

4. **Brainy Enough.**—What kind of women make the best wives? The woman who is brainy enough to be a companion, wise enough to be a counsellor, skilled enough in the domestic virtues to be a good housekeeper, and loving enough to guide in true paths the children with whom the home may be blessed.

5. **Found the Right Husband.**—The best wife is the woman who has found the right husband, a husband who understands her. A man will have the best wife when he rates

67

that wife as queen among women. Of all women she should always be to him the dearest. This sort of man will not only praise the dishes made by his wife, but will actually eat them.

PUNISHMENT OF WIFE BEATERS IN NEW ENGLAND IN THE EARLY DAYS.

6. **Bank Account.**—He will allow his life-companion a bank account, and will exact no itemized bill at the end of the month. Above all, he will pay the Easter bonnet bill without a word, never bring a friend to dinner without first telephoning home,—short, he will comprehend that the [180]woman who makes the best wife is the woman whom, by his indulgence of her ways and whims, he makes the best wife. So after all, good husbands have the most to do with making good wives.

7. **Best Home Maker.**—A woman to be the best home maker needs to be devoid of intensive "nerves." She must be neat and systematic, but not too neat, lest she destroy the comfort she endeavors to create. She must be distinctly amiable, while firm. She should have no "career," or desire for a career, if she would fill to perfection the home sphere. She must be affectionate, sympathetic and patient, and fully appreciative of the worth and dignity of her sphere.

8. **Know Nothing Whatsoever About Cooking or Sewing or Housekeeping.**—I am inclined to make my answer to this question somewhat concise, after the manner of a text without the sermon. Like this: To be the "best wife" depends upon three things: first, an abiding faith with God; second, duty lovingly discharged as daughter, wife and mother; third, self-improvement, mentally, physically, spiritually. With this as a text and as a glittering generality, let me touch upon one or two practical essentials. In the course of every week it is my privilege to meet hundreds of young women,—prospective wives. I am astonished to find that many of these know nothing whatsoever about cooking or sewing or housekeeping. Now, if a woman cannot broil a beefsteak, nor boil the coffee when it is necessary, if she cannot mend the linen, nor patch a coat, if she cannot make a bed, order the dinner, create a lamp-shade, ventilate the house, nor do anything practical in the way of making home actually a home, how can she expect to make even a good wife, not to speak of a better or best wife? I need not continue this sermon. Wise girls will understand.

9. **The Best Keeper of Home.**—As to who is the best keeper of this transition home, memory pictures to me a woman grown white under the old slavery, still bound by it, in that little-out-of-the-way Kansas town, but never so bound that she could not put aside household tasks, at any time, for social intercourse, for religious conversation, for correspondence, for reading, and, above all, for making everyone who came near her feel that her home was the expression of herself, a place for rest, study, and the cultivation of affection. She did not exist for her walls, her carpets, her furniture; they existed for her and all who came to her. She considered herself the equal of all; and everyone else thought her the superior of all.

[181]

Adaptation, Conjugal Affection, and Fatal Errors.

ADVICE TO THE MARRIED AND UNMARRIED.

1. **Marrying for Wealth.**—Those who marry for wealth often get what they marry and nothing else; for rich girls, besides being generally destitute of both industry and economy, are generally extravagant in their expenditures, and require servants enough to dissipate a fortune. They generally have insatiable wants, yet feel that they deserve to be indulged in everything, because they placed their husbands under obligation to them by bringing them a dowry. And then the mere idea of living on the money of a wife, and of being supported by her, is enough to tantalize any man of an independent spirit.

2. **Self-Support.**—What spirited husband would not prefer to support both himself and wife, rather than submit to this perpetual bondage of obligation. To live upon a father, or take a patrimony from him, is quite bad enough; but to run in debt to a wife, and owe her a living, is a little too aggravating for endurance, especially if there be not perfect cordiality between the two, which cannot be the case in money matches. Better live wifeless, or anything else, rather than marry for money.

3. **Money-Seekers.**—Shame on sordid wife-seekers, or, rather, money-seekers; for it is not a wife that they seek, but only filthy lucre! They violate all their other faculties simply to gratify miserly desire. Verily such "have their reward"!

4. **The Penitent Hour.**—And to you, young ladies, let me say with great emphasis, that those who court and marry you because you are rich, will make you rue the day of your pecuniary espousals. They care not for you, but only your money, and when they get that, will be liable to neglect or abuse you, and probably squander it, leaving you destitute and abandoning you to your fate.

5. **Industry the Sign of Nobility.**—Marry a working, industrious young lady, whose constitution is strong, flesh solid, and health unimpaired by confinement, bad habits, or late hours. Give me a plain, home-spun farmer's daughter, and you may have all the rich and fashionable belles of our cities and villages.

AN ILL-MATED COUPLE.

6. **Wasp Waists.**—Marrying small waists is attended with consequences scarcely less disastrous than marrying [183]rich and fashionable girls. An amply developed chest is a sure indication of a naturally vigorous constitution and a strong hold on life; while small waists indicate small and feeble vital organs, a delicate constitution, sickly offspring, and a short life. Beware of them, therefore, unless you wish your heart broken by the early death of your wife and children.

7. **Marrying Talkers.**—In marrying a wit or a talker merely, though the brilliant scintillations of the former, or the garrulity of the latter, may amuse or delight you for the time being, yet you will derive no permanent satisfaction from these qualities, for there will be no common bond of kindred feeling to assimilate your souls and hold each spell-bound at the shrine of the other's intellectual or moral excellence.

8. **The Second Wife.**—Many men, especially in choosing a second wife, are governed by her own qualifications as a housekeeper mainly, and marry industry and economy. Though these traits of character are excellent, yet a good housekeeper may be far from being a good wife. A good housekeeper, but a poor wife, may indeed prepare you a good dinner, and keep her house and children neat and tidy, yet this is but a part of the office of a wife; who, besides all her household duties, has those of a far higher order to perform. She should soothe you with her sympathies, divert your troubled mind, and make the whole family happy by the gentleness of her manners, and the native goodness of her heart. A husband should also likewise do his part.

9. **Do Not Marry a Man With a Low, Flat Head**; for, however fascinating, genteel, polite, tender, plausible or winning he may be, you will repent the day of your espousal.

10. **Healthy Wives and Mothers.**—Let girls romp, and let them range hill and dale in search of flowers, berries, or any other object of amusement or attraction; let them bathe often, skip the rope, and take a smart ride on horseback; often interspersing these amusements with a turn of sweeping or washing, in order thereby to develop their vital organs, and thus lay a substantial physical foundation for becoming good wives and mothers. The wildest romps usually make the best wives, while quiet, still, demure, sedate and sedentary girls are not worth having.

11. **Small Stature.**—In passing, I will just remark, that good size is important in wives and mothers. A small stature is objectionable in a woman, because little women [184]usually have too much activity for their strength, and, consequently, feeble constitutions; hence they die young, and besides, being nervous, suffer extremely as mothers.

12. **Hard Times and Matrimony.**—Many persons, particularly young men, refuse to marry, especially "these hard times," because they cannot support a wife in the style they wish. To this I reply, that a good wife will care less for the style in which she is supported, than for you. She will cheerfully conform to your necessities, and be happy with you in a log-cabin. She will even help you support yourself. To support a good wife, even if she have children, is really less expensive than to board alone, besides being one of the surest means of acquiring property.

13. **Marrying for a Home.**—Do not, however, marry for a home merely, unless you wish to become even more destitute with one than without one; for, it is on the same footing with "marrying for money." Marry a man for his merit, and you take no chances.

14. **Marry to Please No One But Yourself.**—Marriage is a matter exclusively your own; because you alone must abide its consequences. No person, not even a parent, has the least right to interfere or dictate in this matter. I never knew a marriage, made to please another, to turn out any otherwise than most unhappily.

15. **Do Not Marry to Please Your Parents.** Parents cannot love for their children any more than they can eat or sleep, or breathe, or die and go to heaven for them. They may give wholesome advice merely, but should leave the entire decision to the unbiased judgment of the parties themselves, who mainly are to experience the consequences of their choice. Besides, such is human nature, that to oppose lovers, or to speak against the person beloved, only increases their desire and determination to marry.

16. **Run-Away Matches.**—Many a run-away match would never have taken place but for opposition or interference. Parents are mostly to be blamed for these elopements. Their children marry partly out of spite and to be contrary. Their very natures tell them that this interference is unjust—as it really is—and this excites combativeness, firmness, and self-esteem, in combination with the social faculties, to powerful and even blind resistance—which turmoil of the faculties hastens the match. Let the affections of a daughter be once slightly enlisted in your favor, and then let the "old folks" start an opposition, and you may feel sure of your prize. If she did not love you before, she will now, that you are persecuted.[185]

17. **Disinheritance.**—Never disinherit, or threaten to disinherit, a child for marrying against your will. If you wish a daughter not to marry a certain man, oppose her, and she will be sure to marry him; so also in reference to a son.

18. **Proper Training.**—The secret is, however, all in a nutshell. Let the father properly train his daughter, and she will bring her first love-letter to him, and give him an opportunity to cherish a suitable affection, and to nip an improper one in the germ, before it has time to do any harm.

19. **The Fatal Mistakes of Parents.**—*There is, however, one way of effectually preventing an improper match, and that is, not to allow your children to associate with any whom you are unwilling they should marry. How cruel as well as unjust, to allow a daughter to associate with a young man till the affections of both are riveted, and then forbid her marrying him. Forbid all association or consent cheerfully to the marriage.*

20. **An Intemperate Lover.**—Do not flatter yourselves, young women, that you can wean even an occasional wine drinker from his cups by love and persuasion. Ardent spirit at first, kindles up the fires of love into the fierce flames at burning licentiousness, which burn out every element of love and destroy every vestige of pure affection. It over-excites the passions, and thereby finally destroys it,—producing at first, unbridled libertinism, and then an utter barrenness of love; besides reversing the other faculties of the drinker against his own consort, and those of the wife against her drinking husband.

FIRST LOVE, DESERTION AND DIVORCE.

1. **First Love.**—This is the most important direction of all. The first love experiences a tenderness, a purity and unreservedness, an exquisiteness, a devotedness, and a poetry belonging to no subsequent attachment. "Love, like life, has no second spring." Though a second attachment may be accompanied by high moral feeling, and to a devotedness to the object loved; yet, let love be checked or blighted in its first pure emotion, and the beauty of its spring is irrecoverably withered and lost. This does not mean the simple love of children in the first attachment they call love, but rather the mature intelligent love of those of suitable age.

CONSIDERING THE QUESTION.

[187]

2. **Free from Temptations.**—As long as his heart is bound up in its first bundle of love and devotedness—as long as his affections remain reciprocated and uninterrupted—so long temptations cannot take effect. His heart is callous to the charms of others, and the very idea of bestowing his affections upon another is abhorrent. Much more so is animal indulgence, which is morally impossible.

3. **Second Love not Constant.**—But let this first love be broken off, and the flood-gates of passion are raised. Temptations now flow in upon him. He casts a lustful eye upon every passing female, and indulges unchaste imaginations and feelings. Although his conscientiousness or intellect may prevent actual indulgence, yet temptations now take effect, and render him liable to err; whereas before they had no power to awaken improper thoughts or feelings. Thus many young men find their ruin.

4. **Legal Marriage.**—What would any woman give for merely a nominal or legal husband, just to live with and provide for her, but who entertained not one spark of love for her, or whose affections were bestowed upon another? How absurd, how preposterous the doctrine that the obligations of marriage derive their sacredness from legal enactments and injunctions! How it literally profanes this holy of holies, and drags down this heaven-born institution from its original, divine elevation, to the level of a merely human device. Who will dare to advocate the human institution of marriage without the warm heart of a devoted and loving companion!

5. **Legislation.**—But no human legislation can so guard this institution but that it may be broken in spirit, though, perhaps, acceded to in form; for, it is the heart which this institution requires. There must be true and devoted affection, or marriage is a farce and a failure.

6. **The Marriage Ceremony and the Law Governing Marriage** are for the protection of the individual, yet a man and woman may be married by law and yet unmarried in spirit. The law may tie together, and no marriage be consummated. Marriage therefore is Divine, and "whom God hath joined together let no man put asunder." A right marriage means a right state of the heart. A careful study of this work will be a great help to both the unmarried and the married.

7. **Desertion and Divorce.**—For a young man to court a young woman, and excite her love till her affections are riveted, and then (from sinister motives, such as, to marry one richer, or more handsome), to leave her, and try [188]elsewhere, is the very same crime as to divorce her from all that she holds dear on earth—to root up and pull out her imbedded affections, and to tear her from her rightful husband. First love is always constant. The second love brings uncertainty—too often desertions before marriage and divorces after marriage.

8. **The Coquet.**—The young woman to play the coquet, and sport with the sincere affections of an honest and devoted young man, is one of the highest crimes that human nature can commit. Better murder him in body too, as she does in soul and morals, and it is the result of previous disappointment, never the outcome of a sincere first love.

9. **One Marriage.** One evidence that second marriages are contrary to the laws of our social nature, is the fact that almost all step-parents and step-children disagree. Now, what law has been broken, to induce this penalty? The law of marriage; and this is one of the ways in which the breach punishes itself. It is much more in accordance with our natural feelings, especially those of mothers, that children should be brought up by their own parent.

10. **Second Marriage.**—Another proof of this point is, that second marriage is more a matter of business. "I'll give you a home, if you'll take care of my children." "It's a bargain," is the way most second matches are made. There is little of the poetry of first-love, and little of the coyness and shrinking diffidence which characterize the first attachment. Still these remarks apply almost equally to a second attachment, as to second marriage.

11. **The Conclusion of the Whole Matter.**—Let this portion be read and pondered, and also the one entitled, "Marry your First Love if possible," which assigns the cause, and points out the only remedy, of licentiousness. As long as the main cause of this vice exists, and is aggravated by purse-proud, high-born, aristocratic parents and friends, and even by the virtuous and religious, just so long, and exactly in the same ratio will this blighting Sirocco blast the fairest flowers of female innocence and lovliness, and blight our noblest specimens of manliness. No sin of our land is greater.

[189]

CUPID'S CHARM.

Flirting and Its Dangers.
HOW MANY YOUNG GIRLS ARE RUINED.

1. **No Excuse.**—In this country there is no excuse for the young man who seeks the society of the loose and the dissolute. There is at all times and everywhere open to him a society of persons of the opposite sex of his own age and of pure thoughts and lives, whose conversation will refine him and drive from his bosom ignoble and impure thoughts.

2. **The Dangers.**—The young man who may take pleasure in the fact that he is the hero of half a dozen or more [191]engagements and love episodes, little realizes that such constant excitement often causes not only dangerously frequent and long-continued nocturnal emissions, but most painful affections of the testicles. Those who show too great familiarity with the other sex, who entertain lascivious thoughts, continually exciting the sexual desires, always suffer a weakening of power and sometimes the actual diseases of degeneration, chronic inflammation of the gland, spermatorrhœa, impotence, and the like.—Young man, beware; your punishment for trifling with the affections of others may cost you a life of affliction.

3. **Remedy.**—Do not violate the social laws. Do not trifle with the affections of your nature. Do not give others countless anguish, and also do not run the chances of injuring yourself and others for life. The society of refined and pure women is one of the strongest safeguards a young man can have, and he who seeks it will not only find satisfaction, but happiness. Simple friendship and kind affections for each other will ennoble and benefit.

4. **The Time for Marriage.**—When a young man's means permit him to marry, he should then look intelligently for her with whom he expects to pass the remainder of his life in perfect loyalty, and in sincerity and singleness of heart. Seek her to whom he is ready to swear to be ever true.

5. **Breach of Confidence.**—Nothing is more certain, says Dr. Naphey, to undermine domestic felicity, and sap the foundation of marital happiness, than marital infidelity. The risks of disease which a married man runs in impure intercourse are far more serious, because they not only involve himself, but his wife and his children. He should know that there is nothing which a woman will not forgive sooner than such a breach of confidence. He is exposed to the plots and is pretty certain sooner or later to fall into the snares of those atrocious parties who subsist on blackmail. And should he escape these complications, he still must lose self-respect, and carry about with him the burden of a guilty conscience and a broken vow.

6. **Society Rules and Customs.**—A young man can enjoy the society of ladies without being a "flirt." He can escort ladies to parties, public places of interest, social gatherings, etc., without showing special devotion to any one special young lady. When he finds the choice of his heart, then he will be justified to manifest it, and publicly proclaim it by paying her the compliment, exclusive attention. To keep a lady's company six months is a public announcement of an engagement.

A Word to Maidens.

1. **No Young Lady** who is not willing to assume the responsibility of a true wife, and be crowned with the sacred diadem of motherhood, should ever think of getting married. We have too many young ladies to-day who despise maternity, who openly vow that they will never be burdened with children, and yet enter matrimony at the first opportunity. What is the result? Let echo answer, What? Unless a young lady believes that motherhood is noble, is honorable, is divine, and she is willing to carry out that sacred function of her nature, she had a thousand times better refuse every proposal, and enter some honorable occupation and wisely die an old maid by choice.

2. **On the Other Hand, Young Lady**, never enter into the physical relations of marriage with a man until you have conversed with him freely and fully on these relations. Learn distinctly his views and feelings and expectations in regard to that purest and most ennobling of all the functions of your nature, and the most sacred of all intimacies of conjugal love. Your self-respect, your beauty, your glory, your heaven, as a wife, will be more

directly involved in his feelings and views and practices, in regard to that relation, than in all other things. As you would not become a weak, miserable, imbecile, unlovable and degraded wife and mother, in the very prime of your life, come to a perfect understanding with your chosen one, ere you commit your person to his keeping in the sacred intimacies of home. Beware of that man who, under pretence of delicacy, modesty, and propriety, shuns conversation with you on this relation, and on the hallowed function of maternity.

3. **Talk With Your Intended** frankly and openly. Remember, concealment and mystery in him, towards you, on all other subjects pertaining to conjugal union might be overlooked, but if he conceals his views here, rest assured it bodes no good to your purity and happiness as a wife and mother. You can have no more certain assurance that you are to be victimized, your soul and body offered up, *slain*, on the altar of his sensualism, than his unwillingness to converse with you on subjects so vital to your happiness. Unless he is willing to hold his manhood in abeyance to the calls of your nature and to your conditions, and consecrate its passions and its powers to the elevation and happiness of his wife and children, your maiden soul had better return to God unadorned with the diadem of conjugal and maternal love than that you should become the wife of such a man and the mother of his children.[193]

ROMAN LOVE MAKING.

[194]

POPPING THE QUESTION.
Uniformed Men are always Popular with the Ladies.

1. **Making the Declaration.**—There are few emergencies in business and few events in life that bring to man the trying ordeal of "proposing to a lady." We should be glad to help the bashful lover in his hours of perplexity, embarrassment and hesitation, but unfortunately we cannot pop the question for him, nor give him a formula by which [195]he may do it. Different circumstances and different surroundings compel every lover to be original in his form or mode of proposing.

2. **Bashfulness.**—If a young man is very bashful, he should write his sentiments in a clear, frank manner on a neat white sheet of note paper, enclose it in a plain white envelope and find some way to convey it to the lady's hand.

3. **The Answer.**—If the beloved one's heart is touched, and she is in sympathy with the lover, the answer should be frankly and unequivocally given. If the negative answer is necessary, it should be done in the kindest and most sympathetic language, yet definite, positive and to the point, and the gentleman should at once withdraw his suit and continue friendly but not familiar.

4. **Saying "No" for "Yes."**—If girls are foolish enough to say "No" when they mean "Yes," they must suffer the consequences which often follow. A man of intelligence and self-respect will not ask a lady twice. It is begging for recognition and lowers his dignity, should he do so. A lady is supposed to know her heart sufficiently to consider the question to her satisfaction before giving an answer.

5. **Confusion of Words and Misunderstanding.**—Sometimes a man's happiness, has depended on his manner of popping the question. Many a time the girl has said "No" because the question was so worded that the affirmative did not come from the mouth naturally; and two lives that gravitated toward each other with all their inward force have been thrown suddenly apart, because the electric keys were not carefully touched.

6. **Scriptural Declaration.**—The church is not the proper place to conduct a courtship, yet the following is suggestive and ingenious.

A young gentleman, familiar with the Scriptures, happening to sit in a pew adjoining a young lady for whom he conceived a violent attachment, made his proposal in this way: He politely handed his neighbor a Bible open, with a pin stuck in the following text: Second Epistle of John, verse 5:

"And I beseech thee, lady, not as though I wrote a new commandment unto thee, but that we had from the beginning, that we love one another."

SEALING THE ENGAGEMENT.
From the Most Celebrated Painting in the German Department at the World's Fair.

She returned it, pointing to the second chapter of Ruth, verse 10: "Then she fell on her face, and bowed herself to the ground, and said unto him. Why have I found grace in [197]thine eyes that thou shouldest take knowledge of me, seeing I am a stranger?"

He returned the book, pointing to the 13th verse of the Third Epistle of John: "Having many things to write unto you, I would not write to you with paper and ink, but trust to come unto you and speak face to face, that your joy may be full."

From the above interview a marriage took place the ensuing month in the same church.

7. How Jenny was Won.

On a sunny Summer morning,
Early as the dew was dry,
Up the hill I went a berrying;
Need I tell you—tell you why?
Farmer Davis had a daughter,
And it happened that I knew,
On each sunny morning, Jenny
Up the hill went berrying too.
Lonely work is picking berries,
So I joined her on the hill:
"Jenny, dear," said I, "your basket's
Quite too large for one to fill."
So we stayed—we two—to fill it,
Jenny talking—I was still.—
Leading where the hill was steepest,
Picking berries up the hill.
"This is up-hill work," said Jenny;
"So is life," said I; "shall we
Climb it each alone, or, Jenny,
Will you come and climb with me?"
Redder than the blushing berries
Jenny's cheek a moment grew,
While without delay she answered,
"I will come and climb with you."
[198]

8. A Romantic Way for Proposing.—In Peru they have a romantic way of popping the question. The suitor appears on the appointed evening, with a gaily dressed troubadour, under the balcony of his beloved. The singer steps before her flower-bedecked window, and sings her beauties in the name of her lover. He compares her size to that of a pear-tree, her lips to two blushing rose-buds, and her womanly form to that of a dove. With assumed harshness the lady asks her lover: "Who are you, and what do you want?" He answers with ardent confidence: "Thy love I do adore, The stars live in the harmony of love, and why should not we, too, love each other?" Then the proud beauty gives herself away: she takes her flower-wreath from her hair and throws it down to her lover, promising to be his forever.

A PERUVIAN BEAUTY.

[199]

The Wedding.
THE BRIDE.

1. The Proper Time.—Much has been printed in various volumes regarding the time of the year, the influence of the seasons, etc., as determining the proper time to set for the wedding day. Circumstances must govern these things. To be sure, it is best to avoid extremes of heat and cold. Very hot weather is debilitating, and below zero is uncomfortable.

2. The Lady Should Select the Day.—There is one element in the time that is of great importance, physically, especially to the lady. It is the day of the month, and it is hoped that every lady who contemplates marriage is informed upon the great facts of ovulation. By reading page [200]245 she will understand that it is to her advantage to select a wedding day about fifteen or eighteen days after the close of menstruation in the month chosen, since it is not best that the first child should be conceived during the excitement or irritation of first attempts at congress; besides modest brides naturally do not wish to become large with child before the season of congratulation and visiting on their return from the "wedding tour" is over.

Again, it is asserted by many of the best writers on this subject, that the mental condition of either parent at the time of intercourse will be stamped upon the embryo; hence it is not only best, but wise, that the first-born should not be conceived until several months after marriage, when the husband and wife have nicely settled in their new home, and become calm in their experience of each other's society.

3. **The "Bridal Tour"** is considered by many newly-married couples as a necessary introduction to a life of connubial joy. There is, in our opinion, nothing in the custom to recommend it. After the excitement and overwork before and accompanying a wedding, the period immediately following should be one of *rest*.

Again, the money expended on the ceremony and a tour of the principal cities, etc., might, in most cases, be applied to a multitude of after-life comforts of far more lasting value and importance. To be sure, it is not pleasant for the bride, should she remain at home, to pass through the ordeal of criticism and vulgar comments of acquaintants and friends, and hence, to escape this, the young couple feel like getting away for a time. Undoubtedly the best plan for the great majority, after this most eventful ceremony, is to enter their future home at once, and there to remain in comparative privacy until the novelty of the situation is worn off.

4. **If the Conventional Tour** is taken, the husband should remember that his bride cannot stand the same amount of tramping around and sight-seeing that he can. The female organs of generation are so easily affected by excessive exercise of the limbs which support them, that at this critical period it would be a foolish and costly experience to drag a lady hurriedly around the country on an extensive and protracted round of sight-seeing or visiting. Unless good common-sense is displayed in the manner of spending the "honeymoon," it will prove very untrue to its name. In many cases it lays the foundation for the wife's first and life-long "backache."

[201]
Advice to Newly Married Couples.
THE HONEY-MOON.

1. **"Be Ye Fruitful and Multiply"** is a Bible commandment which the children of men habitually obey. However they may disagree on other subjects, all are in accord on this; the barbarous, the civilized, the high, the low, the fierce, the gentle—all unite in the desire which finds its accomplishment in the reproduction of their kind. Who [202]shall quarrel with the Divinely implanted instinct, or declare it to be vulgar or unmentionable? It is during the period of the honeymoon that the intensity of this desire, coupled with the greatest curiosity, is at its height, and the unbridled license often given the passions at this time is attended with the most dangerous consequences.

2. **Consummation of Marriage.**—The first time that the husband and wife cohabit together after the ceremony has been performed is called the consummation of marriage. Many grave errors have been committed by people in this, when one or both of the contracting parties were not physically or sexually in a condition to carry out the marriage relation. A marriage, however, is complete without this in the eyes of the law, as it is a maxim taken from the Roman civil statutes that consent, not cohabitation, is the binding element in the ceremony. Yet, in most States of the U.S., and in some other countries; marriage is legally declared void and of no effect where it is not possible to consummate the marriage relation. A divorce may be obtained provided the injured party begins the suit.

3. **Test of Virginity.**—The consummation of marriage with a virgin is not necessarily attended with a flow of blood, and the absence of this sign is not the slightest presumption against her former chastity. The true test of virginity is modesty void of any disagreeable familiarity. A sincere Christian faith is one of the best recommendations.

4. **Let Every Man Remember** that the legal right of marriage does not carry with it the moral right to injure for life the loving companion he has chosen. Ignorance may be the cause, but every man before he marries should know something of the physiology and the laws of health, and we here give some information which is of very great importance to every newly-married man.

5. **Sensuality.**—Lust crucifies love. The young sensual husband is generally at fault. Passion sways and the duty to bride and wife is nor thought of, and so a modest young wife is often actually forced and assaulted by the unsympathetic haste of her husband. An amorous man in that way soon destroys his own love, and thus is laid the foundation for many difficulties that soon develop trouble and disturb the happiness of both.

6. **Abuse After Marriage.**—Usually marriage is consummated within a day or two after the ceremony, but this is [203]gross injustice to the bride. In most cases she is nervous, timid, and exhausted by the duties of preparation for the wedding, and in no way in a condition, either in body or mind, for the vital change which the married relation bring upon her. Many a young husband often lays the foundation of many diseases of the womb and of the nervous system in gratifying his unchecked passions without a proper regard for his wife's exhausted condition.

7. **The First Conjugal Approaches** are usually painful to the new wife, and no enjoyment to her follows. Great caution and kindness should be exercised. A young couple rushing together in their animal passion soon produce a nervous and irritating condition which ere long brings apathy, indifference, if not dislike. True love and a high regard for each other will temper passion into moderation.

8. **Were the Above Injunctions Heeded** fully and literally it would be folly to say more, but this would be omitting all account of the bridegroom's new position, the power of his passion, and the timidity of the fair creature who is wondering what fate has in store for her trembling modesty. To be sure, there are some women who are possessed of more forward natures and stronger desires than others. In such cases there may be less trouble.

9. **A Common Error.**—The young husband may have read in some treatise on physiology that the hymen in a virgin is the great obstacle to be overcome. He is apt to conclude that this is all, that some force will be needed to break it down, and that therefore an amount of urgency even to the degree of inflicting considerable pain is justifiable. This is usually wrong. It rarely constitutes any obstruction, and, even when its rupturing may be necessary, it alone seldom causes suffering.

There are sometimes certain deformities of the vagina, but no woman should knowingly seek matrimonial relations when thus afflicted.

We quote from Dr. C. A. Huff the following:

10. **"What Is It, then, that Usually Causes** distress to many women, whether a bride or a long-time wife?" The answer is, Simply those conditions of the organs in which they are not properly prepared, by anticipation and desire, to receive a foreign body. The modest one craves only refined and platonic love at first, and if husbands, new and old, would only realize this plain truth, wife-torturing would cease and the happiness of each one of all human pairs vastly increase.[204]

11. **The Conditions of the Female** organs depend upon the state of the mind just as much as in the case of the husband. The male, however, being more sensual, is more quickly roused. She is far less often or early ready. In its unexcited state the vagina is lax, its walls are closed together, and their surfaces covered by but little lubricating secretion. The chaster one of the pair has no desire that this sacred vestibule to the great arcana of procreation shall be immediately and roughly invaded. This, then, is the time for all approaches by the husband to be of the most delicate, considerate, and refined description possible. The quietest and softest demeanor, with gentle and re-assuring words, are all that should be attempted at first. The wedding day has probably been one of fatigue, and it is foolish to go farther.

12. **For More Than One Night** it will be wise, indeed, if the wife's confidence shall be as much wooed and won by patient, delicate, and prolonged courting, as before the marriage engagement. How long should this period of waiting be can only be decided by the circumstances of any case. The bride will ultimately deny no favor which is sought with full deference to her modesty, and in connection with which bestiality is not exhibited. Her

nature is that of delicacy; her affection is of a refined character; if the love and conduct offered to her are a careful effort to adapt roughness and strength to her refinement and weakness, her admiration and responsive love will be excited to the utmost.

13. **When That Moment Arrives** when the bride finds she can repose perfect confidence in the kindness of her husband, that his love is not purely animal, and that no violence will be attempted, the power of her affection for him will surely assert itself; the mind will act on those organs which nature has endowed to fulfil the law of her being, the walls of the vagina will expand, and the glands at the entrance will be fully lubricated by a secretion of mucous which renders congress a matter of comparative ease.

14. **When This Responsive Enlargement** and lubrication are fully realized, it is made plain why the haste and force so common to first and subsequent coition is, as it has been justly called, nothing but "legalized rape." Young husband! Prove your manhood, not by yielding to unbridled lust and cruelty, but by the exhibition of true power in *self-control* and patience with the helpless being confided to your care! Prolong the delightful season of courting into and *through* wedded life, and rich shall be your reward.[205]

15. **A Want of Desire** may often prevail, and may be caused by loss of sleep, study, constant thought, mental disturbance, anxiety, self-abuse, excessive use of tobacco or alcoholic drink, etc. Overwork may cause debility; a man may not have an erection for months, yet it may not be a sign of debility, sexual lethargy or impotence. Get the mind and the physical constitution in proper condition, and most all these difficulties will disappear. Good athletic exercise by walking, riding, or playing croquet, or any other amusement, will greatly improve the condition. A good rest, however, will be necessary to fully restore the mind and the body, then the natural condition of the sexual organs will be resumed.

16. **Having Twins.**—Having twins is undoubtedly hereditary and descends from generation to generation, and persons who have twins are generally those who have great sexual vigor. It is generally the result of a second cohabitation immediately following the first, but some parents have twins who cohabit but once during several days.

17. **Proper Intercourse.**—The right relation of a newly-married couple will rather increase than diminish love. To thus offer up the maiden on the altar of love and affection only swells her flood of joy and bliss; whereas, on the other hand, sensuality humbles, debases, pollutes, and never elevates. Young husbands should wait for an *invitation to the banquet*, and they will be amply paid by the very pleasure sought. Invitation or permission delights, and possession by force degrades. The right-minded bridegroom will postpone the exercise of his nuptial rights for a few days, and allow his young wife to become rested from the preparation and fatigue of the wedding, and become accustomed to the changes in her new relations of life.

18. **Rightly Beginning Sexual Life.**—Intercourse promotes all the functions of the body and mind, but rampant lust and sexual abuses soon destroy the natural pleasures of intercourse, and unhappiness will be the result. Remember that *intercourse* should not become the polluted purpose of marriage. To be sure, rational enjoyment benefits and stimulates love, but the pleasure of each other's society, standing together on all questions of mutual benefit, working hand in hand and shoulder to shoulder in the battle of life, raising a family of beautiful children, sharing each other's joys and sorrows, are the things that bring to every couple the best, purest, and noblest enjoyment that God has bestowed upon man.[206]

A TURKISH HAREM.

Sexual Proprieties and Improprieties.

1. To have offspring is not to be regarded as a luxury, but as a great primary necessity of health and happiness, of which every fully-developed man and woman should have a fair share, while it cannot be denied that the ignorance of the necessity of sexual intercourse to the health and virtue of both man and woman is the most fundamental error in medical and moral philosophy.

2. In a state of pure nature, where man would have his sexual instincts under full and natural restraint, there would be little, if any, licentiousness, and children would be the result of natural desire, and not the accidents of lust.

3. This is an age of sensuality; unnatural passions are cultivated and indulged. Young people in the course of their engagement often sow the seed of serious excesses. This habit

of embracing, sitting on the lover's lap, leaning on his breast, long and uninterrupted periods of secluded companionship, have become so common that it is amazing how a young lady can safely arrive at the wedding day. While this conduct may safely terminate with the wedding day, yet it cultivates the tendency which often results in excessive indulgencies after the honey-moon is over.

4. **Separate Beds.**—Many writers have vigorously championed as a reform the practice of separate beds for husband and wife. While we would not recommend such separation, it is no doubt very much better for both husband and wife, in case the wife is pregnant. Where people are reasonably temperate, no such ordinary precautions as [207]separate sleeping places may be necessary. But in case of pregnancy it will add rest to the mother and add vigor to the unborn child. Sleeping together, however, is natural and cultivates true affection, and it is physiologically true that in very cold weather life is prolonged by husband and wife sleeping together.

5. **The Authority of the Wife.**—Let the wife judge whether she desires a separate couch or not. She has the superior right to control her own person. In such diseases as consumption, or other severe or lingering diseases, separate beds should always be insisted upon.

6. **The Time for Indulgence.**—The health of the generative functions depends upon exercise, just the same as any other vital organ. Intercourse should be absolutely avoided just before or after meals, or just after mental excitement or physical exercise. No wife should indulge her husband when he is under the influence of alcoholic stimulants, for idiocy and other serious maladies are liable to be visited upon the offspring.

7. **Restraint during Pregnancy.**—There is no question but what moderate indulgence during the first few months of pregnancy does not result in serious harm; but people who excessively satisfy their ill-governed passions are liable to pay a serious penalty.

8. **Miscarriage.**—If a woman is liable to abortion or miscarriage, absolute abstinence is the only remedy. No sexual indulgence during pregnancy can be safely tolerated.

9. It is better for people not to marry until they are of proper age. It is a physiological fact that men seldom reach the full maturity of their virile power before the age of twenty-five, and the female rarely attains the full vigor of her sexual powers before the age of twenty.

10. **Illicit Pleasures.**—The indulgence of illicit pleasures, says Dr. S. Pancoast, sooner or later is sure to entail the most loathsome diseases on their votaries. Among these diseases are Gonorrhœa, Syphilis, Spermatorrhœa (waste of semen by daily and nightly involuntary emissions), Satyriasis (a species of sexual madness, or a sexual diabolism, causing men to commit rape and other beastly acts and outrages, not only on women and children, but men and animals, as sodomy, pederasty, etc.), Nymphomania (causing women to assail every man they meet, and supplicate and excite him to gratify their lustful passions, or who resort to means of sexual pollutions, which is impossible to describe without shuddering), together with spinal diseases and many disorders of the most distressing and disgusting character, [208]filling the bones with rottenness, and eating away the flesh by gangrenous ulcers, until the patient dies, a horrible mass of putridity and corruption.

11. **Sensuality.**—Sensuality is not love, but an unbridled desire which kills the soul. Sensuality will drive away the roses in the cheeks of womanhood, undermine health and produce a brazen countenance that can be read by all men. The harlot may commit her sins in the dark, but her countenance reveals her character and her immorality is an open secret.

12. **Sexual Temperance.**—All excesses and absurdities of every kind should be carefully avoided. Many of the female disorders which often revenge themselves in the cessation of all sexual pleasure are largely due to the excessive practice of sexual indulgence.

13. **Frequency.**—Some writers claim that intercourse should never occur except for the purpose of childbearing; but such restraint is not natural and consequently not conducive to health. There are many conditions in which the health of the mother and offspring must be respected. It is now held that it is nearer a crime than a virtue to prostitute woman to the degradation of breeding animals by compelling her to bring into life more offspring than can be born healthy, or be properly cared for and educated.

14. In this work we shall attempt to specify no rule, but simply give advice as to the health and happiness of both man and wife. A man should not gratify his own desires at the expense of his wife's health, comfort or inclination. Many men no doubt harass their wives and force many burdens upon their slender constitutions. But it is a great sin and no true husband will demand unreasonable recognition. The wife when physically able, however, should bear with her husband. Man is naturally sensitive on this subject, and it takes but little to alienate his affections and bring discord into the family.

15. The best writers lay down the rule for the government of the marriage-bed, that sexual indulgence should only occur about once in a week or ten days, and this of course applies only to those who enjoy a fair degree of health. But it is a hygienic and physiological fact that those who indulge only once a month receive a far greater degree of the intensity of enjoyment than those who indulge their passions more frequently. Much pleasure is lost by excesses where much might be gained by temperance, giving rest to the organs for the accumulation of nervous force.[209]

How to Perpetuate the Honey-Moon.

1. **Continue Your Courtship.**—Like causes produce like effects.

2. **Neglect of Your Companion.**—Do not assume a right to neglect your companion more after marriage than you did before.

3. **Secrets.**—Have no secrets that you keep from your companion. A third party is always disturbing.

4. **Avoid the Appearance of Evil.**—In matrimonial matters it is often that the mere appearance contains all the evil. Love, as soon as it rises above calculation and becomes love, is exacting. It gives all, and demands all.

5. **Once Married, Never Open Your Mind to Any Change.**—If you keep the door of your purpose closed, evil or even desirable changes cannot make headway without help.

6. **Keep Step in Mental Development.**—A tree that grows for forty years may take all the sunlight from a tree that stops growing at twenty.

7. **Keep a Lively Interest in the Business of the Home.**—Two that do not pull together are weaker than either alone.

8. **Gauge Your Expenses by Your Revenues.**—Love must eat. The sheriff often levies on Cupid long before he takes away the old furniture.

9. **Start From Where Your Parents Started Rather than from Where They Now Are.**—Hollow and showy boarding often furnishes the too strong temptation, while the quietness of a humble home would cement the hearts beyond risk.[210]

10. **Avoid Debt.**—Spend your own money, but earn it first, then it will not be necessary to blame any one for spending other people's.

11. **Do Not Both Get Angry at the Same Time.**—Remember, it takes two to quarrel.

12. **Do Not Allow Yourself Ever to Come to an Open Rupture.**—Things unsaid need less repentance.

13. **Study to Conform Your Tastes and Habits to the Tastes and Habits of Your Companion.**—If two walk together, they must agree.

How to Be a Good Wife.

1. **Reverence Your Husband.**—He sustains by God's order a position of dignity as head of a family, head of the woman. Any breaking down of this order indicates a mistake in the union, or a digression from duty.

2. **Love Him.**—A wife loves as naturally as the sun shines. Love is your best weapon. You conquered him with that in the first place. You can reconquer by the same means.

3. **Do Not Conceal Your Love from Him.**—If he is crowded with care, and too busy to seem to heed your love, you need to give all the greater attention to securing his knowledge of your love. If you intermit he will settle down into a hard, cold life with increased rapidity. Your example will keep the light on his conviction. The more he neglects the fire on the hearth, the more carefully must you feed and guard it. It must not be allowed to go out. Once out you must sit ever in darkness and in the cold.

4. **Cultivate the Modesty and Delicacy of Your Youth.**—The relations and familiarity of wedded life may seem to tone down the sensitive and retiring instincts of girlhood, but nothing can compensate for the loss of these. However, much men may admire the public performance of gifted women, they do not desire that boldness and dash in a wife. The holy blush of a maiden's modesty is more powerful in hallowing and governing a home than the heaviest armament that ever a warrior bore.

5. **Cultivate Personal Attractiveness.**—This means the storing of your mind with a knowledge of passing events, and with a good idea of the world's general advance. If you read nothing, and make no effort to make yourself attractive, you will soon sink down into a dull hack of stupidity. If [211]your husband never hears from you any words of wisdom, or of common information, he will soon hear nothing from you. Dress and gossips soon wear out. If your memory is weak, so that it hardly seems worth while to read, that is additional reason for reading.

TALKING BEFORE MARRIAGE.

6. **Cultivate Physical Attractiveness.**—When you were encouraging the attentions of him whom you now call husband, you did not neglect any item of dress or appearance [212]that could help you. Your hair was always in perfect training. You never greeted him with a ragged or untidy dress or soiled hands. It is true that your "market is made," but you cannot afford to have it "broken." Cleanliness and good taste will attract now as they did formerly. Keep yourself at your best. Make the most of physical endowments. Neatness and order break the power of poverty.

7. **Study Your Husband's Character.**—He has his peculiarities. He has no right to many of them, and you need to know them; thus you can avoid many hours of friction. The good pilot steers around the sunken rocks that lie in the channel. The engineer may remove them, not the pilot. You are more pilot than engineer. Consult his tastes. It is more important to your home, that you should please him than anybody else.

8. **Practice Economy.**—Many families are cast out of peace into grumbling and discord by being compelled to fight against poverty. When there are no great distresses to be endured or accounted for, complaint and fault-finding are not so often evoked. Keep your husband free from the annoyance of disappointed creditors, and he will be more apt to keep free from annoying you. To toil hard for bread, to fight the wolf from the door, to resist impatient creditors, to struggle against complaining pride at home, is too much to ask of one man. A crust that is your own is a feast, while a feast that is purloined from unwilling creditors is a famine.

How to Be a Good Husband.

1. **Show Your Love.**—All life manifests itself. As certainly as a live tree will put forth leaves in the spring, so certainly will a living love show itself. Many a noble man toils early and late to earn bread and position for his wife. He hesitates at no weariness for her sake. He justly thinks that such industry and providence give a better expression of his love than he could by caressing her and letting the grocery bills go unpaid. He fills the cellar and pantry. He drives and pushes his business. He never dreams that he is actually starving his wife to death. He may soon have a woman left to superintend his home, but his wife is dying. She must be kept alive by the same process that called her into being. Recall and repeat the little attentions and delicate compliments that once made you so agreeable, and that fanned her love into a consuming flame. It is not beneath the dignity of the skillful physician to study all the [214]little symptoms, and order all the little round of attentions that check the waste of strength and brace the staggering constitution. It is good work for a husband to cherish his wife.

TALKING AFTER MARRIAGE.

2. **Consult with Your Wife.**—She is apt to be as right as you are, and frequently able to add much to your stock of wisdom. In any event she appreciates your attentions.

3. **Study to Keep Her Young.**—It can be done. It is not work, but worry, that wears. Keep a brave, true heart between her and all harm.

4. **Help to Bear Her Burdens.**—Bear one another's burdens, and so fulfill the law of love. Love seeks opportunities to do for the loved object. She has the constant care of

your children. She is ordained by the Lord to stand guard over them. Not a disease can appear in the community without her taking the alarm. Not a disease can come over the threshold without her instantly springing into the mortal combat. If there is a deficiency anywhere, it comes out of her pleasure. Her burdens are everywhere. Look for them, that you may lighten them.

5. **Make Yourself Helpful by Thoughtfulness.**—Remember to bring into the house your best smile and sunshine. It is good for you, and it cheers up the home. There is hardly a nook in the house that has not been carefully hunted through to drive out everything that might annoy you. The dinner which suits, or ought to suit you, has not come on the table of itself. It represents much thoughtfulness and work. You can do no more manly thing than find some way of expressing, in word or look, your appreciation of it.

6. **Express Your Will, Not by Commands, but by Suggestions.**—It is God's order that you should be the head of the family. You are clothed with authority. But this does not authorize you to be stern and harsh, as an officer in the army. Your authority is the dignity of love. When it is not clothed in love it ceases to have the substance of authority. A simple suggestion that may embody a wish, an opinion or an argument, becomes one who reigns over such a kingdom as yours.

7. **Seek to Refine Your Nature.**—It is no slander to say that many men have wives much more refined than themselves. This is natural in the inequalities of life. Other qualities may compensate for any defect here. But you need have no defect in refinement. Preserve the gentleness and refinement of your wife as a rich legacy for your children, and in so doing you will lift yourself to higher levels.[215]

8. **Be a Gentleman as well as a Husband.**—The signs and bronze and calluses of toil are no indications that you are not a gentleman. The soul of gentlemanliness is a kindly feeling toward others, that prompts one to secure their comfort. That is why the thoughtful peasant lover is always so gentlemanly, and in his love much above himself.

9. **Stay at Home.**—Habitual absence during the evenings is sure to bring sorrow. If your duty or business calls you, you have the promise that you will be kept in all your ways. But if you go out to mingle with other society, and leave your wife at home alone, or with the children and servants, know that there is no good in store for you. She has claims upon you that you can not afford to allow to go to protest. Reverse the case. You sit down alone after having waited all day for your wife's return, and think of her as reveling in gay society, and see if you can keep out all the doubts as to what takes her away. If your home is not as attractive as you want it, you are a principal partner. Set yourself about the work of making it attractive.

10. **Take Your Wife with You into Society.**—Seclusion begets morbidness. She needs some of the life that comes from contact with society. She must see how other people appear and act. It often requires an exertion for her to go out of her home, but it is good for her and for you. She will bring back more sunshine. It is wise to rest sometimes. When the Arab stops for his dinner he unpacks his camel. Treat your wife with as much consideration.

[217]
Cause of Family Troubles.
TIRED OF LIFE.

1. **Much Better to Be Alone.**—He who made man said it is not good for him to be alone; but it is much better to be alone, than it is to be in some kinds of company. Many couples who felt unhappy when they were apart, have been utterly miserable when together; and scores who have been ready to go through fire and water to get married, have been willing to run the risk of fire and brimstone to get divorced. It is by no means certain that because persons are wretched before marriage they will be happy after it. The wretchedness of many homes, and the prevalence of immorality and divorce is a sad commentary on the evils which result from unwise marriages.

2. **Unavoidable Evils.**—There are plenty of unavoidable evils in this world, and it is mournful to think of the multitudes who are preparing themselves for needless disappointments, and who yet have no fear, and are unwilling to be instructed, cautioned or

warned. To them the experience of mature life is of little account compared with the wisdom of ardent and enthusiastic youth.

3. **Matrimonial Infelicity.**—One great cause of matrimonial infelicity is the hasty marriages of persons who have no adequate knowledge of each other's characters. Two strangers become acquainted, and are attracted to each other, and without taking half the trouble to investigate or inquire that a prudent man would take before buying a saddle horse, they are married. In a few weeks or months it is perhaps found that one of the parties was married already, or possibly that the man is drunken or vicious, or the woman anything but what she should be. Then begins the bitter part of the experience: shame, disgrace, scandal, separation, sin and divorce, all come as the natural results of a rash and foolish marriage. A little time spent in honest, candid, and careful preliminary inquiry and investigation, would have saved the trouble.

4. **The Climax.**—It has been said that a man is never utterly ruined until he has married a bad woman. So the climax of woman's miseries and sorrows may be said to come only when she is bound with that bond which should be her chiefest blessing and her highest joy, but which may prove her deepest sorrow and her bitterest curse.

5. **The Folly of Follies.**—There are some lessons which people are very slow to learn, and yet which are based upon [218]the simple principles of common-sense. A young lady casts her eye upon a young man. She says, "I mean to have that man." She plies her arts, engages his affections, marries him, and secures for herself a life of sorrow and disappointment, ending perhaps in a broken up home or an early grave. Any prudent, intelligent person of mature age, might have warned or cautioned her; but she sought no advice, and accepted no admonition. A young man may pursue a similar course with equally disastrous results.

6. **Hap-Hazard.**—Many marriages are undoubtedly arranged by what may be termed the accident of locality. Persons live near each other, become acquainted, and engage themselves to those whom they never would have selected as their companions in life if they had wider opportunities of acquaintance. Within the borders of their limited circle they make a selection which may be wise or may be unwise. They have no means of judging, they allow no one else to judge for them. The results are sometimes happy and sometimes unhappy in the extreme. It is well to act cautiously in doing what can be done but once. It is not a pleasant experience for a person to find out a mistake when it is too late to rectify it.

7. **We All Change.**—When two persons of opposite sex are often thrown together they are very naturally attracted to each other, and are liable to imbibe the opinion that they are better fitted for life-long companionship than any other two persons in the world. This may be the case, or it may not be. There are a thousand chances against such a conclusion to one in favor of it. But even if at the present moment these two persons were fitted to be associated, no one can tell whether the case will be the same five or ten years hence. Men change; women change; they are not the same they were ten years ago; they are not the same they will be ten years hence.

8. **The Safe Rule.**—Do not be in a hurry; take your time, and consider well before you allow your devotion to rule you. Study first your character, then study the character of her whom you desire to marry. Love works mysteriously, and if it will bear careful and cool investigation, it will no doubt thrive under adversity. When people marry they unite their destinies for the better or the worse. Marriage is a contract for life and will never bear a hasty conclusion. *Never be in a hurry!*

[219]

Jealousy—Its Cause and Cure.

Trifles, light as air
Are to the jealous confirmations strong,
As proofs of holy writ.—SHAKESPEARE.
Nor Jealousy
Was understood, the injur'd lover's hell.—MILTON.
O, beware, my lord, of jealousy;

It is the green-eyed monster which doth mock
The meat it feeds on.—SHAKESPEARE.

1. **Definition.**—Jealousy is an accidental passion, for which the faculty indeed is unborn. In its nobler form and in its nobler motives it arises from love, and in its lower form it arises from the deepest and darkest Pit of Satan.

2. **How Developed.**—Jealousy arises either from weakness, which from a sense of its own want of lovable qualities is not convinced of being sure of its cause, or from distrust, which thinks the beloved person capable of infidelity. Sometimes all these motives may act together.

3. **Noblest Jealousy.**—The noblest jealousy, if the term noble is appropriate, is a sort of ambition or pride of the loving person who feels it is an insult that another one should assume it as possible to supplant his love, or it is the highest degree of devotion which sees a declaration of its object in the foreign invasion, as it were, of his own altar. Jealousy is always a sign that a little more wisdom might adorn the individual without harm.

4. **The Lowest Jealousy.**—The lowest species of jealousy is a sort of avarice of envy which, without being capable of love, at least wishes to possess the object of its jealousy alone by the one party assuming a sort of property right over the other. This jealousy, which might be called the Satanic, is generally to be found with old withered "husbands," whom the devil has prompted to marry young women and who forthwith dream night and day of cuck-old's horns. These Argus-eyed keepers are no longer capable of any feeling that could be called love, they are rather as a rule heartless house-tyrants, and are in constant dread that some one may admire or appreciate his unfortunate slave.

5. **Want of Love.**—The general conclusion will be that jealousy is more the result of wrong conditions which cause uncongenial unions, and which through moral corruption, artificially create distrust, than a necessary accompaniment of love.

SEEKING THE LIFE OF A RIVAL.

[221]

6. **Result of Poor Opinion.**—Jealousy is a passion with which those are most afflicted who are the least worthy of love. An innocent maiden who enters marriage will not dream of getting jealous; but all her innocence cannot secure her against the jealousy of her husband if he has been a libertine. Those are wont to be the most jealous who have the consciousness that they themselves are most deserving of jealousy. Most men in consequence of their present education and corruption have so poor an opinion not only of the male, but even of the female sex, that they believe every woman at every moment capable of what they themselves have looked for among all and have found among the most unfortunate, the prostitutes. No libertine can believe in the purity of woman; it is contrary to nature. A libertine therefore cannot believe in the loyalty of a faithful wife.

7. **When Justifiable.**—There may be occasions where jealousy is justifiable. If a woman's confidence has been shaken in her husband, or a husband's confidence has been shaken in his wife by certain signs or conduct, which have no other meaning but that of infidelity, then there is just cause for jealousy. There must, however, be certain proof as evidence of the wife's or husband's immoral conduct. Imaginations or any foolish absurdities should have no consideration whatever, and let everyone have confidence until his or her faith has been shaken by the revelation of absolute facts.

8. **Caution and Advice.**—No couple should allow their associations to develop into an engagement and marriage if either one has any inclination to jealousy. It shows invariably a want of sufficient confidence, and that want of confidence, instead of being diminished after marriage, is liable to increase, until by the aid of the imagination and wrong interpretation the home is made a hell and divorce a necessity. Let it be remembered, there can be no true love without perfect and absolute confidence. Jealousy is always the sign of weakness or madness. Avoid a jealous disposition, for it is an open acknowledgment of a lack of faith.

[222]

The Improvement of Offspring.

83

Why Bring Into the World Idiots, Fools, Criminals and Lunatics?

The Mother's Good Night Prayer.

1. **The Right Way.**—When mankind will properly love and marry and then rightly generate, carry, nurse and educate their children, will they in deed and in truth carry out [223]the holy and happy purpose of their Creator. See those miserable and depraved scape-goats of humanity, the demented simpletons, the half-crazy, unbalanced multitudes which infest our earth, and fill our prisons with criminals and our poor-houses with paupers. Oh! the boundless capabilities and perfections of our God-like nature and, alas! its deformities! All is the result of the ignorance or indifference of parents. As long as children are the accidents of lust instead of the premeditated objects of love, so long will the offspring deteriorate and the world be cursed with deformities, monstrosities, unhumanities and cranks.

2. **Each After Its Kind.**—"Like parents like children." "In their own image beget" they them. In what other can they? "How can a corrupt tree bring forth good fruit?" How can animal propensities in parents generate other than depraved children, or moral purity beget beings other than as holy by nature as those at whose hands they received existence and constitution?

3. **As Are the Parents**, physically, mentally and morally when they stamp their own image and likeness upon progeny, so will be the constitution of that progeny.

4. **"Just as the Twig Is Bent the Tree's Inclined."**—Yet the bramble cannot be bent to bear delicious peaches, nor the sycamore to bear grain. Education is something, but *parentage* is *everything*; because it *"dyes in the wool,"* and thereby exerts an influence on character almost infinitely more powerful than all other conditions put together.

5. **Healthy and Beautiful Children.**—Thoughtless mortal! Before you allow the first goings forth of love, learn what the parental conditions in you mean, and you will confer a great boon upon the prospective bone of your bone, and flesh of your flesh! If it is in your power to be the parent of beautiful, healthy, moral and talented children instead of diseased and depraved, is it not your imperious duty then, to impart to them that physical power, moral perfection, and intellectual capability, which shall ennoble their lives and make them good people and good citizens?

6. **Pause and Tremble.**—Prospective parents! Will you trifle with the dearest interests of your children? Will you in matters thus momentous, head-long rush

"Where angels dare not tread?"

Seeking only mere animal indulgence?—Well might cherubim shrink from assuming responsibilities thus momentous! Yet, how many parents tread this holy ground completely unprepared, and almost as thoughtlessly and ignorantly as brutes—entailing even loathsome diseases and [224]sensual propensities upon the fruit of their own bodies. Whereas they are bound, by obligations the most imperious, to bestow on them a good physical organization, along with a pure, moral, and strong intellectual constitution, or else not to become parents! Especially since it is easier to generate human angels than devils incarnate.

7. **Hereditary Descent.**—This great law of things, "Hereditary Descent," fully proves and illustrates in any required number and variety of cases, showing that progeny inherits the constitutional natures and characters, mental and physical, of parents, including pre-dispositions to consumption, insanity, all sorts of disease, etc., as well as longevity, strength, stature, looks, disposition, talents,—all that is constitutional. From what other source do or can they come? Indeed, who can doubt a truth as palpable as that children inherit some, and if some, therefore all, the physical and mental nature and constitution of parents, thus becoming almost their fac-similes?

8. **Illustrations.**—A whaleman was severely hurt by a harpooned and desperate whale turning upon the small boat, and, by his monstrous jaws, smashing it to pieces, one of which, striking him in his right side, crippled him for life. When sufficiently recovered, he married, according to previous engagement, and his daughter, born in due time, and closely resembling him in looks, constitution and character, has a weak and sore place corresponding in location with that of the injury of her father. Tubercles have been found in the lungs of infants at birth, born of consumptive parents,—a proof, clear and

84

demonstrative, that children inherit the several states of parental physiology existing at the time they received their physiological constitution. The same is true of the transmission of those diseases consequent on the violation of the law of chastity, and the same conclusion established thereby.

9. **Parent's Participation.**—Each parent furnishing an indispensable portion of the materials of life, and somehow or other, contributes parentally to the formation of the constitutional character of their joint product, appears far more reasonable, than to ascribe, as many do, the whole to either, some to paternity, others to maternity. Still this decision go which way it may, does not affect the great fact that children inherit both the physiology and the mentality existing in parents at the time they received being and constitution.

10. **Illegitimates or Bastards** also furnish strong proof of the correctness of this our leading doctrine. They are generally lively, sprightly, witty, frolicsome, knowing, [225]quick of perception, apt to learn, full of passion, quick-tempered, impulsive throughout, hasty, indiscreet, given to excesses, yet abound in good feeling, and are well calculated to enjoy life, though in general sadly deficient in some essential moral elements.

11. **Character of Illegitimates.**—Wherein, then, consists this difference? First, in "novelty lending an enchantment" rarely experienced in sated wedlock, as well as in power of passion sufficient to break through all restraint, external and internal; and hence their high wrought organization. They are usually wary and on the alert, and their parents drank "stolen waters." They are commonly wanting in moral balance, or else delinquent in some important moral aspect; nor would they have ever been born unless this had been the case, for the time being at least, with their parents. Behold in these, and many other respects easily cited, how striking the coincidence between their characters on the one hand, and, on the other, those parental conditions necessarily attendant on their origin.

12. **Children's Condition** depends upon parents' condition at the time of the sexual embrace. Let parents recall, as nearly as may be their circumstances and states of body and mind at this period, and place them by the side of the physical and mental constitutions of their children, and then say whether this law is not a great practical truth, and if so, its importance is as the happiness and misery it is capable of affecting! The application of this mighty engine of good or evil to mankind, to the promotion of human advancement, is the great question which should profoundly interest all parents.

13. **The Vital Period.**—The physical condition of parents at the vital period of transmission of life should be a perfect condition of health in both body and mind, and a rigorous condition of all the animal organs and functions.

14. **Muscular Preparation.**—Especially should parents cultivate their muscular system preparatory to the perfection of this function, and of their children; because, to impart strength and stamina to offspring they must of necessity both possess a good muscular organization, and also bring it into vigorous requisition at this period. For this reason, if for no other, let those of sedentary habits cultivate muscular energy preparatory to this time of need.

15. **The Seed.**—So exceedingly delicate are the seeds of life, that, unless planted in a place of perfect security, they must all be destroyed, and our race itself extinguished. And what place is as secure as that chosen, where they can [226]be reached only with the utmost difficulty, and than only at the peril of even life itself? Imperfect seed sown in poor ground means a sickly harvest.

16. **Healthy People—Most Children.**—The most healthy classes have the most numerous families; but that, as luxury enervates society, it diminishes the population, by enfeebling parents, nature preferring none rather than those too weakly to live and be happy, and thereby rendering that union unfruitful which is too feeble to produce offspring sufficiently strong to enjoy life. Debility and disease often cause barrenness. Nature seems to rebel against sickly offspring.

17. **Why Children Die.**—Inquire whether one or both the parents of those numerous children that die around us, have not weak lungs, or a debilitated stomach, or a diseased liver, or feeble muscles, or else use them but little, or disordered nerves, or some other debility or form of disease. The prevalence of summer complaints, colic, cholera infantum, and other affections of these vital organs of children is truly alarming, sweeping

them into their graves by the million. Shall other animals rear nearly all their young, and shall man, constitutionally by far the strongest of them all, lose half or more of his? Is this the order of nature? No, but their death-worm is born in and with them, and by parental agency.

18. **Grave-Yard Statistics.**—Take grave-yard statistics in August, and then say, whether most of the deaths of children are not caused by indigestion, or feebleness of the bowels, liver, etc., or complaints growing out of them? Rather, take family statistics from broken-hearted parents! And yet, in general, those very parents who thus suffer more than words can tell, were the first and main transgressors, because they entailed those dyspeptic, heart, and other kindred affections so common among American parents upon their own children, and thereby almost as bad as killed them by inches; thus depriving them of the joys of life, and themselves of their greatest earthly treasure!

19. **All Children May Die.**—Children may indeed die whose parents are healthy, but they almost must whose parents are essentially ailing in one or more of their vital organs; because, since they inherit this organ debilitated or diseased, any additional cause of sickness attacks this part first, and when it gives out, all go by the board together.

20. **Parents Must Learn and Obey.**—How infinitely more virtuous and happy would your children be if you should be healthy in body, and happy in mind, so as to beget in[227]them a constitutionally healthy and vigorous physiology, along with a serene and happy frame of mind! Words are utterly powerless in answer, and so is everything but a lifetime of consequent happiness or misery! Learn and obey, then, the laws of life and health, that you may both reap the rich reward yourself, and also shower down upon your children after you, blessings many and most exalted. Avoid excesses of all kinds, be temperate, take good care of the body and avoid exposures and disease, and your children will be models of health and beauty.

21. **The Right Condition.**—The great practical inference is, that those parents who desire intellectual and moral children, must love each other; because, this love, besides perpetually calling forth and cultivating their higher faculties, awakens them to the highest pitch of exalted action in that climax, concentration, and consummation of love which propagates their existing qualities, the mental endowment of offspring being proportionate to the purity and intensity of parental love.

22. **The Effects.**—The children of affectionate parents receive existence and constitution when love has rendered the mentality of their parents both more elevated and more active than it is by nature, of course the children of loving parents are both more intellectual and moral by nature than their parents. Now, if these children and their companions also love one another, this same law which renders the second generation better than the first, will of course render the third still better than the second, and thus of all succeeding generations.

23. **Animal Impulse.**—You may preach and pray till doomsday—may send out missionaries, may circulate tracts and Bibles, and multiply revivals and all the means of grace, with little avail; because, as long as mankind go on, as now, to propagate by animal impulse, so long must their offspring be animal, sensual, devilish! But only induce parents cordially to love each other, and you thereby render their children constitutionally talented and virtuous. Oh! parents, by as much as you prefer the luxuries of concord to the torments of discord, and children that are sweet dispositioned and highly intellectual to those that are rough, wrathful, and depraved, be entreated to "*love one another.*"

[229]

Too Many Children.
JUST HOME FROM SCHOOL.

1. **Lessening Pauperism.**—Many of the agencies for lessening pauperism are afraid of tracing back its growth to the frequency of births under wretched conditions. One begins to question whether after all sweet charity or dignified philanthropy has not acted with an unwise reticence. Among the problems which defy practical handling this is the most complicated. The pauperism which arises from marriage is the result of the worst elements of character legalized. In America, where the boundaries of wedlock are practically

boundless, it is not desirable, even were it possible, that the state should regulate marriage much further than it now does; therefore must the sociologist turn for aid to society in his struggle with pauperism.

2. **Right Physical and Spiritual Conditions of Birth.**—Society should insist upon the right spiritual and physical conditions for birth. It should be considered more than "a pity" when another child is born into a home too poor to receive it. The underlying selfishness of such an event should be recognized, for it brings motherhood under wrong conditions of health and money. Instead of each birth being the result of mature consideration and hallowed love, children are too often born as animals are born. To be sure the child has a father whom he can call by name. Better that there had never been a child.

3. **Wrong Results.**—No one hesitates to declare that it is want of self-respect and morality which brings wrong results outside of marriage, but it is also the want of them which begets evil inside the marriage relation. Though there is nothing more difficult than to find the equilibrium between self-respect and self-sacrifice, yet on success in finding it depends individual and national preservation. The fact of being wife and mother or husband and father should imply dignity and joyousness, no matter how humble the home.

4. **Difference of Opinion amongst Physicians.**—In regard to teaching, the difficulties are great. As soon as one advances beyond the simplest subjects of hygiene, one is met with the difference of opinions among physicians. When each one has a different way of making a mustard plaster, no wonder that each has his own notions about everything else. One doctor recommends frequent births, another advises against them.

5. **Different Natures.**—If physiological facts are taught to a large class, there are sure to be some in it whose impressionable natures are excited by too much plain [230]speaking, while there are others who need the most open teaching in order to gain any benefit. Talks to a few persons generally are wiser than popular lectures. Especially are talks needed by mothers and unmothered girls who come from everywhere to the city.

6. **Boys and Young Men.**—It is not women alone who require the shelter of organizations and instruction, but boys and young men. There is no double standard of morality, though the methods of advocating it depend upon the sex which is to be instructed. Men are more concerned with the practical basis of morality than with its sentiment, and with the pecuniary aspects of domestic life than with its physical and mental suffering. We all may need medicine for moral ills, yet the very intangibleness of purity makes us slow to formulate rules for its growth. Under the guidance of the wise in spirit and knowledge, much can be done to create a higher standard of marriage and to proportion the number of births according to the health and income of parents.

7. **For the Sake of the State.**—If the home exists primarily for the sake of the individual, it exists secondarily for the sake of the state. Therefore, any home into which are continually born the inefficient children of inefficient parents, not only is a discomfort in itself, but it also furnishes members for the armies of the unemployed, which are tinkering and hindering legislation and demanding by the brute force of numbers that the state shall support them.

8. **Opinions From High Authorities.**—In the statements and arguments made in the above we have not relied upon our own opinions and convictions, but have consulted the best authorities, and we hereby quote some of the highest authorities upon this subject.

9. **Rev. Leonard Dawson.**—"How rapidly conjugal prudence might lift a nation out of pauperism was seen in France.—Let them therefore hold the maxim that the production of offspring with forethought and providence is rational nature. It was immoral to bring children into the world whom they could not reasonably hope to feed, clothe and educate."

10. **Mrs. Fawcett.**—"Nothing will permanently offset pauperism while the present reckless increase of population continues."

11. **Dr. George Napheys.**—"Having too many children unquestionably has its disastrous effects on both mother and [231]children as known to every intelligent physician. Two-thirds of all cases of womb disease, says Dr. Tilt, are traceable to child-bearing in feeble women. There are also women to whom pregnancy is a nine months' torture, and others to whom it is nearly certain to prove fatal. Such a condition cannot be discovered before marriage—The detestable crime of abortion is appallingly rife in our day. It is abroad in our

land to an extent which would have shocked the dissolute women of pagan Rome—This wholesale, fashionable murder, how are we to stop it? Hundreds of vile men and women in our large cities subsist by this slaughter of the innocent."

12. **Rev. H. R. Haweis.**—"Until it is thought a disgrace in every rank of society, from top to bottom of social scale, to bring into the world more children than you are able to provide for, the poor man's home, at least, must often be a purgatory—his children dinnerless, his wife a beggar—himself too often drunk—here, then, are the real remedies: first, control the family growth according to the family means of support."

13. **Montague Cookson.**—"The limitation of the number of the family—is as much the duty of married persons as the observance of chastity is the duty of those that are unmarried."

14. **John Stuart Mill.**—"Every one has aright to live. We will suppose this granted. But no one has a right to bring children into life to be supported by other people. Whoever means to stand upon the first of these rights must renounce all pretension to the last. Little improvement can be expected in morality until the production of a large family is regarded in the same light as drunkenness or any other physical excess."

15. **Dr. T. D. Nicholls.**—"In the present social state, men and women should refrain from having children unless they see a reasonable prospect of giving them suitable nurture and education."

16. **Rev. M. J. Savage.**—"Some means ought to be provided for checking the birth of sickly children."

17. **Dr. Stockham.**—"Thoughtful minds must acknowledge the great wrong done when children are begotten under adverse conditions. Women must learn the laws of life so as to protect themselves, and not be the means of bringing sin-cursed, diseased children into the world. The remedy is in the prevention of pregnancy, not in producing abortion."

[232]
Small Families and the Improvement of the Race.

1. **Married People Must Decide for Themselves.**—It is the fashion of those who marry nowadays to have few children, often none. Of course this is a matter which married people must decide for themselves. As is stated in an earlier chapter, sometimes this policy is the wisest that can be pursued.

2. **Diseased People.**—Diseased people who are likely to beget only a sickly offspring, may follow this course, and so may thieves, rascals, vagabonds, insane and drunken persons, and all those who are likely to bring into the world beings that ought not to be here. But why so many well-to-do folks should pursue a policy adapted only to paupers and criminals, is not easy to explain. Why marry at all if not to found a family that shall live to bless and make glad the earth after father and mother are gone? It is not wise to rear too many children, nor is it wise to have too few. Properly brought up, they will make home a delight and parents happy.

3. **Population Limited.**—Galton, in his great work on hereditary genius, observes that "the time may hereafter arrive in far distant years, when the population of this earth shall be kept as strictly within bounds of number and suitability of race, as the sheep of a well-ordered moor, or the plants in an orchard-house; in the meantime, let us do what we can to encourage the multiplication of the races best [233]fitted to invent and conform to a high and generous civilization."

4. **Shall Sickly People Raise Children?**—The question whether sickly people should marry and propagate their kind, is briefly alluded to in an early chapter of this work. Where father and mother are both consumptive the chances are that the children will inherit physical weakness, which will result in the same disease, unless great pains are taken to give them a good physical education, and even then the probabilities are that they will find life a burden hardly worth living.

5. **No Real Blessing.**—Where one parent is consumptive and the other vigorous, the chances are just half as great. If there is a scrofulous or consumptive taint in the blood,

beware! Sickly children are no comfort to their parents, no real blessing. If such people marry, they had better, in most cases, avoid parentage.

6. **Welfare of Mankind.**—The advancement of the welfare of mankind is a most intricate problem: all ought to refrain from marriage who cannot avoid abject poverty for their children; for poverty is not only a great evil, but tends to its own increase by leading to recklessness in marriage. On the other hand, as Mr. Galton has remarked, if the prudent avoid marriage, while the reckless marry, the inferior members will tend to supplant the better members of society.

7. **Preventives.**—Remember that the thousands of preventives which are advertised in papers, private circulars, etc., are not only inefficient, unreliable and worthless, but positively dangerous, and the annual mortality of females in this country from this cause alone is truly horrifying. Study nature, and nature's laws alone will guide you safely in the path of health and happiness.

8. **Nature's Remedy.**—Nature in her wise economy has prepared for overproduction, for during the period of pregnancy and nursing, and also most of the last half of each menstrual month, woman is naturally sterile; but this condition may become irregular and uncertain on account of stimulating drinks or immoral excesses.

[234]

The Generative Organs.

THE MALE GENERATIVE ORGANS AND THEIR STRUCTURE AND ADAPTATION.

1. The reproductive organs in man are the penis and testicles and their appendages.

2. The penis deposits the seminal life germ of the male. It is designed to fulfill the seed planting mission of human life.

3. In the accompanying illustration all the parts are named.

4. **Urethra.**—The urethra performs the important mission of emptying the bladder, and is rendered very much larger by the passion, and the semen is propelled along through it by little layers of muscles on each side meeting [235]above and below. It is this canal that is inflamed by the disease known as gonorrhœa.

5. **Prostrate Gland.**—The prostrate gland is located just before the bladder. It swells in men who have previously overtaxed it, thus preventing all sexual intercourse, and becomes very troublesome to void urine. This is a very common trouble in old age.

6. **The Penal Gland.**—The penal gland, located at the end of the penis, becomes unduly enlarged by excessive action and has the consistency of India rubber. It is always enlarged by erection. It is this gland at the end that draws the semen forward. It is one of the most essential and wonderful constructed glands of the human body.

7. **Female Magnetism.**—When the male organ comes in contact with female magnetism, the natural and proper excitement takes place. When excited without this female magnetism it becomes one of the most serious injuries to the human body. The male organ was made for a high and holy purpose, and woe be to him who pollutes his manhood by practicing the secret vice. He pays the penalty in after years either by the entire loss of sexual power, or by the afflictions of various urinary diseases.

8. **Nature Pays** all her debts, and when there is an abuse of organ, penalties must follow. If the hand is thrust into the fire it will be burnt.

THE FEMALE SEXUAL ORGANS.

ANATOMY OR STRUCTURE OF THE FEMALE ORGANS OF GENERATION.

1. The generative or reproductive organs of the human female are usually divided into the internal and external. Those regarded as internal are concealed from view and protected within the body. Those that can be readily perceived are termed external. The entrance of the vagina may be stated as the line of demarcation of the two divisions.[236]

Impregnated Egg. In the first formation of Embryo.

89

2. **Hymen or Vaginal Valve.**—This is a thin membrane of half moon shape stretched across the opening of the vagina. It usually contains before marriage one or more small openings for the passage of the menses. This membrane has been known to cause much distress in many females at the first menstrual flow. The trouble resulting from the openings in the hymen not being large enough to let the flow through and consequently blocking up the vaginal canal, and filling the entire [237]internal sexual organs with blood; causing paroxysms and hysterics and other alarming symptoms. In such cases the hymen must be ruptured that a proper discharge may take place at once.

3. **Unyielding Hymen.**—The hymen is usually ruptured by the first sexual intercourse, but sometimes it is so unyielding as to require the aid of a knife before coition can take place.

4. **The presence of the Hymen** was formerly considered a test of virginity, but this theory is no longer held by competent authorities, as disease or accidents or other circumstances may cause its rupture.

5. **The Ovaries.**—The ovaries are little glands for the purpose of forming the female ova or egg. They are not fully developed until the period of puberty, and usually are about the size of a large chestnut. The are located in the broad ligaments between the uterus and the Fallopian tubes. During pregnancy the ovaries change position; they are brought farther into the abdominal cavity as the uterus expands.

6. **Office of the Ovary.**—The ovary is to the female what the testicle is to the male. It is the germ vitalizing organ and the most essential part of the generative apparatus. The ovary is not only an organ for the formation of the ova, but is also designed for their separation when they reach maturity.

7. **Fallopian Tubes.**—These are the ducts that lead from the ovaries to the uterus. They are entirely detached from the glands or ovaries, and are developed on both sides of the body.

8. **Office of the Fallopian Tubes.**—The Fallopian tubes have a double office: receiving the ova from the ovaries and conducting it into the uterus, as well as receiving the spermatic fluid of the male and conveying it from the uterus in the direction of the ovaries, the tubes being the seat of impregnation.

OVUM.

9. **Sterility In Females.**—Sterility in the female is sometimes caused by a morbid adhesion of the tube to a portion of the ovary. By what power the mouth of the tube is directed toward a particular portion of an ovary from which the ovum is about to be discharged, remains entirely unknown, as does also the precise nature of the cause which effects this movement.

[238]
THE MYSTERIES OF THE FORMATION OF LIFE.
Ripe Ovum from the Ovary.

1. **Scientific Theories.**—Darwin, Huxley, Haeckel, Tyndall, Meyer, and other renowned scientists, have tried to find the *missing link* between man and animal; they have also exhausted their genius in trying to fathom the mysteries of the beginning of life, or find where the animal and mineral kingdoms unite to form life; but they have added to the vast accumulation of theories only, and the world is but little wiser on this mysterious subject.

2. **Physiology.**—Physiology has demonstrated what physiological changes take place in the germination and formation of life, and how nature expresses the intentions of reproduction by giving animals distinctive organs with certain secretions for this purpose, etc. All the different stages of development can be easily determined, but how and why life takes place under such special condition and under no other, is an unsolved mystery.

3. **Ovaries.**—The ovaries are the essential parts of the generative system of the human female in which ova are matured. There are two ovaries, one on each side of the uterus, and connected with it by the Fallopian tubes. They are egg-shaped, about an inch in diameter, and furnish the [239]germs or ovules. These germs or ovules are very small, measuring about 1/120 of an inch in diameter.

90

4. **Development.**—The ovaries develop with the growth of the female, so that finally at the period of puberty they ripen and liberate an ovum or germ vesicle, which is carried into the uterine cavity of the Fallopian tubes. By the aid of the microscope we find that these ova are composed of granular substance, in which is found a miniature yolk surrounded by a transparent membrane called the zona pellucida. This yolk contains a germinal vesicle in which can be discovered a nucleus, called the germinal spot. The process of the growth of the ovaries is very gradual, and their function of ripening and discharging one ovum monthly into the Fallopian tubes and uterus, is not completed until between the twelfth and fifteenth years.

5. **What Science Knows.**—After the sexual embrace we know that the sperm is lifted within the genital passages or portion of the vagina and mouth of the uterus. The time between the deposit of the semen and fecundation varies according to circumstances. If the sperm-cell travels to the ovarium it generally takes from three to five days to make the journey. As Dr. Pierce says: "The transportation is aided by the ciliary processes (little hairs) of the mucous surface of the vaginal and uterine walls, as well as by its own vibratile movements. The action of the cilia, under the stimulus of the sperm, seems to be from without, inward. Even if a minute particle of sperm, less than a drop, be left upon the margin of the external genitals of the female, it is sufficient in amount to impregnate, and can be carried, by help of these cilia, to the ovaries."

6. **Conception.**—After intercourse at the proper time the liability to conception is very great. If the organs are in a healthy condition, conception must necessarily follow, and no amount of prudence and the most rigid precautions often fail to prevent pregnancy.

7. **Only One Absolutely Safe Method.**—There is only one absolutely safe method to prevent conception, entirely free from danger and injury to health, and one that is in the reach of all; that is to refrain from union altogether.

[240]

PREVENTION OF CONCEPTION.
THE PATIENT MOTHER.

1. The question is always asked, "Can Conception be prevented at all times?" Certainly, this is possible; but such an interference with nature's laws is inadmissible, and perhaps never to be justified in any case whatever, except in cases of deformity or disease.

2. If the parties of a marriage are both feeble and so adapted to each other that their children are deformed, insane or idiots, then to beget offspring would be a flagrant wrong; if the mother's health is in such a condition as to forbid the right of laying the burden of motherhood upon her, then medical aid may safely come to her relief. If the man, however, respects his wife, he ought to come to her relief without the counsel of a physician.[241]

3. **Forbearance.**—Often before the mother has recovered from the effects of bearing, nursing and rearing one child, ere she has regained proper tone and vigor of body and mind, she is unexpectedly overtaken, surprised by the manifestation of symptoms which again indicate pregnancy. Children thus begotten cannot become hardy and long-lived. By the love that parents may feel for their posterity, by the wishes for their success, by the hopes for their usefulness, by every consideration for their future well-being, let them exercise precaution and forbearance until the wife becomes sufficiently healthy and enduring to bequeath her own rugged, vital stamina to the child she bears in love.

4. **Impostors.**—During the past few years hundreds of books and pamphlets have been written on the subject, claiming that new remedies had been discovered for the prevention of conception, etc., but these are all money making devices to deceive the public, and enrich the pockets of miserable and unprincipled impostors.

5. **The Follies of Prevention.**—Dr. Pancoast, an eminent authority, says: "The truth is, there is no medicine taken internally capable of preventing conception, and the person who asserts to the contrary, not only speaks falsely, but is both a knave and a fool. It is true enough that remedies may be taken to produce abortion after conception occurs; but those who prescribe and those who resort to such desperate expedients, can only be placed in the category of lunatics and assassins!"

91

6. **Patent Medicines.**—If nature does not promptly respond, there are many patent medicines which when taken at the time the monthly flow is to begin, will produce the desired result. Let women beware; for it is only a question of a few years when their constitution, complexion, and health will be a sorry evidence of their folly. The woman who continually takes a drug to prevent conception, cannot retain her natural complexion; her eyes will become dull, her cheeks flabby, and she will show various evidences of poor health, and her sexual organs will soon become permanently impaired and hopelessly diseased.

7. **Foolish Dread of Children.**—What is more deplorable and pitiable than an old couple childless. Young people dislike the care and confinement of children and prefer society and social entertainments and thereby do great injustice and injury to their health and fit themselves in later years to visit infirmities and diseases upon their children. The vigilant and rigid measures which have to be resorted to in order to prevent conception for a period of years unfits many a wife for the production of healthy children.[242]

8. **Having Children** under proper circumstances never ruins the health and happiness of any woman. In fact, womanhood is incomplete without them. She may have a dozen or more, and still have better health than before marriage. It is having them too close together, and when she is not in a fit state, that her health gives way. Sometimes the mother is diseased; the outlet from the womb, as a result of laceration by a previous child-birth, is frequently enlarged, thus allowing conception to take place very readily, and hence she has children in rapid succession.

Besides the wrong to the mother in having children in such rapid succession, it is a great injustice to the babe in the womb and the one at the breast that they should follow each other so quickly that one is conceived while the other is nursing. One takes the vitality of the other; neither has sufficient nourishment, and both are started in life stunted and incomplete.

9. **"The Desirability and Practicability** of limiting offspring," says Dr. Stockham, "are the subject of frequent inquiry. Fewer and better children are desired by right-minded parents. Many men and women, wise in other things of the world, permit generation as a chance result of copulation, without thought of physical or mental conditions to be transmitted to the child. Coition, the one important act of all others, carrying with it the most vital results, is usually committed for selfish gratification. Many a drunkard owes his life-long appetite for alcohol to the fact that the inception of his life could be traced to a night of dissipation on the part of his father. Physical degeneracy and mental derangements are too often caused by the parents producing offspring while laboring under great mental strain or bodily fatigue. Drunkenness and licentiousness are frequently the heritage of posterity. Future generations demand that such results be averted by better pre-natal influences. The world is groaning under the curse of chance parenthood. It is due to posterity that procreation be brought under the control of reason and conscience.

10. **"It Has Been Feared that a Knowledge** of means to prevent conception would, if generally diffused, be abused by women; that they would to so great an extent escape motherhood as to bring about social disaster. This fear is not well founded. The maternal instinct is inherent and sovereign in woman. Even the pre-natal influences of a murderous intent on the part of parents scarcely ever [243]eradicate it. With this natural desire for children, we believe few women would abuse the knowledge or privilege of controlling conception. Although women shrink from forced maternity, and from the bearing of children under the great burden of suffering, as well as other adverse conditions, it is rare to find a woman who is not greatly disappointed if she does not, some time in her life, wear the crown of motherhood.

"An eminent lady teacher, in talking to her pupils, once said: 'The greatest calamity that can befall a woman is never to have a child. The next greatest calamity is to have one only.' From my professional experience I am happy to testify that more women seek to overcome causes of sterility than to obtain knowledge of limiting the size of the family or means to destroy the embryo. Also, if consultation for the latter is sought, it is usually at the instigation of the husband. Believing in the rights of unborn children, and in the maternal instinct, I am consequently convinced that no knowledge should be withheld that will secure proper conditions for the best parenthood.

11. **"Many of the Means Used to Prevent** conception are injurious, and often lay the foundation for a train of physical ailments. Probably no one means is more serious in its results than the practice of withdrawal, or the discharge of the semen externally to the vagina. The act is incomplete and unnatural, and is followed by results similar to and as disastrous as those consequent upon *masturbation*. In the male it may result in impotence, in the female in sterility. In both sexes many nervous symptoms are produced, such as headache, defective vision, dyspepsia, insomnia, loss of memory, etc. Very many cases of uterine diseases can be attributed solely to this practice. The objection to the use of the syringe is that if the sperm has passed into the uterus the fluid cannot reach it. A cold fluid may, in some instances, produce contractions to throw it off, but cannot be relied upon."

12. **Is It Ever Right to Prevent Conception?** We submit the following case of the *Juke* family, mostly of New York State, as related by R. L. Dugdale, when a member of the Prison Association, and let the reader judge for himself:

"It was traced out by painstaking research that from one woman called Margaret, who, like Topsy, merely 'growed' without pedigree as a pauper in a village on the upper Hudson, about eighty-five years ago, there descended 673 [244]children, grandchildren, and great-grandchildren, of whom 200 were criminals of the dangerous class, 280 adult paupers, and fifty prostitutes, while 300 children of her lineage died prematurely. The last fact proves to what extent in this family nature was kind to the rest of humanity in saving it from a still larger aggregation of undesirable and costly members, for it is estimated that the expense to the State of the descendants of Maggie was over a million dollars, and the State itself did something also towards preventing a greater expense by the restrain exercised upon the criminals, paupers, and idiots of the family during a considerable portion of their lives."

13. **The Legal Aspect.**—By the Revised Statutes of the United States it is provided "that no obscene, * * * or lascivious book, picture, or any article or thing designed or intended for the prevention of conception or producing of abortion shall be carried in the mail, and any person who shall knowingly deposit or cause to be deposited for mailing or delivery any of the hereinbefore mentioned things shall be guilty of misdemeanor," etc. In New Jersey, Oregon, South Carolina, Texas and District of Columbia we find no local law against abortion. Nine states, viz.: New Hampshire, Connecticut, New York, Indiana, Wisconsin, Dakotas, Wyoming and California punish the woman upon whom the abortion is attempted; while Massachusetts, New York, Ohio, Indiana, Michigan, Nebraska, Kansas and California punish the advertising or furnishing of means for the prevention of conception; and Ohio makes it a crime to even have such means in one's possession. There is exception made in favor of every case where the early birth of the infant is necessary to save the life of the mother. It will be noticed that the common law punishes the furnishing or advertising of means for the prevention of conception, and hence regards it as a crime. There is, however, no ban of the civil law on Nature's law as laid down by Nature's God and discovered by medical science, which we here make known.

14. **Is Nature's Method Reliable?**—Dr. Cowan says: "Sexual excitement hastens the premature ripening and meeting of the germ cell with the sperm cell, and impregnation may result, although intercourse occurs only in the specified two weeks' absence of the egg from the uterus."

This is just possible under certain peculiar circumstances of diseased conditions, or after long separation of husband and wife. However, it seldom happens, and married people in normal health, temperate in the sexual relation, desirous of controlling the size of their family, can usually depend upon this law.

[245]

15. **Moderation.**—Continence, self-control, a willingness to deny himself—that is what is required from the husband. But a thousand voices reach us from suffering women in all parts of the land that this will not suffice; that men refuse thus to restrain themselves; that it leads to a loss of domestic happiness and to illegal amour, or it is injurious physically and morally; that, in short, such advice is useless because impracticable.

16. **Nature's Method.**—To such we reply that Nature herself has provided, to some extent, against over-production, and that it is well to avail ourselves of her provision. It is well known that women, when nursing, rarely become pregnant, and for this reason, if for

no other, women should nurse their own children, and continue the period until the child is at least nine months or a year old. However, the nursing, if continued too long, weakens both the mother and the child, and, moreover, ceases to accomplish the end for which we now recommend it.

17. **Another Provision of Nature.**—For a certain period between her monthly illness, every woman is sterile. Conception may be avoided by refraining from coition except for this particular number of days, and there will be no evasion of natural intercourse, no resort to disgusting practices, and nothing degrading. The following facts have been established, without a doubt: The Graafian Vesicle, containing the egg in the ovary, enlarges during menstruation and bursts open to let the egg escape usually on the first day after the flow ceases, and seldom, if ever, later than the fourth day. It then takes from two to six days for the egg to pass down through the Fallopian tube into the womb, where it remains from two to six days, when, if not impregnated, it passes down through the vagina from the body. After the egg has passed from the body, conception is not possible until after the next menstrual flow.

The period, therefore, from after the sixteenth to within three days of the following menstrual discharge is one of almost absolute safety. We say within three days of the next menstruation, because the male seminal fluid may be retained there till the egg leaves the ovary, and in that way impregnation might follow. Impregnation would, however, rarely occur if the period was extended to from the twelfth day after menstruation close up to one day before it began again.

The above is the only physiological method (and it is no secret to a great many people) by which conception can be limited, without the employment of such means as involve danger and serious evils.

18. **Warning.**—Let women be warned in the most emphatic manner against the employment of the secret methods constantly advertised by quacks. Such means are the almost certain cause of painful uterine diseases and of shortened life. They are productive of more misery by far than over-production itself.

[246]

[1]New Revelation for Women.

VAGINAL CLEANLINESS.

1. The above Syringe has a patent tube known as the vaginal cleanser. This keeps the sides of the vagina apart and permits the water to thoroughly clean and cleanse the organ. It will be found a great relief in both health and sickness, and in many cases cure barrenness and other diseases of the womb. It can be used the same as any other syringe. The tube can be procured at almost any drug store and applied to either bulb or fountain syringe. Many women are barren on account of an acid secretion in the vagina. The cleanser is almost a certain remedy and cure.

2. **Cleanliness.**—Cleanliness is next to godliness. Without cleanliness the human body is more or less defiled and repulsive. A hint to the wise is sufficient. The vagina should be cleansed with the same faithfulness as any other portion of the body.

3. **Temperature of the Water.**—Those not accustomed to use vaginal injections would do well to use water milk-warm at the commencement; after this the temperature may be varied according to circumstances. In case of local inflammation use hot water. The indiscriminate use of cold water injections will be found rather injurious than beneficial, and a woman in feeble health will always find warm water invigorating and preferable.

[247]

4. **Leucorrhœa.**—In case of persistent leucorrhœa use the temperature of water from seventy-two to eighty-five degrees Fahrenheit.

5. **The Cleanser** will greatly stimulate the health and spirits of any woman who uses it. Pure water injections have a stimulating effect, and it seems to invigorate the entire body.

6. **Salt and Water Injections.**—This will cure mild cases of leucorrhœa. Add a teaspoonful of salt to a pint and a half of water at the proper temperature. Injections may be repeated daily if deemed necessary.

7. **Soap and Water.**—Soap and water is a very simple domestic remedy, and will many times afford relief in many diseases of the womb. It seems it thoroughly cleanses the parts. A little borax or vinegar may be used the same as salt water injections. (See No. 6.)

8. **Sterile Women** desiring offspring should seek sexual union soon after the appearance of the menses, and not use the vaginal cleanser till several days later. Those not desiring offspring should avoid copulation until the ovum has passed the generative tract.

9. **Holes in the Tubes.**—Most of the holes in the tubes of syringes are too small. See that they are sufficiently large to produce thorough cleansing.

10. **Injections During the Monthly Flow.**—Of course it is not proper to arrest the flow, and the injections will stimulate a healthy action of the organs. The injections may be used daily throughout the monthly flow with much comfort and benefit. If the flow is scanty and painful the injections may be as warm as they can be comfortably borne. If the flowing is immoderate, then cool water may be used. A woman will soon learn her own condition and can act accordingly.

11. **Bloom and Grace of Youth.**—The regular bathing of the body will greatly improve woman's beauty. Remember that a perfect complexion depends upon the healthy action of all the organs. Vaginal injections are just as important as the bath. A beautiful woman must not only be cleanly, but robust and healthy. There can be no perfect beauty without good health.

[248]

IMPOTENCE AND STERILITY.
Trying On a New Dress.

1. Actual impotence during the period of manhood is a very rare complaint, and nature very unwillingly, and only after the absolute neglect of sanitary laws, gives up the power of reproduction.

2. Not only sensual women, but all without exception, feel deeply hurt, and are repelled by the husband whom they may previously have loved dearly, when, after entering the married state, they find that he is impotent. The more inexperienced and innocent they were at the time of marriage, the longer it often is before they find that something is lacking in the husband; but, once knowing this, the wife infallibly has a feeling of contempt and aversion for him; though there are many happy families where this defect exists. It is often very uncertain who is the weak one, and no cause for separation should be sought.

3. Unhappy marriages, barrenness, divorces, and perchance an occasional suicide, may be prevented by the experienced physician, who can generally give correct information, comfort, and consolation, when consulted on these delicate matters.

4. When a single man fears that he is unable to fulfill the duties of marriage, he should not marry until his fear is dispelled. The suspicion of such a fear strongly tends to bring about the very weakness which he dreads. Go to a good physician (not to one of those quacks whose [249]advertisements you see in the papers; they are invariably unreliable), and state the case fully and freely.

5. Diseases, malformation, etc., may cause impotence. In case of malformation there is usually no remedy, but in case of disease it is usually within the reach of a skillful physician.

6. Self-abuse and spermatorrhœa produce usually only temporary impotence and can generally be relieved by carrying out the instructions given elsewhere in this book.

7. Excessive indulgences often enfeeble the powers and often result in impotence. Dissipated single men, professional libertines, and married men who are immoderate, often pay the penalty of their violations of the laws of nature, by losing their vital power. In such cases of excess there may be some temporary relief, but as age advances the effects of such indiscretion will become more and more manifest.

8. The condition of sterility in man may arise either from a condition of the secretion which deprives it of its fecundating powers or it may spring from a malformation which prevents it reaching the point where fecundation takes place. The former condition is most common in old age, and is a sequence of venereal disease, or from a change in the structure

or functions of the glands. The latter has its origin in a stricture, or in an injury, or in that condition technically known as hypospadias, or in debility.

9. It can be safely said that neither self-indulgence nor spermatorrhœa often leads to permanent sterility.

10. It is sometimes, however, possible, even where there is sterility in the male, providing the secretion is not entirely devoid of life properties on part of the husband, to have children, but these are exceptions.

11. No man need hesitate about matrimony on account of sterility, unless that condition arises from a permanent and absolute degeneration of his functions.

12. Impotence from mental and moral causes often takes place. Persons of highly nervous organization may suffer incapacity in their sexual organs. The remedy for these difficulties is rest and change of occupation.

13. **Remedies in case of Impotence on account of former Private Diseases, or Masturbation, or other causes.**—First build up the body by taking some good stimulating tonics. The general health is the most essential feature to be considered, in order to secure restoration of the sexual powers. Constipation must be carefully avoided. If the [250]kidneys do not work in good order, some remedy for their restoration must be taken. Take plenty of out-door exercise, avoid horseback riding or heavy exhaustive work.

14. **Food and Drinks which Weaken Desire.**—All kinds of food which cause dyspepsia or bring on constipation, diarrhœa, or irritate the bowels, alcoholic beverages, or any indigestible compound, has the tendency to weaken the sexual power. Drunkards and tipplers suffer early loss of vitality. Beer drinking has a tendency to irritate the stomach and to that extent affects the private organs.

15. **Coffee.**—Coffee drank excessively causes a debilitating effect upon the sexual organs. The moderate use of coffee can be recommended, yet an excessive habit of drinking very strong coffee will sometimes wholly destroy vitality.

16. **Tobacco.**—It is a hygienic and physiological fact that tobacco produces sexual debility and those who suffer any weakness from that source should carefully avoid the weed in all its forms.

17. **Drugs which Stimulate Desire.**—There are certain medicines which act locally on the membranes and organs of the male, and the papers are full of advertisements of "Lost Manhood Restored", etc., but in every case they are worthless or dangerous drugs and certain to lead to some painful malady or death. All these patent medicines should be carefully avoided. People who are troubled with any of these ailments should not attempt to doctor themselves by taking drugs, but a competent physician should be consulted. Eating rye, corn, or graham bread, oatmeal, cracked wheat, plenty of fruit, etc. is a splendid medicine. If that is not sufficient, then a physician should be consulted.

18. **Drugs which Moderate Desire.**—Among one of the most common domestic remedies is camphor. This has stood the test for ages. Small doses of half a grain in most instances diminishes the sensibility of the organs of sex. In some cases it produces irritation of the bladder. In that case it should be at once discontinued. On the whole a physician had better be consulted. The safest drug among domestic remedies is a strong tea made out of hops. Saltpeter, or nitrate of potash, taken in moderate quantities, are very good remedies.

[251]

19. **Strictly   Speaking** there   is   a   distinction   made between *impotence* and *sterility.Impotence* is a loss of power to engage in the sexual act and is common to men. It may be imperfection in the male organ or a lack of sufficient sexual vigor to produce and maintain erection. *Sterility* is a total loss of capacity in the reproduction of the species, and is common to women.

There are, however, very few causes of barrenness that cannot be removed when the patient is perfectly developed. Sterility, in a female, most frequently depends upon a weakness or irritability either in the ovaries or the womb, and anything having a strengthening effect upon either organ will remove the disability. (See page 249.)

20. **"Over-Indulgence** in intercourse," says Dr. Hoff, "is sometimes the cause of barrenness; this is usually puzzling to the interested parties, inasmuch as the practices which,

96

in their opinion, should be the source of a numerous progeny, have the very opposite effect. By greatly moderating their ardor, this defect may be remedied."

21. **"Napoleon and Josephine.**—A certain adaptation between the male and female has been regarded as necessary to conception, consisting of some mysterious influence which one sex exerts over the other, neither one, however, being essentially impotent or sterile. The man may impregnate one woman and not another, and the woman will conceive by one man and not by another. In the marriage of Napoleon Bonaparte and Josephine no children were born, but after he had separated from the Empress and wedded Maria Louisa of Austria, an heir soon came. Yet Josephine had children by Beauharnais, her previous husband. But as all is not known as to the physical condition of Josephine during her second marriage, it cannot be assumed that mere lack of adaptability was the cause of unfruitfulness between them. There may have been some cause that history has not recorded, or unknown to the state of medical science of those days. There are doubtless many cases of apparently causeless unfruitfulness in marriage that even physicians, with a knowledge of all apparent conditions in the parties, cannot explain; but when, as elsewhere related in this volume, impregnation by artificial means is successfully practised, it is useless to attribute barrenness to purely psychological and adaptative influences."

[252]
Producing Boys or Girls at Will.

1. **Can the Sexes be Produced at Will?**—This question has been asked in all ages of the world. Many theories have been advanced, but science has at last replied with some authority. The following are the best known authorities which this age of science has produced.

2. **The Agricultural Theory.**—The agricultural theory, as it may be called, because adopted by farmers, is that impregnation occurring within four days of the close of the female monthlies produces a girl, because the ovum is yet immature; but that when it occurs after the fourth day from its close, gives a boy, because this egg is now mature; whereas after about the eighth day this egg dissolves and passes off, so that impregnation is thereby rendered impossible, till just before the mother's next monthly.—*Sexual Science.*

3. **Queen Bees Lay Female Eggs First**, and male afterwards. So with hens; the first eggs laid after the tread give females, the last males. Mares shown the stallion late in their periods drop horse colts rather than fillies.—*Napheys.*

4. **If You Wish Females**, give the male at the first sign of heat; if males, at its end.—*Prof. Thury.*

5. **On Twenty-two Successive Occasions** I desired to have heifers, and succeeded in every case. I have made in all twenty-nine experiments, after this method, and succeeded in every one, in producing the sex I desired.—*A Swiss Breeder.*

6. **This Thury Plan** has been tried on the farms of the Emperor of the French with unvarying success.

7. **Conception in the First Half** of the time between the menstrual periods produces females, and males is the latter.—*London Lancet.*

8. **Intercourse** in from two to six days after cessation of the menses produces girls, in from nine to twelve, boys.—*Medical Reporter.*

9. **The Most Male Power** and passion creates boys; female girls. This law probably causes those agricultural facts just cited thus: Conception right after menstruation give girls, because the female is then the most impassioned; later, boys, because her wanting sexual warmth leaves him the most vigorous. Mere sexual excitement, a wild, fierce, furious rush of passion, is not only not sexual vigor, but in its inverse ratio; and a genuine insane fervor caused by weakness; just as a like nervous excitability indicates weak nerves instead of strong. Sexual power is deliberate, not wild; cool, not impetuous; while all false excitement diminishes effectiveness.—*Fowler.*

[253]
ABORTION OR MISCARRIAGE.
HEALTHY CHILDREN.

1. **Abortion or Miscarriage** is the expulsion of the child from the womb previous to six months; after that it is called premature birth.

2. **Causes.**—It may be due to a criminal act of taking medicine for the express purpose of producing miscarriage or it may be caused by certain medicines, severe sickness or nervousness, syphilis, imperfect semen, lack of room in the pelvis and abdomen, lifting, straining, violent cold, sudden mental excitement, excessive sexual intercourse, dancing, tight lacing, the use of strong purgative medicines, bodily fatigue, late suppers, and fashionable amusements.

3. **Symptoms.**—A falling or weakness and uneasiness in the region of the loins, thighs and womb, pain in the small [254]of the back, vomiting and sickness of the stomach, chilliness with a discharge of blood accompanied with pain in the lower portions of the abdomen. These may take place in a single hour, or it may continue for several days. If before the fourth month, there is not so much danger, but the flow of blood is generally greater. If miscarriage is the result of an accident, it generally takes place without much warning, and the service of a physician should at once be secured.

4. **Home Treatment.**—A simple application of cold water externally applied will produce relief, or cold cloths of ice, if convenient, applied to the lower portions of the abdomen. Perfect quiet, however, is the most essential thing for the patient. She should lie on her back and take internally a teaspoonful of paregoric every two hours; drink freely of lemonade or other cooling drinks, and for nourishment subsist chiefly on chicken broth, toast, water gruel, fresh fruits, etc. The principal homeopathic remedies for this disease are ergot and cimicifuga, given in drop-doses of the tinctures.

5. **Injurious Effects.**—Miscarriage is a very serious difficulty, and the health and the constitution may be permanently impaired. Any one prone to miscarriage should adopt every measure possible to strengthen and build up the system; avoid going up stairs or doing much heavy lifting or hard work.

6. **Prevention.**—Practice the laws of sexual abstinence, take frequent sitz-baths, live on oatmeal, graham bread, and other nourishing diet. Avoid highly seasoned food, rich gravies, late suppers and the like.

[255]

The Murder of the Innocents.

AN INDIAN FAMILY. The Savage Indian Teaches Us Lessons of Civilization.

1. **Many Causes.**—Many causes have operated to produce a corruption of the public morals so deplorable; prominent among which may be mentioned the facility with which divorces may be obtained in some of the States, the constant promulgation of false ideas of marriage and its duties by means of books, lectures, etc., and the distribution through the mails of impure publications. But an influence not less powerful than any of these is the growing devotion of fashion and luxury of this age, and the idea which practically obtains to so great an extent that pleasure, instead of the health or morals, is the great object of life.

2. **A Monstrous Crime.**—The abiding interest we feel in the preservation of the morals of our country, constrains us to raise our voice against the daily increasing practice of [256]infanticide, especially before birth. The notoriety this monstrous crime has obtained of late, and the hecatombs of infants that are annually sacrificed to Moloch, to gratify an unlawful passion, are a sufficient justification for our alluding to a painful and delicate subject, which should "not even be named," only to correct and admonish the wrong-doers.

3. **Localities in Which It Is Most Prevalent.**—We may observe that the crying sin of infanticide is most prevalent in those localities where the system of moral education has been longest neglected. This inhuman crime might be compared to the murder of the innocents, except that the criminals, in this case, exceed in enormity the cruelty of Herod.

4. **Shedding Innocent Blood.**—If it is a sin to take away the life even of an enemy; if the crime of shedding innocent blood cries to heaven for vengeance; in what language can we characterize the double guilt of those whose souls are stained with the innocent blood of their own unborn, unregenerated offspring?

5. **The Greatness of the Crime.**—The murder of an infant before its birth, is, in the sight of God and the law, as great a crime as the killing of a child after birth.

6. **Legal Responsibility.**—Every State of the Union has made this offense one of the most serious crimes. The law has no mercy for the offenders that violate the sacred law of human life. It is murder of the most cowardly character and woe to him who brings this curse upon his head, to haunt him all the days of his or her life, and to curse him at the day of his death.

7. **The Product of Lust.**—Lust pure and simple. The only difference between a marriage of this character and prostitution is, that society, rotten to its heart, pulpits afraid to cry aloud against crime and vice, and the church conformed to the world, have made such a profanation of marriage respectable. To put it in other words, when two people determine to live together as husband and wife, and evade the consequences and responsibilities of marriage, they are simply engaged in prostitution without the infamy which attaches to that vice and crime.

8. **Outrageous Violation of All Law.**—The violation of all law, both natural and revealed, is the cool and villainous contract by which people entering into the marital relation engage in defiance of the laws of God and the laws of the commonwealth, that they shall be unincumbered with a family of children. "Disguise the matter as you will," says Dr. Pomeroy, "yet the fact remains that the first and [257]specific object of marriage is the rearing of a family." "Be fruitful and multiply and replenish the earth," is God's first word to Adam after his creation.

9. **The National Sin.**—The prevention of offspring is preeminently the sin of America. It is fast becoming the national sin of America, and if it is not checked, it will sooner or later be an irremediable calamity. The sin has its roots in a low and perverted idea of marriage, and is fostered by false standards of modesty.

10. **The Sin of Herod.**—Do these same white-walled sepulchres of hell know that they are committing the damning sin of Herod in the slaughter of the innocents, and are accessories before the fact to the crime of murder? Do women in all circles of society, when practicing these terrible crimes realize the real danger? Do they understand that it is undermining their health, and their constitution, and that their destiny, if persisted in, is a premature grave just as sure as the sun rises in the heavens? Let all beware, and let the first and only purpose be, to live a life guiltless before God and man.

11. **The Crime of Abortion.**—From the moment of conception a new life commences; a new individual exists; another child is added to the family. The mother who deliberately sets about to destroy this life, either by want of care, or by taking drugs, or using instruments, commits as great a crime, and is just as guilty as if she strangled her new-born infant or as if she snatched from her own breast her six months' darling and dashed out its brains against the wall. Its blood is upon her head, and as sure as there is a God and a judgment, that blood will be required of her. The crime she commits is murder, child murder—the slaughter of a speechless, helpless being, whom it is her duty, beyond all things else, to cherish and preserve.

12. **Dangerous Diseases.**—We appeal to all such with earnest and with threatening words. If they have no feeling for the fruit of their womb, if maternal sentiment is so callous in their breasts, let them know that such produced abortions are the constant cause of violent and dangerous womb diseases, and frequently of early death; that they bring on mental weakness, and often insanity; that they are the most certain means to destroy domestic happiness which can be adopted. Better, far better, to bear a child every year for twenty years than to resort to such a wicked and injurious step; better to die, if need be, in the pangs of child-birth, than to live with such a weight of sin on the conscience.

[258]

The Unwelcome Child.[2]

1. **Too Often the Husband** thinks only of his personal gratification; he insists upon what he calls his rights (?); forces on his wife an *unwelcome child*, and thereby often alienates her affections, if he does not drive her to abortion.

Dr Stockham reports the following case: "A woman once consulted me who was the mother of five children, all born within ten years. These were puny, scrofulous, nervous and irritable. She herself was a fit subject for doctors and drugs. Every organ in her body seemed diseased, and every function perverted. She was dragging out a miserable existence. Like other physicians, I had prescribed in vain for her many maladies. One day she chanced to inquire how she could safely prevent conception. This led me to ask how great was the danger. She said: 'Unless my husband is absent from home, few nights have been exempt since we were married, except it may be three or four immediately after confinement.'

"'And yet your husband loves you?'

"'O, yes, he is kind and provides for his family. Perhaps I might love him but for this. While now—(will God forgive me?)—*I detest, I loathe him*, and if I knew how to support myself and children, I would leave him.'

"'Can you talk with him upon this subject?'

"'I think I can.'

"' Then there is hope, for many women cannot do that. Tell him I will give you treatment to improve your health, and if he will wait until you can respond, *take time for the act, have it entirely mutual from first to last*, the demand will not come so frequent.'

"'Do you think so?'

"'The experience of many proves the truth of this statement.'

"Hopefully she went home, and in six months I had the satisfaction of knowing my patient was restored to health, and a single coition in a month gave the husband more satisfaction than the many had done previously, that the creative power was under control, and that my lady could proudly say 'I love,' where previously she said 'I hate.'

"If husbands will listen, a few simple instructions will [259]appeal to their *common sense*, and none can imagine the gain to themselves, to their wives and children, and their children's children. Then it may not be said of the babes that the 'Death borders on their birth, and their cradle stands in the grave.'"

2. **Wives! Be Frank and True** to your husbands on the subject of maternity, and the relation that leads to it. Interchange thoughts and feelings with them as to what nature allows or demands in regard to these. Can maternity be natural when it is undesigned by the father or undesired by the mother? Can a maternity be natural, healthful, ennobling to the mother, to the child, to the father, and to the home, when no loving, tender, anxious forethought presides over the relation in which it originated?—when the mother's nature loathed and repelled it, and the father's only thought was his own selfish gratification; the feelings and conditions of the mother, and the health, character and destiny of the child that may result being ignored by him. Wives! let there be a perfect and loving understanding between you and your husbands on these matters, and great will be your reward.

3. **A Woman Writes:**—"There are few, very few, wives and mothers who could not reveal a sad, dark picture in their own experience in their relations to their husbands and their children. Maternity, and the relation in which it originates, are thrust upon them by their husbands, often without regard to their spiritual or physical conditions, and often in contempt of their earnest and urgent entreaties. No joy comes to their heart at the conception and birth of their children, except that which arises from the consciousness that they have survived the sufferings wantonly and selfishly inflicted upon them."

4. **Husband, When Maternity** is imposed on your wife without her consent, and contrary to her appeal, how will her mind necessarily be affected towards her child? It was conceived in dread and in bitterness of spirit. Every stage of its fœtal development is watched with feeling of settled repugnance. In every step of its ante-natal progress the child meets only with grief and indignation in the mother. She would crush out its life, if she could. She loathed its conception; she loathed it in every stage of its ante-natal development. Instead of fixing her mind on devising ways and means for the healthful and happy organization and [260]development of her child before it is born, and for its postnatal comfort and support, her soul may be intent on its destruction, and her thoughts devise plans to kill it. In this, how often is she aided by others! There are those, and they are called men and women, whose profession is to devise ways to kill children before they are born. Those who do this would not hesitate (but for the consequences) to kill them after they are born, for the state of mind that would justify and instigate *ante-natal* child-murder would justify and instigate *post-natal* child-murder. Yet, public sentiment consigns the murderer of

post-natal children to the dungeon or the gallows, while the murderers of ante-natal children are often allowed to pass in society as honest and honorable men and women.

5. **The Following is an Extract** from a letter written by one who has proudly and nobly filled the station of a wife and mother, and whose children and grandchildren surround her and crown her life with tenderest love and respect:

"It has often been a matter of wonder to me that men should, so heedlessly, and so injuriously to themselves, their wives and children, and their homes, demand at once, as soon as they get legal possession of their wives, the gratification of a passion, which, when indulged merely for the sake of the gratification of the moment, must end in the destruction of all that is beautiful, noble and divine in man or woman. I have often felt that I would give the world for a friendship with man that should show no impurity in its bearing, and for a conjugal relation that would, at all times, heartily and practically recognize the right of the wife to decide for herself when she should enter into the relation that leads to maternity."

6. **Timely Advice.**—Here let me say that on no subject should a man and woman, as they are being attracted into conjugal relations, be more open and truthful with each other than on this. No woman, who would save herself and the man she loves from a desecrated and wretched home, should enter into the physical relations of marriage with a man until she understands what he expects of her as to the function of maternity, and the relation that leads to it. If a woman is made aware that the man who would win her as a wife regards her and the marriage relation only as the means of a legalized gratification of his passions, and she sees fit to live with him as a wife, with such a prospect before her, she must take the consequences of a course so [261]degrading and so shameless. If she sees fit to make an offering of her body and soul on the altar of her husband's sensuality, she must do it; but she has a right to know to what base uses her womanhood is to be put, and it is due to her, as well as to himself, that he should tell beforehand precisely what he wants and expects of her.

Too frequently, man shrinks from all allusion, during courtship, to his expectations in regard to future passional relations. He fears to speak of them, lest he should shock and repel the woman he would win as a wife. Being conscious, it may be, of an intention to use power he may acquire over her person for his own gratification, he shuns all interchange of views with her, lest she should divine the hidden sensualism of his soul, and his intention to victimize her person to it the moment he shall get the license. A woman had better die at once than enter into or continue in marriage with a man whose highest conception of the relation is, that it is a means of licensed animal indulgence. In such a relation, body and soul are sacrificed.

7. **One Distinctive Characteristic** of a true and noble husband is a feeling of manly pride in the physical elements of his manhood. His physical manhood, as well as his soul, is dear to the heart of his wife, because through this he can give the fullest expression of his manly power. How can you, my friend, secure for your person the loving care and respect of your wife? There is but one way: so manifest yourself to her, in the hours of your most endearing intimacies, that all your manly power shall be associated only with all that is generous, just and noble in you, and with purity, freedom and happiness in her. Make her feel that all which constitutes you a man, and qualifies you to be her husband and the father of her children, belongs to her, and is sacredly consecrated to the perfection and happiness of her nature. Do this, and the happiness of your home is made complete. Your *body* will be lovingly and reverently cared for, because the wife of your bosom feels that it is the sacred symbol through which a noble, manly love is ever speaking to her, to cheer and sustain her.

8. **Woman is Ever Proud,** and justly so, of the manly passion of her husband, when she knows it is controlled by a love for her, whose manifestations have regard only to her elevation and happiness. The power which, when bent only on selfish indulgence, becomes a source of more shame, degradation, disease and wretchedness, to [262]women and to children than all other things put together, does but ennoble her, add grace and glory to her being, and concentrate and vitalize the love that encircles her as a wife when it is controlled by wisdom and consecrated to her highest growth and happiness, and that of her children. It lends enchantment to her person, and gives a fascination to her smiles, her words and her caresses, which ever breathe of purity and of heaven, and make her all lovely as a wife and mother to her husband and the father of her child. *Manly passion is to the conjugal love of the wife*

like the sun to the rose-bud, that opens its petals, and causes them to give out their sweetest fragrance and to display their most delicate tints; or like the frost, which chills and kills it ere it blossoms in its richness and beauty.

9. **A Diadem of Beauty.**—Maternity, when it exists at the call of the wife, and is gratefully received, but binds her heart more tenderly and devotedly to her husband. As the father of her child, he stands before her invested with new beauty and dignity. In receiving from him the germ of a new life, she receives that which she feels is to add new beauty and glory to her as a woman—a new grace and attraction to her as a wife. She loves and honors him, because he has crowned her with the glory of a mother. Maternity, to her, instead of being repulsive, is a diadem of beauty, a crown of rejoicing; and deep, tender, and self-forgetting are her love and reverence for him who has placed it on her brow. How noble, how august, how beautiful is maternity when thus bestowed and received!

10. **Conclusion.**—Would you, then, secure the love and trust of your wife, and become an object of her ever-growing tenderness and reverence? Assure her, by all your manifestations, and your perfect respect for the functions of her nature, that your passion shall be in subjection of her wishes. It is not enough that you have secured in her heart respect for your spiritual and intellectual manhood. To maintain your self-respect in your relations with her, to perfect your growth and happiness as a husband, you must cause your *physical* nature to be tenderly cherished and reverenced by her in all the sacred intimacies of home. No matter how much she reverences your intellectual or your social power, if by reason of your uncalled-for passional manifestations you have made your physical manhood disagreeable, how can you, in her presence, preserve a sense of manly pride and dignity as a husband?

[263]

Heredity and the Transmission of Diseases.
HEALTH AND DISEASE.

1. **Bad Habits.**—It is known that the girl who marries the man with bad habits, is, in a measure, responsible for the evil tendencies which these habits have created in the children; and young people are constantly warned of the danger in marrying when they know they come from families troubled with chronic diseases or insanity. To be sure the warnings have had little effect thus far in preventing such marriages, and it is doubtful whether they will, unless the prophecy of an extremist writing for one of our periodicals comes to pass—that the time is not far distant when such marriages will be a crime punishable by law.[264]

2. **Tendency in the Right Direction.**—That there is a tendency in the right direction must be admitted, and is perhaps most clearly shown in some of the articles on prison reform. Many of them strongly urge the necessity of preventive work as the truest economy, and some go so far as to say that if the present human knowledge of the laws of heredity were acted upon for a generation, reformatory measures would be rendered unnecessary.

3. **Serious Consequences.**—The mother who has ruined her health by late hours, highly-spiced food, and general carelessness in regard to hygienic laws, and the father who is the slave of questionable habits, will be very sure to have children either mentally or morally inferior to what they might otherwise have had a right to expect. But the prenatal influences may be such that evils arising from such may be modified to a great degree.

4. **Formation of Character.**—I believe that pre-natal influences may do as much in the formation of character as all the education that can come after, and that the mother may, in a measure, "will" what that influence shall be, and that, as knowledge on the subject increases, it will be more and more under their control. In that, as in everything else, things that would be possible with one mother would not be with another, and measures that would be successful with one would produce opposite results from the other.

5. **Inheriting Disease.** Consumption—that dread foe of modern life—is the most frequently encountered of all affections as the result of inherited predispositions. Indeed, some of the most eminent physicians have believed it is never produced in any other way. Heart disease, disease of the throat, excessive obesity, affections of the skin, asthma, disorders of the brain and nervous system, gout, rheumatism and cancer, are all hereditary. A

tendency to bleed frequently, profusely and uncontrollably, from trifling wounds, is often met with as a family affection.

6. **Mental Derangements.**—Almost all forms of mental derangements are hereditary—one of the parents or near relation being afflicted. Physical or bodily weakness is often hereditary, such as scrofula, gout, rheumatism, rickets, consumption, apoplexy, hernia, urinary calculi, hemorrhoids or piles, cataract, etc. In fact, all physical weakness, if ingrafted in either parent, is transmitted from parents to offspring, and is often more strongly marked in the latter than in the former.

7. **Marks and Deformities.**—Marks and deformities are all transmissible from parents to offspring, equally with [265]diseases and peculiar proclivities. Among such blemishes may be mentioned moles, hair-lips, deficient or supernumerary fingers, toes, and other characteristics. It is also asserted that dogs and cats that have accidentally lost their tails, bring forth young similarly deformed. Blumenbach tells of a man who had lost his little finger, having children with the same deformity.

8. **Caution.**—Taking facts like these into consideration, how very important is it for persons, before selecting partners for life, to deliberately weigh every element and circumstances of this nature, if they would insure a felicitous union, and not entail upon their posterity disease, misery and despair. Alas! in too many instances matrimony is made a matter of money, while all earthly joys are sacrificed upon the accursed altars of lust and mammon.

[266]
Preparation for Maternity.

1. **Woman Before Marriage.**—It is not too much to say that the life of women before marriage ought to be adjusted with more reference to their duties as mothers than to any other one earthly object. It is the continuance of the race which is the chief purpose of marriage. The passion of amativeness is probably, on the whole, the most powerful of all human impulses. Its purpose, however, is rather to subserve the object of continuing the species, than merely its own gratification.

2. **Exercise.**—Girls should be brought up to live much in the open air, always with abundant clothing against wet and cold. They should be encouraged to take much active exercise; as much, if they want to, as boys. It is as good for little girls to run and jump, to ramble in the woods, to go boating, to ride and drive, to play and "have fun" generally, as for little boys.

3. **Preserve the Sight.**—Children should be carefully prevented from using their eyes to read or write, or in any equivalent exertion, either before breakfast, by dim daylight, or by artificial light. Even school studies should be such that they can be dealt with by daylight. Lessons that cannot be learned without lamp-light study are almost certainly excessive. This precaution should ordinarily be maintained until the age of puberty is reached.

4. **Bathing.**—Bathing should be enforced according to constitutions, not by an invariable rule, except the invariable rule of keeping clean. Not necessarily every day, nor necessarily in cold water; though those conditions are doubtless often right in case of abundant physical health and strength.

5. **Wrong Habits.**—The habit of daily natural evacuations should be solicitously formed and maintained. Words or figures could never express the discomforts and wretchedness which wrong habits in this particular have locked down upon innumerable women for years and even for life.

6. **Dress.**—Dress should be warm, loose, comely, and modest rather than showy; but it should be good enough to satisfy a child's desires after a good appearance, if they are reasonable. Children, indeed, should have all their reasonable desires granted as far as possible; for nothing makes them reasonable so rapidly and so surely as to treat them reasonably.

[267]
7. **Tight Lacing.**—Great harm is often done to maidens for want of knowledge in them, or wisdom and care in their parents. The extremes of fashions are very prone to violate not only taste, but physiology. Such cases are tight lacing, low necked dresses, thin

shoes, heavy skirts. And yet, if the ladies only knew, the most attractive costumes are not the extremes of fashion, but those which conform to fashion enough to avoid oddity, which preserve decorum and healthfulness, whether or no; and here is the great secret of successful dress—vary fashion so as to suit the style of the individual.

8. **Courtship and Marriage.**—Last of all, parental care in the use of whatever influence can be exerted in the matter of courtship and marriage. Maidens, as well as youths, must, after all, choose for themselves. It is their own lives which they take in their hands as they enter the marriage state, and not their parents'; and as the consequences affect them primarily it is the plainest justice that with the responsibility should be joined the right of choice. The parental influence, then, must be indirect and advisory. Indirect, through the whole bringing up of their daughter; for if they have trained her aright, she will be incapable of enduring a fool, still more a knave.

9. **A Young Woman and a Young Man Had Better Not Be Alone Together Very Much until They Are Married.**—This will be found to prevent a good many troubles. It is not meant to imply that either sex, or any member of it, is worse than another, or bad at all, or anything but human. It is simply the prescription of a safe general rule. It is no more an imputation than the rule that people had better not be left without oversight in presence of large sums of other folks' money. The close personal proximity of the sexes is greatly undesirable before marriage. Kisses and caresses are most properly the monopoly of wives. Such indulgences have a direct and powerful physiological effect. Nay, they often lead to the most fatal results.

10. **Ignorance before Marriage.**—At some time before marriage those who are to enter into it ought to be made acquainted with some of the plainest common-sense limitations which should govern their new relations to each other. Ignorance in such matters has caused an infinite amount of disgust, pain, and unhappiness. It is not necessary to specify particulars here: see other portions of this work.

[269]

Impregnation.
A HEALTHY MOTHER.

1. **Conception or Impregnation.**—Conception or impregnation takes place by the union of the male sperm and female sperm. Whether this is accomplished in the ovaries, the oviducts or the uterus, is still a question of discussion and investigation by physiologists.

2. **Passing Off The Ovum.**—"With many woman," says Dr. Stockham in her Tokology, "the ovum passes off within twenty-four or forty-eight hours after menstruation begins. Some, by careful observation, are able to know with certainty when this takes place. It is often accompanied with malaise, nervousness, headache or actual uterine pain. A minute substance like the white of an egg; with a fleck of blood in it, can frequently be seen upon the clothing. Ladies who have noticed this phenomenon testify to its recurring very regularly upon the same day after menstruation. Some delicate women have observed it as late as the fourteenth day."

3. **Calculations.**—Conception is more liable to take place either immediately before or immediately after the period, and, on that account it is usual when calculating the date at which to expect labor, to count from the day of disappearance of the last period. The easiest way to make a calculation is to count back three months from the date of the last period and add seven days; thus we might say that the date was the 18th of July; counting back brings us to the 18th of April, and adding the seven days will bring us to the 25th day of April, the expected time.

4. **Evidence of Conception.**—Very many medical authorities, distinguished in this line, have stated their belief that women never pass more than two or three days at the most beyond the forty weeks conceded to pregnancy—that is two hundred and eighty days or ten lunar months, or nine calendar months and a week. About two hundred and eighty days will represent the average duration of pregnancy, counting from the last day of the last period. Now it must be borne in mind, that there are many disturbing elements which might cause the young married woman to miss a time. During the first month of pregnancy there is no sign by which the condition may be positively known. The missing of a period, especially in

a person who has been regular for some time, may lead one to suspect it; but there are many attendant causes in married life, the little annoyances of household duties, embarrassments, and the enforced gayety which naturally surrounds the bride, and [270]these should all be taken into consideration in the discussion as to whether or not she is pregnant. But then, again, there are some rare cases who have menstruated throughout their pregnancy; and also cases where menstruation was never established and pregnancy occurred. Nevertheless, the non-appearance of the period, with other signs, may be taken as presumptive evidence.

5. **"Artificial Impregnation.**—It may not be generally known that union is not essential to impregnation; it is possible for conception to occur without congress. All that is necessary is that seminal animalcules enter the womb and unite there with the egg or ovum. It is not essential that the semen be introduced through the medium of the male organ, as it has been demonstrated repeatedly that by means of a syringe and freshly obtained and healthy semen, impregnation can be made to follow by its careful introduction. There are physicians in France who make a specialty of "Artificial Impregnation," as it is called, and produce children to otherwise childless couples, being successful in many instances in supplying them as they are desired."

Signs and Symptoms of Pregnancy.

1. **The First Sign.**—The first sign that leads a lady to suspect that she is pregnant is her ceasing-to-be-unwell. This, provided she has just before been in good health, is a strong symptom of pregnancy; but still there must be others to corroborate it.

2. **Abnormal Condition.**—Occasionally, women menstruate during the entire time of gestation. This, without doubt, is an abnormal condition, and should be remedied, as disastrous consequences may result. Also, women have been known to bear children who have never menstruated. The cases are rare of pregnancy taking place where menstruation has never occurred, yet it frequently happens that women never menstruate from one pregnancy to another. In these cases this symptom is ruled out for diagnostic purposes.

3. **May Proceed from Other Causes.**—But a ceasing-to-be-unwell may proceed from other causes than that of pregnancy, such as disease or disorder of the womb or of other[271]organs of the body—especially of the lungs—it is not by itself alone entirely to be depended upon; although, as a single sign, it is, especially if the patient be healthy, one of the most reliable of all the other signs of pregnancy.

4. **Morning Sickness.**—If this does not arise from a disordered stomach, it is a trustworthy sign of pregnancy. A lady who has once had morning-sickness can always for the future distinguish it from each and from every other sickness; it is a peculiar sickness, which no other sickness can simulate. Moreover, it is emphatically a morning-sickness—the patient being, as a rule, for the rest of the day entirely free from sickness or from the feeling of sickness.

Embryo of Twenty Days, Laid Open.

b, the Back: *a a a*, Covering, and pinned to Back.

5. **A Third Symptom.**—A third symptom is shooting, throbbing and lancinating pains in, and enlargement of the breasts, with soreness of the nipples, occurring about the second month. In some instances, after the first few months, a small quantity of watery fluid or a little milk, may be squeezed out of them. This latter symptom, in a first pregnancy, is valuable, and can generally be relied on as fairly conclusive of pregnancy. Milk in the breast, however small it may be in quantity, especially in a first pregnancy, is a reliable sign, indeed, we might say, a certain sign, of pregnancy.

6. **A Dark Brown Areola or Mark** around the nipple is one of the distinguishing signs of pregnancy—more especially of a first pregnancy. Women who have had large families, seldom, even when they are not pregnant, lose this mark entirely; but when they are pregnant it is more intensely dark—the darkest brown—especially if they be brunettes.

7. **Quickening.**—Quickening is one of the most important signs of pregnancy, and one of the most valuable, as at the moment it occurs, as a rule, the motion of the child is first felt, whilst, at the same time, there is a sudden increase in the size of the abdomen. Quickening is a proof that nearly half the time of pregnancy has passed. If there be a[272]liability to miscarry, quickening makes matters more safe, as there is less likelihood of a

105

miscarriage after than before it. A lady at this time frequently feels faint or actually faints away; she is often giddy, or sick, or nervous, and in some instances even hysterically; although, in rare cases, some women do not even know the precise time when they quicken.

8. **Increased Size and Hardness of the Abdomen.**—This is very characteristic of pregnancy. When a lady is not pregnant the abdomen is soft and flaccid; when she is pregnant, and after she has quickened, the abdomen; over the region of the womb, is hard and resisting.

Embryo at Thirty Days. *a*, the Head; *b*, the Eyes; *d*, the Neck;*e*, the Chest; *f*, the Abdomen.

9. **Excitability of Mind.**—Excitability of mind is very common in pregnancy, more especially if the patient be delicate; indeed, excitability is a sign of debility, and requires plenty of good nourishment, but few stimulants.

10. **Eruptions on the Skin.**—Principally on the face, neck, or throat, are tell-tales of pregnancy, and to an experienced matron, publish the fact that an acquaintance thus marked is pregnant.

[273]

11. **The Fœtal Heart.**—In the fifth month there is a sign which, if detected, furnishes indubitable evidence of conception, and that is the sound of the child's heart. If the ear be placed on the abdomen, over the womb, the beating of the fœtal heart can sometimes be heard quite plainly, and by the use of an instrument called the stethoscope, the sounds can be still more plainly heard. This is a very valuable sign, inasmuch as the presence of the child is not only ascertained, but also its position, and whether there are twins or more.

OUR KING.

[274]

Diseases of Pregnancy.

1. **Costive State of the Bowels.**—A costive state of the bowels is common in pregnancy; a mild laxative is therefore occasionally necessary. The mildest must be selected, as a strong purgative is highly improper, and even dangerous. Calomel and all other preparations of mercury are to be especially avoided, as a mercurial medicine is apt to weaken the system, and sometimes even to produce a miscarriage. Let me again urge the importance of a lady, during the whole period of pregnancy, being particular as to the state of her bowels, as costiveness is a fruitful cause of painful, tedious and hard labors.

2. **Laxatives.**—The best laxatives are castor oil, salad oil, compound rhubarb pills, honey, stewed prunes, stewed rhubarb, Muscatel raisins, figs, grapes, roasted apples, baked pears, stewed Normandy pippins, coffee, brown-bread and treacle. Scotch oatmeal made with new milk or water, or with equal parts of milk and water.

3. **Pills.**—When the motions are hard, and when the bowels are easily acted upon, two, or three, or four pills made of Castile soap will frequently answer the purpose; and if they will, are far better than any other ordinary laxative. The following is a good form. Take of:

Castile Soap, five scruples;

Oil of Caraway, six drops;

To make twenty-four pills. Two, or three, or four to be taken at bedtime, occasionally.

4. **Honey.**—A teaspoonful of honey, either eaten at breakfast or dissolved in a cup of tea, will frequently, comfortably and effectually, open the bowels, and will supersede the necessity of taking laxative medicine.

5. **Nature's Medicines.**—Now, Nature's medicines—exercise in the open air, occupation, and household duties—on the contrary, not only at the time open the bowels, but keep up a proper action for the future; hence their inestimable superiority.[275]

6. **Warm Water Injections.**—An excellent remedy for costiveness of pregnancy is an enema, either of warm water, or of Castile soap and water, which the patient, by means of a

self-injecting enema-apparatus, may administer to herself. The quantity of warm water to be used, is from half a pint to a pint; the proper heat is the temperature of new milk; the time for administering it is early in the morning, twice or three times a week.

7. **Muscular Pains of the Abdomen.**—The best remedy is an abdominal belt constructed for pregnancy, and adjusted with proper straps and buckles to accomodate the gradually increasing size of the womb. This plan often affords great comfort and relief; indeed, such a belt is indispensably necessary.

8. **Diarrhœa.**—Although the bowels in pregnancy are generally costive, they are sometimes in an opposite state, and are relaxed. Now, this relaxation is frequently owing to there having been prolonged constipation, and Nature is trying to relieve herself by purging. Do not check it, but allow it to have its course, and take a little rhubarb or magnesia. The diet should be simple, plain, and nourishing, and should consist of beef tea, chicken broth, arrowroot, and of well-made and well-boiled oatmeal gruel. Butcher's meat, for a few days, should not be eaten; and stimulants of all kinds must be avoided.

9. **Fidgets.**—A pregnant lady sometimes suffers severely from "fidgets"; it generally affects her feet and legs, especially at night, so as to entirely destroy her sleep; she cannot lie still; she every few minutes moves, tosses and tumbles about—first on one side, then on the other. The causes of "fidgets" are a heated state of the blood; an irritable condition of the nervous system, prevailing at that particular time; and want of occupation. The treatment of "fidgets" consists of: sleeping in a well-ventilated apartment, with either window or door open; a thorough ablution of the whole body every morning, and a good washing with tepid water of the face, neck, chest, arms and hands every night; shunning hot and close rooms; taking plenty of out-door exercise; living on a bland, nourishing, but not rich diet; avoiding meat at night, and substituting in lieu thereof, either a cupful of arrow-root made with milk, or of well-boiled oatmeal gruel.

10. **Exercise.**—If a lady, during the night, have the "fidgets," she should get out of bed; take a short walk up and down the room, being well protected by a dressing-gown; empty her bladder; turn her pillow, so as to have [276]the cold side next the head; and then lie down again; and the chances are that she will now fall asleep. If during the day she have the "fidgets," a ride in an open carriage; or a stroll in the garden, or in the fields; or a little housewifery, will do her good, and there is nothing like fresh air, exercise, and occupation to drive away "the fidgets."

11. **Heartburn.**—Heartburn is a common and often a distressing symptom of pregnancy. The acid producing the heartburn is frequently much increased by an overloaded stomach. An abstemious diet ought to be strictly observed. Great attention should be paid to the quality of the food. Greens, pastry, hot buttered toast, melted butter, and everything that is rich and gross, ought to be carefully avoided. Either a teaspoonful of heavy calcined magnesia, or half a teaspoonful of carbonate of soda—the former to be preferred if there be constipation—should occasionally be taken in a wine-glassful of warm water. If these do not relieve—the above directions as to diet having been strictly attended to—the following mixture ought to be tried. Take of:

Carbonate of Ammonia, half a drachm;

Bicarbonate of Soda, a drachm and a half;

Water, eight ounces;

To make a mixture: Two tablespoonfuls to be taken twice or three times a day, until relief be obtained.

12. **Wind in the Stomach and Bowels.**—This is a frequent reason why a pregnant lady cannot sleep at night. The two most frequent causes of flatulence are, first, the want of walking exercise during the day, and second, the eating of a hearty meal just before going to bed at night. The remedies are, of course, in each instance, self-evident.

13. **Swollen Legs from Enlarged Veins (Varicose Veins.)**—The veins are frequently much enlarged and distended, causing the legs to be greatly swollen and very painful, preventing the patient from taking proper walking exercise. Swollen legs are owing to the pressure of the womb upon the blood-vessels above. Women who have had large families are more liable than others to varicose veins. If a lady marry late in life, or if she be very heavy in pregnancy—carrying the child low down—she is more likely to have distention

of the veins. The best plan will be for her to wear during the day an elastic stocking, which ought to be made on purpose for her, in order that it may properly fit the leg and foot.

14. **Stretching of the Skin of the Abdomen.**—This is frequently, in a first pregnancy, distressing, from the [277]soreness it causes. The best remedy is to rub the abdomen, every night and morning, with warm camphorated oil, and to wear a belt during the day and a broad flannel bandage at night, both of which should be put on moderately but comfortably tight. The belt must be secured in its situation by means of properly adjusted straps.

15. **Before the Approach of Labor.**—The patient, before the approach of labor, ought to take particular care to have the bowels gently opened, as during that state a costive state greatly increases her sufferings, and lengthens the period of her labor. A gentle action is all that is necessary; a violent one would do more harm than good.

16. **Swollen and Painful Breasts.**—The breasts are, at times, during pregnancy, much swollen and very painful and, now and then, they cause the patient great uneasiness as she fancies that she is going to have either some dreadful tumor or a gathering of the bosom. There need, in such a case, be no apprehension. The swelling and the pain are the consequences of the pregnancy, and will in due time subside without any unpleasant result. For treatment she cannot do better than rub them well, every night and morning, with equal parts of Eau de Cologne and olive oil, and wear a piece of new flannel over them; taking care to cover the nipples with soft linen, as the friction of the flannel might irritate them.

17. **Bowel Complaints.**—Bowel complaints, during pregnancy, are not unfrequent. A dose either of rhubarb and magnesia, or of castor oil, are the best remedies, and are generally, in the way of medicine, all that is necessary.

17. **Cramps.**—Cramps of the legs and of the thighs during the latter period, and especially at night, are apt to attend pregnancy, and are caused by the womb pressing upon the nerves which extend to the lower extremities. Treatment.—Tightly tie a handkerchief, folded like a neckerchief, round the limb a little above the part affected, and let it remain on for a few minutes. Friction by means of the hand either with opodeldoc or with laudanum, taking care not to drink the lotion by mistake, will also give relief.

A PRECIOUS FLOWER.

19. **The Whites.**—The whites during pregnancy, especially during the latter months, and particularly if the lady have had many children, are frequently troublesome, and are, in a measure, occasioned by the pressure of the womb on the parts below, causing irritation. The best way, therefore, to obviate such pressure is for the patient to lie down a great part of each day either on a bed or a sofa. She ought to retire early to rest; she should sleep on a hard[279]mattress and in a well-ventilated apartment, and should not overload her bed with clothes. A thick, heavy quilt at these times, and indeed at all times, is particularly objectionable; the perspiration cannot pass readily through it as through blankets, and thus she is weakened. She ought to live on plain, wholesome, nourishing food; and she must abstain from beer and wine and spirits. The bowels ought to be gently opened by means of a Seidlitz powder, which should occasionally be taken early in the morning.

20. **Irritation and Itching of the External Parts.**—This a most troublesome affection, and may occur at any time, but more especially during the latter period of the pregnancy. Let her diet be simple and nourishing; let her avoid stimulants of all kinds. Let her take a sitz-bath of warm water, considerably salted. Let her sit in the bath with the body thoroughly covered.

21. **Hot and inflamed.**—The external parts, and the passage to the womb (vagina), in these cases, are not only irritable and itching, but are sometimes hot and inflamed, and are covered either with small pimples, or with a whitish exudation of the nature of aphtha (thrush), somewhat similar to the thrush on the mouth of an infant; then, the addition of glycerine to the lotion is a great improvement and usually gives much relief.

22. [3]**Biliousness** is defined by some one as piggishness. Generally it may be regarded as *overfed*. The elements of the bile are in the blood in excess of the power of the liver to eliminate them. This may be caused either from the superabundance of the materials from which the bile is made or by inaction of the organ itself. Being thus retained the system is *clogged*. It is the result of either too much food in quantity or too rich in quality. Especially is

it caused by the excessive use of *fats and sweets*. The simplest remedy is the best. A plain, light diet with plenty of acid fruits, avoiding fats and sweets, will ameliorate or remove it. Don't force the appetite. Let hunger demand food. In the morning the sensitiveness of the stomach may be relieved by taking before rising a cup of hot water, hot milk, hot lemonade, rice or barley water, selecting according to preference. For this purpose many find coffee made from browned wheat or corn the best drink. Depend for a time upon liquid food that can be taken up by absorbents. The juice of lemons and other acid fruits is usually grateful, and [280]assists in assimilating any excess in nutriment. These may be diluted according to taste. With many, an egg lemonade proves relishing and acceptable.

23. **Deranged Appetite.**—Where the appetite fails, let the patient go without eating for a little while, say for two or three meals. If, however, the strength begins to go, try the offering of some unexpected delicacy; or give small quantities of nourishing food, as directed in case of morning sickness.

24. **Piles.**—For cases of significance consult a physician. As with constipation, so with piles, its frequent result, fruit diet, exercise, and sitz-bath regimen will do much to prevent the trouble. Frequent local applications of a cold compress, and even of ice, and tepid water injections, are of great service. Walking or standing aggravate this complaint. Lying down alleviates it. Dr. Shaw says, "There is nothing in the world that will produce so great relief in piles as fasting. If the fit is severe, live a whole day, or even two, if necessary, upon pure soft cold water alone. Give then very lightly of vegetable food."

25. **Toothache.**—There is a sort of proverb that a woman loses one tooth every time she has a child. Neuralgic toothache during pregnancy is, at any rate, extremely common, and often has to be endured. It is generally thought not best to have teeth extracted during pregnancy, as the shock to the nervous system has sometimes caused miscarriage. To wash out the mouth morning and night with cold or lukewarm water and salt is often of use. If the teeth are decayed, consult a good dentist in the early stages of pregnancy, and have the offending teeth properly dressed. Good dentists, in the present state of the science, extract very few teeth, but save them.

26. **Salivation.**—Excessive secretion of the saliva has usually been reckoned substantially incurable. Fasting, cold water treatment, exercise and fruit diet may be relied on to prevent, cure or alleviate it, where this is possible, as it frequently is.

27. **Headache.**—This is, perhaps, almost as common in cases of pregnancy as "morning sickness." It may be from determination of blood to the head, from constipation or indigestion, constitutional "sick headache," from neuralgia, from a cold, from rheumatism. Correct living will prevent much headache trouble; and where this does not answer the purpose, rubbing and making magnetic passes over the [281]head by the hand of some healthy magnetic person will often prove of great service.

28. **Liver-Spots.**—These, on the face, must probably be endured, as no trustworthy way of driving them off is known.

29. **Jaundice.**—See the doctor.

30. **Pain on the Right Side.**—This is liable to occur from about the fifth to the eighth month, and is attributed to the pressure of the enlarging womb upon the liver. Proper living is most likely to alleviate it. Wearing a wet girdle in daytime or a wet compress at night, sitz-baths, and friction with the wet hand may also be tried. If the pain is severe a mustard poultice may be used. Exercise should be carefully moderated if found to increase the pain. If there is fever and inflammation with it, consult a physician. It is usually not dangerous, but uncomfortable only.

31. **Palpitation of the Heart.**—To be prevented by healthy living and calm, good humor. Lying down will often gradually relieve it, so will a compress wet with water, as hot as can be borne, placed over the heart and renewed as often as it gets cool.

32. **Fainting.**—Most likely to be caused by "quickening," or else by tight dress, bad air, over-exertion, or other unhealthy living. It is not often dangerous. Lay the patient in an easy posture, the head rather low than high, and where cool air may blow across the face; loosen the dress if tight; sprinkle cold water on the face and hands.

33. **Sleeplessness.**—Most likely to be caused by incorrect living, and to be prevented and cured by the opposite. A glass or two of cold water drank deliberately on going to bed

often helps one to go to sleep; so does bathing the face and hands and the feet in cold water. A short nap in the latter part of the forenoon can sometimes be had, and is of use. Such a nap ought not to be too long, or it leaves a heavy feeling; it should be sought with the mind in a calm state, in a well-ventilated though darkened room, and with the clothing removed, as at night. A similar nap in the afternoon is not so good, but is better than nothing. The tepid sitz-bath on going to bed will often produce sleep, and so will gentle percussion given by an attendant with palms of the hand over the back for a few minutes on retiring. To secure sound sleep do not read, write or severely tax the mind in the evening.[282]

MORNING SICKNESS.

1. A pregnant woman is especially liable to suffer many forms of dyspepsia, nervous troubles, sleeplessness, etc.

2. **Morning Sickness** is the most common and is the result of an irritation in the womb, caused by some derangement, and it is greatly irritated by the habit of indulging in sexual gratification during pregnancy. If people would imitate the lower animals and reserve the vital forces of the mother for the benefit of her unborn child, it would be a great boon to humanity. Morning sickness may begin the next day after conception, but it usually appears from two to three weeks after the beginning of pregnancy and continues with more or less severity from two to four months.

3. **Home Treatment for Morning Sickness.**—Avoid all highly seasoned and rich food. Also avoid strong tea and coffee. Eat especially light and simple suppers at five o'clock and no later than six. Some simple broths, such as will be found in the cooking department of this book will be very nourishing and soothing. Coffee made from brown wheat or corn is an excellent remedy to use. The juice of lemons reduced with water will sometimes prove very effectual. A good lemonade with an egg well stirred is very nourishing and toning to the stomach.

4. **Hot Fomentation** on the stomach and liver is excellent, and warm and hot water injections are highly beneficial.

5. A little powdered magnesia at bed time, taken in a little milk, will often give almost permanent relief.

6. Avoid corsets or any other pressure upon the stomach. All garments must be worn loosely. In many cases this will entirely prevent all stomach disturbances.

[283]

Relation of Husband and Wife During Pregnancy.

1. **Miscarriage.**—If the wife is subject to miscarriage every precaution should be employed to prevent its happening again. Under such exceptional circumstances the husband should sleep apart the first five months of pregnancy; after that length of time, the ordinary relation may be assumed. If miscarriage has taken place, intercourse should be avoided for a month or six weeks at least after the accident.

2. **Impregnation**—Impregnation is the only mission of intercourse, and after that has taken place, intercourse can subserve no other purpose than sensual gratification.

3. **Woman Must Judge.**—Every man should recognize the fact that woman is the sole umpire as to when, how frequent, and under what circumstances, connection should take place. Her desires should not be ignored, for her likes and dislikes are—as seen in another part of this book—easily impressed upon the unborn child. If she is strong and healthy there is no reason why passion should not be gratified with moderation and caution during the whole period of pregnancy, but she must be the sole judge and her desires supreme.

4. **Voluntary Instances.**—No voluntary instances occur through the entire animal kingdom. All females repel with force and fierceness the approaches of the male. The human family is the only exception. A man that loves his wife, however, will respect her under all circumstances and recognize her condition and yield to her wishes.

[284]

A Private Word to the Expectant Mother

Elizabeth Cady Stanton, in a lecture to ladies, thus strongly states her views regarding maternity and painless childbirth:

"We must educate our daughters to think that motherhood is grand, and that God never cursed it. And this curse, if it be a curse, may be rolled off, as man has rolled away the curse of labor; as the curse has been rolled from the descendants of Ham. My mission is to preach this new gospel. If you suffer, it is not because you are cursed of God, but because you violate His laws. What an incubus it would take from woman could she be educated to know that the pains of maternity are no curse upon her kind. We know that among the Indians the squaws do not suffer in childbirth. They will step aside from the ranks, even on the march, and return in a short time to them with the newborn child. What an absurdity then, to suppose that only enlightened Christian women are cursed. But one word of fact is worth a volume of philosophy; let me give you some of my own experience. I am the mother of seven children. My girlhood was spent mostly in the open air. I early imbibed the idea that a girl was just as good as a boy, and I carried it out. I would walk five miles before breakfast or [285]ride ten on horseback. After I was married I wore my clothing sensibly. Their weight hung entirely on my shoulders. I never compressed my body out of its natural shape. When my first four children were born, I suffered very little. I then made up my mind that it was totally unnecessary for me to suffer at all; so I dressed lightly, walked every day, lived as much as possible in the open air, ate no condiments or spices, kept quiet, listened to music, looked at pictures, and took proper care of myself. The night before the birth of the child I walked three miles. The child was born without a particle of pain. I bathed it and dressed it, and it weighed ten and one-half pounds. That same day I dined with the family. Everybody said I would surely die, but I never had a relapse or a moment's inconvenience from it. I know this is not being delicate and refined, but if you would be vigorous and healthy, in spite of the diseases of your ancestors, and your own disregard of nature's laws, try it."

Shall Pregnant Women Work?

1. **Over-worked Mothers.**—Children born of over-worked mothers, are liable to be a dwarfed and puny race. However, their chances are better than those of the children of inactive, dependent, indolent mothers who have neither brain nor muscle to transmit to son or daughter. The truth seems to be that excessive labor, with either body or mind, is alike injurious to both men and women, and herein lies the sting of that old curse. This paragraph suggests all that need be said on the question whether pregnant women should or should not labor.

2. **Foolishly Idle.**—At least it is certain that they should not be foolishly idle; and on the other hand, it is equally certain that they should be relieved from painful laborious occupations that exhaust and unfit them for happiness. Pleasant and useful physical and intellectual occupation, however, will not only do no harm, but positive good.

3. **The Best Man and the Best Woman.**—The best man is he who can rear the best child, and the best woman is she who can rear the best child. We very properly extol to the skies Harriet Hosmer, the artist, for cutting in marble the statue of a Zenobia, how much more should we sing praises to the man and the woman who bring into the world a noble boy or girl. The one is a piece of lifeless beauty, the other a piece of life including all beauty, all possibilities.

[286]

Words for Young Mothers.

The act of nursing is sometimes painful to the mother, especially before the habit is fully established. The discomfort is greatly increased if the skin that covers the nipples is tender and delicate. The suction pulls it off, leaving them in a state in which the necessary pressure of the child's lips cause intense agony. This can be prevented in a great measure, says Elizabeth Robinson Scovil, in *Ladies' Home Journal*, if not entirely, by bathing the nipples twice a day for six weeks before the confinement with powdered alum dissolved in alcohol;

or salt dissolved in brandy. If there is any symptom of the skin cracking when the child begins to nurse, they should be painted with a mixture of tannin and glycerine. This must be washed off before the baby touches them and renewed when it leaves them. If they are [287]very painful, the doctor will probably order morphia added to the mixture. A rubber nipple shield to be put on at the time of nursing, is a great relief. If the nipples are retracted or drawn inward, they can be drawn out painlessly by filling a pint bottle with boiling water, emptying it and quickly applying the mouth over the nipple. As the air in the bottle cools, it condenses, leaving a vacuum and the nipple is pushed out by the air behind it.

When the milk accumulates or "cakes" in the breast in hard patches, they should be rubbed very gently, from the base upwards, with warm camphorated oil. The rubbing should be the lightest, most delicate stroking, avoiding pressure. If lumps appear at the base of the breast and it is red, swollen and painful, cloths wrung out of cold water should be applied and the doctor sent for. While the breast is full and hard all over, not much apprehension need be felt. It is when lumps appear that the physician should be notified, that he may, if possible, prevent the formation of abscesses.

While a woman is nursing she should eat plenty of nourishing food—milk, oatmeal, cracked wheat, and good juicy, fresh meat, boiled, roasted, or broiled, but not fried. Between each meal, before going to bed, and once during the night, she should take a cup of cocoa, gruel made with milk, good beef tea, mutton broth, or any warm, nutritive drink. Tea and coffee are to be avoided. It is important to keep the digestion in order and the bowels should be carefully regulated as a means to this end. If necessary, any of the laxative mineral waters can be used for this purpose, or a teaspoonful of compound licorice powder taken at night. Powerful cathartic medicines should be avoided because of their effect upon the baby. The child should be weaned at nine months old, unless this time comes in very hot weather, or the infant is so delicate that a change of food would be injurious. If the mother is not strong her nurseling will sometimes thrive better upon artificial food than on its natural nourishment. By gradually lengthening the interval between the nursing and feeding the child, when it is hungry, the weaning can be accomplished without much trouble.

A young mother should wear warm underclothing, thick stockings and a flannel jacket over her night dress, unless she is in the habit of wearing an under vest. If the body is not protected by warm clothing there is an undue demand upon the nervous energy to keep up the vital heat, and nerve force is wasted by the attempt to compel the system to do what ought to be done for it by outside means.

[288]
How to Have Beautiful Children.

1. **Parental Influence.**—The art of having handsome children has been a question that has interested the people of all ages and of all nationalities. There is no longer a question as to the influence that parents may and do exert upon their offspring, and it is shown in other parts of this book that beauty depends largely on the condition of health at the time of conception. It is therefore of no little moment that parents should guard carefully their own health as well as that of their children, that they may develop a vigorous constitution. There cannot be beauty without good health.

2. **Marrying Too Early.**—We know that marriage at too early an age, or too late in life, is apt to produce imperfectly [289]developed children, both mentally and physically. The causes are self-evident: A couple marrying too young, they lack maturity and consequently will impart weakness to their offspring; while on the other hand persons marrying late in life fail to find that normal condition which is conducive to the health and vigor of offspring.

3. **Crossing of Temperaments and Nationalities.**—The crossing of temperaments and nationalities beautifies offspring. If young persons of different nationalities marry, their children under proper hygienic laws are generally handsome and healthy. For instance, an American and German or an Irish and German uniting in marriage, produces better looking children than those marrying in the same nationality. Persons of different temperaments uniting in marriage, always produces a good effect upon offspring.

112

4. The Proper Time.—To obtain the best results, conception should take place only when both parties are in the best physical condition. If either parent is in any way indisposed at the time of conception the results will be seen in the health of the child. Many children brought in the world with diseases or other infirmities stamped upon their feeble frames show the indiscretion and ignorance of parents.

5. During Pregnancy.—During pregnancy the mother should take time for self improvement and cultivate an interest for admiring beautiful pictures or engravings which represent cheerful and beautiful figures. Secure a few good books illustrating art, with some fine representations of statues and other attractive pictures. The purchase of several illustrated art journals might answer the purpose.

6. What to Avoid.—Pregnant mothers should avoid thinking of ugly people, or those marked by any deformity or disease; avoid injury, fright and disease of any kind. Also avoid ungraceful position and awkward attitude, but cultivate grace and beauty in herself. Avoid difficulty with neighbors or other trouble.

7. Good Care.—She should keep herself in good physical condition, and the system well nourished, as a want of food always injures the child.

8. The Improvement of the Mind.—The mother should read suitable articles in newspapers or good books, keep her mind occupied. If she cultivates a desire for intellectual improvement, the same desire will be more or less manifested in the growth and development of the child.[290]

9. Like Produces Like, everywhere and always—in general forms and in particular features—in mental qualities and in bodily conditions—in tendencies of thought and in habits of action. Let this grand truth be deeply impressed upon the hearts of all who desire or expect to become parents.

10. Heredity.—Male children generally inherit the peculiar traits and diseases of the mother and female children those of the father.

11. Advice.—"Therefore it is urged that during the period of utero-gestation, especial pains should be taken to render the life of the female as harmonious as possible, that her surroundings should all be of a nature calculated to inspire the mind with thoughts of physical and mental beauties and perfections, and that she should be guarded against all influences, of whatever character, having a deteriorating tendency."

[292]
Education of the Child in the Womb.
"A lady once interviewed a prominent college president and asked him when the education of a child should begin. 'Twenty-five years before it is born,' was the prompt reply."

No better answer was ever given to that question. Every mother may well consider it.
THE BEAUTIFUL BUTTERFLY.

1. The Unborn Child Affected by the Thoughts and the Surroundings of the Mother.—That the child is affected in the womb of the mother, through the influences apparently connected with objects by which she is surrounded, appears to have been well known in ancient days, as well as at the present time.

2. Evidences.—Many evidences are found in ancient history, especially among the refined nations, showing that certain expedients were resorted to by which their females, during the period of utero-gestation, were surrounded by the superior refinements of the age, with the hope of thus making upon them impressions which should have the effect of communicating certain desired qualities to the offspring. For this reason apartments were adorned with statuary and paintings, and special pains were taken not only to convey favorable impressions, but also to guard against unfavorable ones being made, upon the mind of the pregnant woman.

3. Hankering after Gin.—A certain mother while pregnant, longed for gin, which could not be gotten; and her child cried incessantly for six weeks till gin was given it, which it eagerly clutched and drank with ravenous greediness, stopped crying, and became healthy.

4. Begin to Educate Children at Conception, and continue during their entire carriage. Yet maternal study, of little account before the sixth, after it, is most promotive of talents; which, next to goodness are the father's joy and the mother's pride. What pains are taken after they are born, to render them prodigies of learning, by the best of schools and teachers from their third year; whereas their mother's study, three months before their birth, would improve their intellects infinitely more.

5. **Mothers, Does God Thus Put** the endowment of your darlings into your moulding power? Then tremble in view of its necessary responsibilities, and learn how to wield them for their and your temporal and eternal happiness.[293]

6. **Qualities of the Mind.**—The qualities of the mind are perhaps as much liable to hereditary transmission as bodily configuration.

Memory, intelligence, judgment, imagination, passions, diseases, and what is usually called genius, are often very markedly traced in the offspring.—I have known mental impressions forcibly impressed upon the offspring at the time of conception, as concomitant of some peculiar eccentricity, idiosyncracy, morbidness, waywardness, irritability, or proclivity of either one or both parents.

7. **The Plastic Brain.**—The plastic brain of the fœtus is prompt to receive all impressions. It retains them, and they become the characteristics of the child and the man. Low spirits, violent passions, irritability, frivolity, in the pregnant woman, leave indelible marks on the unborn child.

8. **Formation of Character.**—I believe that pre-natal influences may do as much in the formation of character as all the education that can come after, and that mothers may, in a measure, "will," what that influence shall be, and that, as knowledge on the subject increases, it will be more and more under their control. In that, as in everything else, things that would be possible with one mother would not be with another, and measures that would be successful with one would produce opposite results from the other.

9. **A Historical Illustration.**—A woman rode side by side with her soldier husband, and witnessed the drilling of troops for battle. The scene inspired her with a deep longing to see a battle and share in the excitements of the [294]conquerors. This was but a few months before her boy was born, and his name was Napoleon.

10. **A Musician.**—The following was reported by Dr. F. W. Moffatt, in the mother's own language: "When I was first pregnant, I wished my offspring to be a musician, so, during the period of that pregnancy, settled my whole mind on music, and attended every musical entertainment I possibly could. I had my husband, who has a violin, to play for me by the hour. When the child was born, it was a girl, which grew and prospered, and finally became an expert musician."

11. **Murderous Intent.**—The mother of a young man, who was hung not long ago, was heard to say: "I tried to get rid of him before he was born; and, oh, how I wish now that I had succeeded!" She added that it was the only time she had attempted anything of the sort; but, because of home troubles, she became desperate, and resolved that her burdens should not be made any greater. Does it not seem probable that the murderous intent, even though of short duration, was communicated to the mind of the child, and resulted in the crime for which he was hung?

12. **The Assassin of Garfield.**—Guiteau's father was a man of integrity and considerable intellectual ability. His children were born in quick succession, and the mother was obliged to work very hard. Before this child was born, she resorted to every means, though unsuccessful, to produce abortion. The world knows the result. Guiteau's whole life was full of contradictions. There was little self-controlling power in him; no common sense, and not a vestige of remorse or shame. In his wild imagination, he believed himself capable of doing the greatest work, and of filling the loftiest station in life. Who will dare question that this mother's effort to destroy him while in embryo was the main cause in bringing him to the level of the brutes?

13. **Caution.**—Any attempt, on the part of the mother, to destroy her child before birth, is liable, if unsuccessful, to produce murderous tendencies. Even harboring murderous thoughts, whether toward her own child or not, might be followed by similar results.

"The great King of kings
Hath in the table of His law commanded

That thou shalt do no murder. Wilt thou, then,
Spurn at His edict, and fulfill a man's?
Take heed, for He holds vengeance in His hand
To hurl upon their heads that break his law."—RICHARD III., *Act 1.*

[295]
How to Calculate the Time of Expected Labor.
The Embryo In Sixty Days.

1. The table on the opposite page has been very accurately compiled, and will be very helpful to those who desire the exact time.

2. The duration of pregnancy is from 278 to 280 days, or nearly forty weeks. The count should be made from the beginning of the last menstruation, and add eight days on account of the possibility of it occurring within that period The heavier the child the longer is the duration; the younger the woman the longer time it often requires. The duration is longer in married than in unmarried women; the duration is liable to be longer if the child is a female.

3. **Movement.**—The first movement is generally felt on the 135th day after impregnation.

4. **Growth of the Embryo.**—About the twentieth day the embryo resembles the appearance of an ant or lettuce seed; the 30th day the embryo is as large as a common horse fly; the 40th day the form resembles that of a person; in sixty days the limbs begin to form, and in four months the embryo takes the name of fœtus.

5. Children born after seven or eight months can survive and develop to maturity.

[296]
DURATION OF PREGNANCY.
DIRECTIONS.—Find in the upper horizontal line the date on which the last menstruation ceased; the figure beneath gives the date of expected confinement (280 days).

```
_____ |Jan. | 1  2  3  4  5  6  7  8  9 10 11 12 13 14 15
16 17 18 19 20 21 22 23 24 25 26 27 28 29 30 31 |   |  |Oct. | 8  9 10 11 12 13 14 15 16 17
18 19 20 21 22 23 24 25 26 27 28 29 30 31   1   2   3   4   5   6   7 |Nov. |  |        |
 |   |  |Feb. | 1  2  3  4  5  6  7  8  9 10 11 12 13 14 15 16 17 18 19 20 21 22 23 24 25 26 27
28      |   |  |Nov. | 8  9 10 11 12 13 14 15 16 17 18 19 20 21 22 23 24 25 26 27 28 29 30
 1      2       3       4       5              |Dec. |  |              |
 |   |  |Mar. | 1  2  3  4  5  6  7  8  9 10 11 12 13 14 15 16 17 18 19 20 21 22 23 24 25 26 27
28 19 30 31 |   |  |Dec. | 6  7  8  9 10 11 12 13 14 15 16 17 18 19 20 21 22 23 24 25 26 27
28     29      30      31       1       2       3       4       5  |Jan. |  |        |
 |   |  |Apr. | 1  2  3  4  5  6  7  8  9 10 11 12 13 14 15 16 17 18 19 20 21 22 23 24 25 26 27
28 29 30 31 |   |  |Jan. | 6  7  8  9 10 11 12 13 14 15 16 17 18 19 20 21 22 23 24 25 26 27
28     29      30      31       1       2       3       4       5  |Feb. |  |        |
 |   |  |May | 1  2  3  4  5  6  7  8  9 10 11 12 13 14 15 16 17 18 19 20 21 22 23 24 25 26 27
28 29 30 31 |   |  |Feb. | 5  6  7  8  9 10 11 12 13 14 15 16 17 18 19 20 21 22 23 24 25 26
27     28       1       2       3       4       5       6       7 |Mar. |  |        |
 |   |  |June | 1  2  3  4  5  6  7  8  9 10 11 12 13 14 15 16 17 18 19 20 21 22 23 24 25 26 27
28 29 30   |   |  |Mar. | 8  9 10 11 12 13 14 15 16 17 18 19 20 21 22 23 24 25 26 27 28 29
30     31       1       2       3       4       5       6              |Apr. |  |        |
 |   |  |July | 1  2  3  4  5  6  7  8  9 10 11 12 13 14 15 16 17 18 19 20 21 22 23 24 25 26 27
28 29 30   |   |  |Apr. | 7  8  9 10 11 12 13 14 15 16 17 18 19 20 21 22 23 24 25 26 27 28
29     30       1       2       3       4       5       6              |May |  |        |
 |   |  |Aug. | 1  2  3  4  5  6  7  8  9 10 11 12 13 14 15 16 17 18 19 20 21 22 23 24 25 26 27
28 29 30 31 |   |  |May | 8  9 10 11 12 13 14 15 16 17 18 19 21 22 23 24 25 26 27 28 29
30     31       1       2       3       4       5       6       7 |June |  |        |
 |   |  |Sept.| 1  2  3  4  5  6  7  8  9 10 11 12 13 14 15 16 17 18 19 20 21 22 23 24 25 26 27
28 29 30   |   |  |June | 8  9 10 11 12 13 14 15 16 17 18 19 21 21 22 23 24 25 26 27 28 29
```

```
30    1    2    3    4    5    6    7         |July  |    |                    |
|    | |Oct. | 1  2  3  4  5  6  7  8  9 10 11 12 13 14 15 16 17 18 19 20 21 22 23 24 25 26 27
28 29 30 31 |    | |July | 8  9 10 11 12 13 14 15 16 17 18 19 20 21 22 23 24 25 26 27 28 29
30   31    1    2    3    4    5    6    7  |Aug.  |    |                    |
|    | |Nov. | 1  2  3  4  5  6  7  8  9 10 11 12 13 14 15 16 17 18 19 20 21 22 23 24 25 26 27
28 29 30    |    | |Aug. | 8  9 10 11 12 13 14 15 16 17 18 19 20 21 22 23 24 25 26 27 28 29
30   31    1    2    3    4    5    6         |Sep.  |    |                    |
|    | |Dec. | 1  2  3  4  5  6  7  8  9 10 11 12 13 14 15 16 17 18 19 20 21 22 23 24 25 26 27
23 29 30 31 |    | |Sep. | 7  8  9 10 11 12 13 14 15 16 17 18 19 20 21 22 23 24 25 26 27 28
29   30    1    2    3    4    5    6    7  |Oct.  |
```

ILLUSTRATION: If menstruation ceased Oct. 11, the confinement will take place July 18.

[297]

The Signs and Symptoms of Labor.

1. Although the majority of patients, a day or two before the labor comes on, are more bright and cheerful, some few are more anxious, fanciful, fidgety and reckless.

2. A few days, sometimes a few hours, before labor commences, the child "falls" as it is called; that is to say, there is a subsidence—a dropping—of the womb lower down the abdomen. This is the reason why she feels lighter and more comfortable, and more inclined to take exercise, and why she can breathe more freely.

3. The only inconvenience of the dropping of the womb is, that the womb presses more on the bladder, and sometimes causes an irritability of that organ, inducing a frequent desire to make water. The wearing the obstetric belt, as so particularly enjoined in previous pages, will greatly mitigate this inconvenience.

4. The subsidence—the dropping—of the womb may then be considered one of the earliest of the precursory symptoms of child-birth, and as the herald of the coming event.

5. She has, at this time, an increased moisture of the vagina—the passage leading to the womb—and of the external parts. She has, at length, slight pains, and then she has a "show," as it is called; which is the coming away of a mucous plug which, during pregnancy, had hermetically sealed up the mouth of the womb. The "show" is generally tinged with a little blood. When a "show" takes place, she may rest assured that labor has actually commenced. One of the early symptoms of labor is a frequent desire to relieve the bladder.

6. She ought not, on any account, unless it be ordered by the medical man, to take any stimulant as a remedy for the shivering. In case of shivering or chills, a cup either of hot tea or of hot gruel will be the best remedy for the shivering; and an extra blanket or two should be thrown over her, and be well tucked around her, in order to thoroughly exclude the air from the body. The extra clothing, as soon as she is warm and perspiring, should be gradually removed, as she ought not to be kept very hot, or it will weaken her, and will thus retard her labor.

7. She must not, on any account, force down—as her female friends or as a "pottering" old nurse may advise—to "grinding pains"; if she does, it will rather retard than forward her labor.[298]

8. During this stage, she had better walk about or sit down, and not confine herself to bed; indeed, there is no necessity for her, unless she particularly desire it, to remain in her chamber.

9. After an uncertain length of time, the pains alter in character. From being "grinding" they become "bearing down," and more regular and frequent, and the skin becomes both hot and perspiring. These may be considered the true labor-pains. The patient ought to bear in mind then that "true labor-pains" are situated in the back, and loins; they come on at regular intervals, rise gradually up to a certain pitch of intensity, and abate as gradually; it is a dull, heavy, deep sort of pain, producing occasionally a low moan from the patient; not sharp or twinging, which would elicit a very different expression of suffering from her.

10. Labor—and truly it maybe called, "labor." The fiat has gone forth that in "sorrow thou shalt bring forth children." Young, in his "Night Thoughts," beautifully expresses the common lot of women to suffer:

"'Tis the common lot;
In this shape, or in that, has fate entailed
The mother's throes on all of women born,
Not more the children than sure heirs of pain."

[299]
Special Safeguards in Confinement.
LOVE OF HOME.

1. Before the confinement takes place everything should be carefully arranged and prepared. The physician should be spoken to and be given the time as near as can be calculated. The arrangement of the bed, bed clothing, the dress for the mother and the expected babe should be arranged for convenient and immediate use.

2. A bottle of sweet oil, or vaseline, or some pure lard should be in readiness. Arrangements should be made for washing all soiled garments, and nothing by way of soiled rags or clothing should be allowed to accumulate.

3. A rubber blanket, or oil or waterproof cloth should be in readiness to place underneath the bottom sheet to be used during labor.

4. As soon as labor pains have begun a fire should be built and hot water kept ready for immediate use. The room should be kept well ventilated and comfortably warm.

5. No people should be allowed in or about the room except the nurse, the physician, and probably members of the family when called upon to perform some duty.[300]

6. During labor no solid food should be taken; a little milk, broth or soup may be given, provided there is an appetite. Malt or spirituous liquors should be carefully avoided. A little wine, however, may be taken in case of great exhaustion. Lemonade, toast, rice water, and tea may he given when desired. Warm tea is considered an excellent drink for the patient at this time.

7. When the pains become regular and intermit, it is time that the physician is sent for. On the physician's arrival he will always take charge of the case and give necessary instructions.

8. In nearly all cases the head of the child is presented first. The first pains are generally grinding and irregular, and felt mostly in the groins and within, but as labor progresses the pains are felt in the abdomen, and as the head advances there is severe pain in the back and hips and a disposition to bear down, but no pressure should be placed upon the abdomen of the patient; it is often the cause of serious accidents. Nature will take care of itself.

9. Conversation should be of a cheerful character, and all allusions to accidents of other child births should be carefully avoided.

10. **Absence of Physician.**—In case the child should be born in the absence of the physician, when the head is born receive it in the hand and support it until the shoulders have been expelled, and steady the whole body until the child is born. Support the child with both hands and lay it as far from the mother as possible without stretching the cord. Remove the mucus from the nostrils and mouth, wrap the babe in warm flannel, make the mother comfortable, give her a drink, and allow the child to remain until the pulsations in the cord have entirely ceased. After the pulsations have entirely ceased then sever the cord. Use a dull pair of scissors, cutting it about two inches from the child's navel, and generally no tying is necessary, and when the physician comes he will give it prompt attention.

11. If the child does not breathe at its arrival, says Dr. Stockham in her celebrated Tokology, a little slapping on the breast and body will often produce respiration, and if this is not efficient, dash cold water on the face and chest; if this fails then close the nostrils with two fingers, breathe into the mouth and then expel the air from the lungs by gentle pressure upon the chest. Continue this as long as any hope of life remains.

12. **After-Birth.**—Usually contractions occur and the after-birth is readily expelled; if not, clothes wrung out in [301]hot water laid upon the bowels will often cause the contraction of the uterus, and the expulsion of the after-birth.

13. If the cord bleeds severely inject cold water into it. This in many cases removes the after-birth.

14. After the birth of the child give the patient a bath, if the patient is not too exhausted, change the soiled quilts and clothing, fix up everything neat and clean and let the patient rest.

15. Let the patient drink weak tea, gruel, cold or hot water, whichever she chooses.

16. After the birth of the baby, the mother should be kept perfectly quiet for the first 24 hours and not allowed to talk or see anyone except her nearest relations, however well she may seem. She should not get out of bed for ten days or two weeks, nor sit up in bed for nine days. The more care taken of her at this time, the more rapid will be her recovery when she does get about. She should go up and down stairs slowly, carefully, and as seldom as possible for six weeks. She should not stand more than is unavoidable during that time, but sit with her feet up and lie down when she has time to rest. She should not work a sewing machine with a treadle for at least six weeks, and avoid any unusual strain or over-exertion. "An ounce of prevention is worth a pound of cure," and carefulness will be well repaid by a perfect restoration to health.

[303]

WHERE DID THE BABY COME FROM?
MY PRICELESS JEWEL.

What will be his fate in life?
Where did you come from, baby dear?
Out of the everywhere into here.
Where did you get the eyes so blue?
Out of the sky, as I came through.
Where did you get that little tear?
I found it waiting when I got here.
What makes your forehead so smooth and high?
A soft hand stroked it as I went by.
What makes your cheek like a warm, white rose?
I saw something better than anyone knows.
Whence that three-cornered smile of bliss?
Three angels gave me at once a kiss.
Where did you get this pretty ear?
God spoke, and it came out to hear.
Where did you get those arms and hands?
Love made itself into hooks and bands.
Feet, whence did you come, you darling things?
From the same box as the cherub's wings.
How did they all come just to be you?
God thought of me, and so I grew.
But how did you come to us, you dear?
God thought about you, and so I am here.—GEORGE MACDONALD.

[304]

Child Bearing Without Pain.
HOW TO DRESS, DIET AND EXERCISE IN PREGNANCY.

1. **Ailments.**—Those ailments to which pregnant women are liable are mostly inconveniences rather than diseases, although they may be aggravated to a degree of danger. No patent nostrums or prescriptions are necessary. If there is any serious difficulty the family physician should be consulted.

2. **Comfort.**—Wealth and luxuries are not a necessity. Comfort will make the surroundings pleasant. Drudgery, overwork and exposure are the three things that tend to

118

make women miserable while in the state of pregnancy, and invariably produce irritable, fretful and feeble children. Dr. Stockham says in her admirable work "Tokology": "The woman who indulges in the excessive gayety of fashionable life, as well as the overworked woman, deprives her child of vitality. She attends parties in a dress that is unphysiological in warmth, distribution and adjustment, in rooms badly ventilated; partakes of a supper of indigestible compounds, and remains into the 'wee, sma' hours,' her nervous system taxed to the utmost."

3. **Exercise.**—A goodly amount of moderate exercise is a necessity, and a large amount of work may be accomplished if prudence is properly exercised. It is overwork, and the want of sufficient rest and sleep that produces serious results.

4. **Dresses.**—A pregnant woman should make her dresses of light material and avoid surplus trimmings. Do not wear anything that produces any unnecessary weight. Let the clothing be light but sufficient in quantity to produce comfort in all kinds of weather.

5. **Garments.**—It is well understood that the mother must breathe for two, and in order to dress healthily the garments should be worn loose, so as to give plenty of room for respiration. Tight clothes only cause disease, or produce frailty or malformation in the offspring.

6. **Shoes.**—Wear a large shoe in pregnancy; the feet may swell and untold discomfort may be the result. Get a good large shoe with a large sole. Give the feet plenty of room. Many women suffer from defects in vision, indigestion, backache, loss of voice, headache, etc., simply [305]as the result of the reflex action of the pressure of tight shoes.

7. **Lacing.**—Many women lace themselves in the first period of their gestation in order to meet their society engagements. All of this is vitally wrong and does great injury to the unborn child as well as to inflict many ills and pains upon the mother.

8. **Corsets.**—Corsets should be carefully avoided, for the corset more than any other one thing is responsible for making woman the victim of more woes and diseases than all other causes put together. About one-half the children born in this country die before they are five years of age, and no doubt this terrible mortality is largely due to this instrument of torture known as the *modern corset.* Tight lacing is the cause of infantile mortality. It slowly but surely takes the lives of tens of thousands, and so effectually weakens and diseases, so as to cause the untimely death of millions more.

9. **Bathing.**—Next to godliness is cleanliness. A pregnant woman should take a sponge or towel-bath two or three times a week. It stimulates and invigorates the entire body. No more than two or three minutes are required. It should be done in a warm room, and the body rubbed thoroughly after each bathing.

10. **The Hot Sitz-Bath.**—This bath is one of the most desirable and healthful baths for pregnant women. It will relieve pain or acute inflammation, and will be a general tonic in keeping the system in a good condition. This may be taken in the middle of the forenoon or just before retiring, and if taken just before retiring will produce invigorating sleep, will quiet the nerves, cure headache, weariness, etc. It is a good plan to take this bath every night before retiring in case of any disorders. A woman who keeps this up during the period of gestation will have a very easy labor and a strong, vigorous babe.

11. **Hot Fomentations.**—Applying flannel cloths wrung out of simple or medicated hot water is a great relief for acute suffering, such as neuralgia, rheumatic pain, biliousness, constipation, torpid liver, colic, flatulency, etc.

12. **The Hot Water-Bag.**—The hot water-bag serves the same purpose as hot fomentations, and is much more convenient. No one should go through the period of gestation without a hot water-bag.

13. **The Cold Compress.**—This is a very desirable and effectual domestic remedy. Take a towel wrung from cold water and apply it to the affected parts; then cover well [306]with several thicknesses of flannel. This is excellent in cases of sore throat, hoarseness, bronchitis, inflammation of the lungs, croup, etc. It is also excellent for indigestion, constipation or distress of the bowels accompanied by heat.

14. **Diet.**—The pregnant woman should eat nutritious, but not stimulating or heating food, and eat at the regular time. Avoid drinking much while eating.

15. **Avoid** salt, pepper and sweets as much as possible.

16. **Eat** all kinds of grains, vegetables and fruits, and avoid salted meat, but eat chicken, steak, fish, oysters, etc.

17. **The Woman Who Eats Indiscriminately** anything and everything the same as any other person, will have a very painful labor and suffer many ills that could easily be avoided by more attention being paid to the diet. With a little study and observation a woman will soon learn what to eat and what to avoid.

Nature Versus Corsets Illustrated.

18. The above cuts are given on page 105; we repeat them here for the benefit of expectant mothers who may be ignorant of the evil effects of the corset.[307]

Displacement of the womb, interior irritation and inflammation, miscarriage and sterility, are some of the many injuries of tight lacing. There are many others, in fact their name is legion, and every woman who has habitually worn a corset and continues to wear it during the early period of gestation must suffer severely during childbirth.

A Contracted Pelvis. Deformity and Insufficient Space.

"The House We Live In" for nine months: showing the ample room provided by Nature when uncontracted by inherited inferiority of form or artificial dressing.

[308]

19. **This is what Dr. Stockham** says: "If women had *common sense*, instead of *fashion sense*, the corset would not exist. There are not words in the English language to express my convictions upon this subject. The corset more than any other one thing is responsible for woman's being the victim of disease and doctors....

"What is the effect upon the child? One-half of the children born in this country die before they are five years of age. Who can tell how much this state of things is due to the enervation of maternal life forces by the one instrument of torture?

"I am a temperance woman. No one can realize more than I the devastation and ruin alcohol in its many tempting forms has brought to the human family. Still I solemnly believe that in weakness and deterioration of health, the corset has more to answer for than intoxicating drinks." When asked how far advanced a woman should be in pregnancy before she laid aside her corset, Dr. Stockham said with emphasis: "*The corset should not be worn for two hundred years before pregnancy takes place.* Ladies, it will take that time at least to overcome the ill-effect of tight garments which you think so essential."

20. **Painless Pregnancy and Child-Birth.**—"Some excellent popular volumes," says Dr. Haff, "have been largely devoted to directions how to secure a comfortable period of pregnancy and painless delivery. After much conning of these worthy efforts to impress a little common sense upon the sisterhood, we are convinced that all may be summed up under the simple heads of: (1) An unconfined and lightly burdened waist; (2) Moderate but persistent outdoor exercise, of which walking is the best form; (3) A plain, unstimulating, chiefly fruit and vegetable diet; (4) Little or no intercourse during the time.

"These are hygienic rules of benefit under any ordinary conditions; yet they are violated by almost every pregnant lady. If they are followed, biliousness, indigestion, constipation, swollen limbs, morning sickness and nausea—all will absent themselves or be much lessened. In pregnancy, more than at any other time, corsets are injurious. The waist and abdomen must be allowed to expand freely with the growth of the child. The great process of *evolution* must have room."

21. **In Addition**, we can do no better than quote the following recapitulation by Dr. Stockham in her famous [309]Tokology: "To give a woman the greatest immunity from suffering during pregnancy, prepare her for a safe and comparatively easy delivery, and insure a speedy recovery, all hygienic conditions must be observed.

"The dress must give:

"1. Freedom of movement;

"2. No pressure upon any part of the body;

"3. No more weight than is essential for warmth, and both weight and warmth evenly distributed.

"These requirements necessitate looseness, lightness and warmth, which can be obtained from the union underclothes, a princess skirt and dress, with a shoe that allows full development and use of the foot. While decoration and elegance are desirable, they should not sacrifice comfort and convenience.

22. **"Let the Diet Be Light**, plain and nutritious. Avoid fats and sweets, relying mainly upon fruits and grain that contain little of the mineral salts. By this diet bilious and inflammatory conditions are overcome, the development of bone in the fœtus lessened, and muscles necessary in labor nourished and strengthened.

23. **"Exercise** should be sufficient and of such a character as will bring into action gently every muscle of the body; but must particularly develop the muscles of the trunk, abdomen and groin, that are specially called into action in labor. Exercise, taken faithfully and systematically, more than any other means assists assimilative processes and stimulates the organs of excretion to healthy action.

24. **"Bathing Must Be Frequent** and regular. Unless in special conditions the best results are obtained from tepid or cold bathing, which invigorates the system and overcomes nervousness. The sitz-bath is the best therapeutic and hygienic measure within the reach of the pregnant woman.

"Therefore, to establish conditions which will overcome many previous infractions of law, *dress* naturally and physiologically; *live* much of the time *out of doors*; have *abundance* of *fresh air* in the house; let *exercise* be *sufficient* and *systematic*; pursue a *diet of fruit*, rice and vegetables; *regular rest* must be faithfully taken; *abstain* from the sexual relation. To those who will commit themselves to this course of life, patiently and persistently carrying it out through the period of gestation, the possibilities of attaining a healthy, natural, painless parturition will be remarkably increased.[310]

25. **"If the First Experiment** should not result in a painless labor, it without doubt will prove the beginning of sound health. Persisted in through years of married life, the ultimate result will be more and more closely approximated, while there will be less danger of diseases after childbirth and better and more vigorous children will be produced.

"Then pregnancy by every true woman will be desired, and instead of being a period of disease, suffering and direful forebodings, will become a period of health, exalted pleasure and holiest anticipations. Motherhood will be deemed the choicest of earth's blessings; women will rejoice in a glad maternity and for any self-denial will be compensated by healthy, happy, buoyant, grateful children."

[311]

A HAPPY MOTHER.

[312]

Solemn Lessons for Parents.
JOAN OF ARC.

1. **Excessive Pleasures and Pains.**—A woman during her time of pregnancy should of all women be most carefully tended, and kept from violent and excessive pleasures and pains; and at that time she should cultivate gentleness, benevolence and kindness.[313]

2. **Hereditary Effects.**—Those who are born to become insane do not necessarily spring from insane parents, or from any ancestry having any apparent taint of lunacy in their blood, but they do receive from their progenitors certain impressions upon their mental and moral, as well as their physical beings, which impressions, like an iron mould, fix and shape their subsequent destinies. Hysteria in the mother may develop insanity in the child, while drunkenness in the father may impel epilepsy, or mania, in the son. Ungoverned passions in the parents may unloose the furies of unrestrained madness in the minds of their children, and the bad treatment of the wife may produce sickly or weak-minded children.

3. **The influence of predominant passion** may be transmitted from the parent to the child, just as surely as similarity of looks. It has been truly said that "the faculties which predominate in power and activity in the parents, when the organic existence of the child commences, determine its future mental disposition." A bad mental condition of the mother may produce serious defects upon her unborn child.

4. **The singular effects** produced on the unborn child by the sudden mental emotions of the mother are remarkable examples of a kind of electrotyping on the sensitive surfaces of living forms. It is doubtless true that the mind's action in such cases may increase

121

or diminish the molecular deposits in the several portions of the system. The precise place which each separate particle assumes in the new organic structure may be determined by the influence of thought or feeling. Perfect love and perfect harmony should exist between wife and husband during this vital period.

5. **An Illustration.**—If a sudden and powerful emotion of a woman's mind exerts such an influence upon her stomach as to excite vomiting, and upon her heart as almost to arrest its motion and induce fainting, can we believe that it will have no effect upon her womb and the fragile being contained within it? Facts and reason then, alike demonstrate the reality of the influence, and much practical advantage would result to both parent and child, were the conditions and extent of its operations better understood.

6. **Pregnant women** should not be exposed to causes likely to distress or otherwise strongly impress their minds. A consistent life with worthy objects constantly kept in mind should be the aim and purpose of every expectant mother.[314]

CASES CITED.

We selected only a few cases to illustrate the above statement. Thousands of cases occur every year that might be cited to illustrate these principles. A mother cannot be too careful, and she should have the hearty co-operation and assistance of her husband. We quote the following cases from Dr. Pancoast's Medical Guide, who is no doubt one of the best authorities on the subject.

1. A woman bitten on the vulva by a dog, bore a child having a similar wound on the glans penis. The boy suffered from epilepsy, and when the fit came on, or during sleep, was frequently heard to cry out, "The dog bites me!"

2. A pregnant woman who was suddenly alarmed from seeing her husband come home with one side of his face swollen and distorted by a blow, bore a girl with a purple swelling upon the same side of the face.

3. A woman, who was forced to be present at the opening of a calf by a butcher, bore a child with all its bowels protruding from the abdomen. She was aware at the time of something going on within the womb.

4. A pregnant woman fell into a violent passion at not being able to procure a particular piece of meat of a butcher; she bled at the nose, and wiping the blood from her lips, bore a child wanting a lip.

5. A woman absent from home became alarmed by seeing a great fire in the direction of her own house, bore a child with a distinct mark of the flame upon its forehead.

6. A woman who had borne healthy children, became frightened by a beggar with a wooden leg and a stumped arm, who threatened to embrace her. Her next child had one stump leg and two stump arms.

7. A woman frightened in her first pregnancy by the sight of a child with a hare lip, had a child with a deformity of the same kind. Her second child had a deep slit, and the third a mark of a similar character or modified hare lips. In this instance the morbid mind of the mother affected several successive issues of her body.

8. A pregnant woman became frightened at a lizard jumping into her bosom. She bore a child with a fleshy excrescence exactly resembling a lizard, growing from the breast, adhering by the head and neck.

[315]

The Care of New-Born Infants.

1. The first thing to be done ordinarily is to give the little stranger a bath by using soap and warm water. To remove the white material that usually covers the child use olive oil, goose oil or lard, and apply it with a soft piece of worn flannel, and when the child is entirely clean rub all off with a fresh piece of flannel.

2. Many physicians in the United States recommend a thorough oiling of the child with pure lard or olive oil, and then rub dry as above stated. By these means water is avoided, and with it much risk of taking cold.

3. The application of brandy or liquor is entirely unnecessary, and generally does more injury than good.[316]

4. If an infant should breathe feebly, or exhibit other signs of great feebleness, it should not be washed at once, but allowed to remain quiet and undisturbed, warmly wrapped up until the vital actions have acquired a fair degree of activity.

5. **Dressing the Navel.**—There is nothing better for dressing the navel than absorbent antiseptic cotton. There needs be no grease or oil upon the cotton. After the separation of the cord the navel should be dressed with a little cosmoline, still using the absorbent cotton. The navel string usually separates in a week's time; it may be delayed for twice this length of time, this will make no material difference, and the rule is to allow it to drop off of its own accord.

6. **The Clothing of the Infant.**—The clothing of the infant should be light, soft and *perfectly* loose. A soft flannel band is necessary *only* until the navel is healed. Afterwards discard bands entirely if you wish your babe to be happy and well. Make the dresses "Mother Hubbard"—Put on first a soft woolen shirt, then prepare the flannel skirts to hang from the neck like a slip. Make one kind with sleeves and one just like it without sleeves, then white muslin skirts (if they are desired), all the same way. Then baby is ready for any weather. In intense heat simply put on the one flannel slip with sleeves, leaving off the shirt. In Spring and Fall the shirt and skirt with no sleeves. In cold weather shirt and both skirts. These garments can be all put on at once, thus making the process of dressing very quick and easy. These are the most approved modern styles for dressing infants, and with long cashmere stockings pinned to the diapers the little feet are free to kick with no old-fashioned pinning blanket to torture the naturally active, healthy child, and retard its development. If tight bands are an injury to grown people, then in the name of pity emancipate the poor little infant from their torture!

7. **The Diaper.**—Diapers should be of soft linen, and great care should be exercised not to pin them too tightly. Never dry them, but always wash them thoroughly before being used again.

8. The band need not be worn after the navel has healed so that it requires no dressing, as it serves no purpose save to keep in place the dressing of the navel. The child's body should be kept thoroughly warm around the chest, bowels and feet. Give the heart and lungs plenty of room to heave.

9. The proper time for shortening the clothes is about three months in Summer and six months in Winter.[317]

10. **Infant Bathing.**—The first week of a child's life it should not be entirely stripped and washed. It is too exhausting. After a child is over a week old it should be bathed every day; after a child is three weeks old it may be put in the water and supported with one hand while it is being washed with the other. Never, however, allow it to remain too long in the water. From ten to twenty minutes is the limit. Use Pears' soap or castile soap, and with a sponge wipe quickly, or use a soft towel.

NURSING.

1. The new-born infant requires only the mother's milk. The true mother will nurse her child if it is a possibility. The infant will thrive better and have many more chances for life.

2. The mother's milk is the natural food, and nothing can fully take its place. It needs no feeding for the first few days as it was commonly deemed necessary a few years ago. The secretions in the mother's breast are sufficient.

3. **Artificial Food.**—Tokology says: "The best artificial food is cream reduced and sweetened with sugar of milk. Analysis shows that human milk contains more cream and sugar and less casein than the milk of animals.[318]

4. Milk should form the basis of all preparations of food. If the milk is too strong, indigestion will follow, and the child will lose instead of gaining strength.

Weaning.—The weaning of the child depends much upon the strength and condition of the mother. If it does not occur in hot weather, from nine to twelve months is as long as any child should be nursed.

123

Food in Weaning.—Infants cry a great deal during weaning, but a few days of patient perseverance will overcome all difficulties. Give the child purely a milk diet, Graham bread, milk crackers and milk, or a little milk thickened with boiled rice, a little jelly, apple sauce, etc., may be safely used. Cracked wheat, oatmeal, wheat germ, or anything of that kind thoroughly cooked and served with a little cream and sugar, is an excellent food.

Milk Drawn from the Breasts.—If the mother suffers considerably from the milk gathering in the breast after weaning the child, withdraw it by taking a bottle that holds about a pint or a quart, putting a piece of cloth wrung out in warm water around the bottle, then fill it with boiling water, pour the water out and apply the bottle to the breast, and the bottle cooling will form a vacuum and will withdraw the milk into the bottle. This is one of the best methods now in use.

Return of the Menses.—If the menses return while the mother is nursing, the child should at once be weaned, for the mother's milk no longer contains sufficient nourishment. In case the mother should become pregnant while the child is nursing it should at once be weaned, or serious results will follow to the health of the child. A mother's milk is no longer sufficiently rich to nourish the child or keep it in good health.

Care of the Bottle.—If the child is fed on the bottle, great care should be taken in keeping it absolutely clean. Never use white rubber nipples. A plain form of bottle with a black rubber nipple is preferable.

CHILDREN should not be permitted to come to the table until two years of age.

Chafing.—One of the best remedies is powdered lycopodium; apply it every time the babe is cleaned; but first wash with pure castile soap; Pears' soap is also good. A preparation of oxide of zinc is also highly recommended. Chafing sometimes results from an acid condition of the stomach; in that case give a few doses of castoria.

Colic.—If an infant is seriously troubled with colic, there is nothing better than camomile or catnip tea. Procure the leaves and make tea and give it as warm as the babe can bear.

[319]

FEEDING INFANTS.

1. The best food for infants is mother's milk; next best is cow's milk. Cow's milk contains about three times as much curd and one-half as much sugar, and it should be reduced with two parts of water.

2. In feeding cow's milk there is too little cream and too little sugar, and there is no doubt no better preparation than Mellin's food to mix it with (according to directions).

3. Children being fed on food lacking fat generally have their teeth come late; their muscles will be flabby and bones soft. Children will be too fat when their food contains too much sugar. Sugar always makes their flesh soft and flabby.

4. During the first two months the baby should be fed every two hours during the day, and two or three times during the night, but no more. Ten or eleven feedings for twenty-four hours are all a child will bear and remain healthy. At three months the child may be fed every three hours instead of every two.

5. Children can be taught regular habits by being fed and put to sleep at the same time every day and evening. Nervous diseases are caused by irregular hours of sleep and diet, and the use of soothing medicines.

6. A child five or six months old should not be fed during the night—from nine in the evening until six or seven in the morning, as overfeeding causes most of the wakefulness and nervousness of children during the night.

7. If a child vomits soon after taking the bottle, and there is an appearance of undigested food in the stool, it is a sign of overfeeding. If a large part of the bottle has been vomited, avoid the next bottle at regular time and pass over one bottle. If the child is nursing the same principles apply.

8. If a child empties its bottle and sucks vigorously its fingers after the bottle is emptied, it is very evident that the child is not fed enough, and should have its food gradually increased.

9. Give the baby a little cold water several times a day.

INFANTILE CONVULSIONS.

Definition.—An infantile convulsion corresponds to a chill in an adult, and is the most common brain affection among children.

Causes.—Anything that irritates the nervous system may cause convulsions in the child, as teething, indigestible food, worms, dropsy of the brain, hereditary constitution, or they may be the accompanying symptom in nearly all the [320]acute diseases of children, or when the eruption is suppressed in eruptive diseases.

Symptoms.—In case of convulsions of a child parents usually become frightened, and very rarely do the things that should be done in order to afford relief. The child, previous to the fit, is usually irritable, and the twitching of the muscles of the face may be noticed, or it may come on suddenly without warning. The child becomes insensible, clenches its hands tightly, lips turn blue, and the eyes become fixed, usually frothing from the mouth with head turned back. The convulsion generally lasts two or three minutes; sometimes, however, as long as ten or fifteen minutes, but rarely.

Remedy.—Give the child a warm bath and rub gently. Clothes wrung out of cold water and applied to the lower and back part of the head and plenty of fresh air will usually relieve the convulsion. Be sure and loosen the clothing around the child's neck. After the convulsion is over, give the child a few doses of potassic bromide, and an injection of castor oil if the abdomen is swollen. Potassic bromide should be kept in the house, to use in case of necessity.

[321]
Pains and Ills in Nursing.
The City Hospital.—A Homeless and Friendless Mother.

1. **Sore Nipples.**—If a lady, during the latter few months of her pregnancy, were to adopt "means to harden the nipples," sore nipples during the period of suckling would not be so prevalent as they are.

2. **Cause.**—A sore nipple is frequently produced by the injudicious custom of allowing the child to have the nipple [322]almost constantly in his mouth. Another frequent cause of a sore nipple is from the babe having the canker. Another cause of a sore nipple is from the mother, after the babe has been sucking, putting up the nipple wet. She, therefore, ought always to dry the nipple, not by rubbing, but by dabbing it with a soft cambric or lawn handkerchief, or with a piece of soft linen rag—one or the other of which ought always to be at hand—every time directly after the child has done sucking, and just before applying any of the following powders or lotions to the nipple.

3. **Remedies.**—One of the best remedies for a sore nipple is the following powder:
Take of—Borax, one drachm; Powdered Starch, seven drachms.
Mix.—A pinch of the powder to be frequently applied to the nipple.
If the above does not cure, try Glycerine by applying it each time after nursing.

4. **Gathered Breast.**—A healthy-woman with a well-developed breast and a good nipple, scarcely, if ever, has a gathered bosom; it is the delicate, the ill-developed breasted and worse-developed nippled lady who usually suffers from this painful complaint. And why? The evil can generally be traced to girlhood. If she be brought up luxuriously, her health and her breasts are sure to be weakened, and thus to suffer, more especially if the development of the bosoms and nipples has been arrested and interfered with by tight stays and corsets. Why, the nipple is by them drawn in, and retained on the level with the breast—countersunk—as though it were of no consequence to her future well-being, as though it were a thing of nought.

5. **Tight Lacers.**—Tight lacers will have to pay the penalties of which they little dream. Oh, the monstrous folly of such proceedings! When will mothers awake from their lethargy! It is high time that they did so! From the mother having "no nipple," the effects of tight lacing, many a home has been made childless, the babe not being able to procure its proper nourishment, and dying in consequence! It is a frightful state of things! But fashion, unfortunately, blinds the eyes and deafens the ears of its votaries!

6. **Bad Breast.**—A gathered bosom, or "bad breast," as it is sometimes called, is more likely to occur after a first confinement and during the first month. Great care, therefore, ought to be taken to avoid such a misfortune. A gathered breast is frequently owing to the carelessness of a [323]mother in not covering her bosoms during the time she is suckling. Too much attention cannot be paid to keeping the breasts comfortably warm. This, during the act of nursing, should be done by throwing either a shawl or a square of flannel over the neck, shoulders, and bosoms.

7. **Another Cause.**—Another cause of gathered breasts arises from a mother sitting up in bed to suckle her babe. He ought to be accustomed to take the bosom while she is lying down; if this habit is not at first instituted, it will be difficult to adopt it afterwards. Good habits may be taught a child from earliest babyhood.

8. **Faintness.**—When a nursing mother feels faint, she ought immediately to lie down and take a little nourishment; a cup of tea with the yolk of an egg beaten up in it, or a cup of warm milk, or some beef-tea, any of which will answer the purpose extremely well. Brandy, or any other spirit we would not recommend, as it would only cause, as soon as the immediate effects of the stimulant had gone off, a greater depression to ensue; not only so, but the frequent taking of brandy might become a habit—a necessity—which would be a calamity deeply to be deplored!

9. **Strong Purgatives.**—Strong purgatives during this period are highly improper, as they are apt to give pain to the infant, as well as to injure the mother. If it be absolutely necessary to give physic, the mildest, such as a dose of castor oil, should be chosen.

10. **Habitually Costive.**—When a lady who is nursing is habitually costive, she ought to eat brown instead of white bread. This will, in the majority of cases, enable her to do without an aperient. The brown bread may be made with flour finely ground all one way; or by mixing one part of bran and three parts of fine wheaten flour together, and then making it in the usual way into bread. Treacle instead of butter, on the brown bread increases its efficacy as an aperient; and raw should be substituted for lump sugar in her tea.

11. **To Prevent Constipation.**—Stewed prunes, or stewed French plums, or stewed Normandy pippins, are excellent remedies to prevent constipation. The patient ought to eat, every morning, a dozen or fifteen of them. The best way to stew either prunes or French plums, is the following:—Put a pound of either prunes or French plums, and two tablespoonfuls of raw sugar, into a brown jar; cover them with water; put them into a slow oven, and stew them for three or four hours. Both stewed rhubarb and stewed [324]pears often act as mild and gentle aperients. Muscatel raisins, eaten at dessert, will oftentimes without medicine relieve the bowels.

12. **Cold Water.**—A tumblerful of cold water, taken early every morning, sometimes effectually relieves the bowels; indeed, few people know the value of cold water as an aperient—it is one of the best we possess, and, unlike drug aperients, can never by any possibility do any harm. An injection of warm water is one of the best ways to relieve the bowels.

13. **Well-Cooked Vegetables.**—Although a nursing mother ought, more especially if she be costive, to take a variety of well-cooked vegetables, such as potatoes, asparagus, cauliflower, French beans, spinach, stewed celery and turnips; she should avoid eating greens, cabbages, and pickles, as they would be likely to affect the babe, and might cause him to suffer from gripings, from pain, and "looseness" of the bowels.

14. **Supersede the Necessity of Taking Physic.**—Let me again—for it cannot be too urgently insisted upon—strongly advise a nursing mother to use every means in the way of diet, etc., to supersede the necessity of taking physic (opening medicine), as the repetition of aperients injures, and that severely, both herself and child. Moreover, the more opening medicine she swallows, the more she requires; so that if she once gets into the habit of regularly taking physic, the bowels will not act without them. What a miserable existence to be always swallowing physic!

[325]

Home Lessons in Nursing Sick Children.
HEALTHY YOUTH AND RIPE OLD AGE.

1. **Mismanagement.**—Every doctor knows that a large share of the ills to which infancy is subject are directly traceable to mismanagement. Troubles of the digestive system are, for the most part due to errors, either in the selection of the food or in the preparation of it.

2. **Respiratory Diseases.**—Respiratory diseases or the diseases of the throat and lungs have their origin, as a rule, in want of care and judgment in matters of clothing, bathing and exposure to cold and drafts. A child should always be dressed to suit the existing temperature of the weather.[326]

3. **Nervous Diseases.**—Nervous diseases are often aggravated if not caused by over-stimulation of the brain, by irregular hours of sleep, or by the use of "soothing" medicines, or eating indigestible food.

4. **Skin Affections.**—Skin affections are generally due to want of proper care of the skin, to improper clothing or feeding, or to indiscriminate association with nurses and children, who are the carriers of contagious diseases.

5. **Permanent Injury.**—Permanent injury is often caused by lifting the child by one hand, allowing it to fall, permitting it to play with sharp instruments, etc.

6. **Rules and Principles.**—Every mother should understand the rules and principles of home nursing. Children are very tender plants and the want of proper knowledge is often very disastrous if not fatal. Study carefully and follow the principles and rules which are laid down in the different parts of this work on nursing and cooking for the sick.

7. **What a Mother Should Know:**

I. INFANT FEEDING.—The care of milk, milk sterilization, care of bottles, preparation of commonly employed infant foods, the general principles of infant feeding, with rules as to quality and frequency.

II. BATHING.—The daily bath; the use of hot, cold and mustard baths.

III. HYGIENE OF THE SKIN. Care of the mouth, eyes and ears. Ventilation, temperature, cleanliness, care of napkins, etc.

IV. TRAINING OF CHILDREN in proper bodily habits. Simple means of treatment in sickness, etc.

8. **The Cry of the Sick Child.**—The cry of the child is a language by which the character of its suffering to some extent may be ascertained. The manner in which the cry is uttered, or the pitch and tone is generally a symptom of a certain kind of disease.

9. **Stomachache.**—The cry of the child in suffering with pain of the stomach is loud, excitable and spasmodic. The legs are drawn up and as the pain ceases, they are relaxed and the child sobs itself to sleep, and rests until awakened again by pain.

10. **Lung Trouble.**—When a child is suffering with an affection of the lungs or throat, it never cries loudly or continuously. A distress in breathing causes a sort of subdued cry and low moaning. If there is a slight cough it is generally a sign that there is some complication with the lungs.[327]

11. **Disease of the Brain.**—In disease of the brain the cry is always sharp, short and piercing. Drowsiness generally follows each spasm of pain.

12. **Fevers.**—Children rarely cry when suffering with fever unless they are disturbed. They should be handled very gently and spoken to in a very quiet and tender tone of voice.

13. **The Chamber of the Sick Room.**—The room of the sick child should be kept scrupulously clean. No noise should disturb the quiet and rest of the child. If the weather is mild, plenty of fresh air should be admitted; the temperature should be kept at about 70 degrees. A thermometer should be kept in the room, and the air should be changed several times during the day. This may be done with safety to the child by covering it up with woolen blankets to protect it from draft, while the windows and doors are opened. Fresh air often does more to restore the sick child than the doctor's medicine. Take the best room in the house. If necessary take the parlor, always make the room pleasant for the sick.

14. **Visitors.**—Carefully avoid the conversation of visitors or the loud and boisterous playing of children in the house. If there is much noise about the house that cannot be avoided, it is a good plan to put cotton in the ears of the patient.

15. **Light in the Room.**—Light has a tendency to produce nervous irritability, consequently it is best to exclude as much daylight as possible and keep the room in a sort of

127

twilight until the child begins to improve. Be careful to avoid any odor coming from a burning lamp in the night. When the child begins to recover, give it plenty of sunlight. After the child begins to get better let in all the sunlight the windows will admit. Take a south room for the sick bed.

16. **Sickness in Summer.**—If the weather is very hot it is a good plan to dampen the floors with cold water, or set several dishes of water in the room, but be careful to keep the patient out of the draft, and avoid any sudden change of temperature.

17. **Bathing.**—Bathe every sick child in warm water once a day unless prohibited by the doctor. If the child has a spasm or any attack of a serious nervous character in absence of the doctor, place him in a hot bath at once. Hot water is one of the finest agencies for the cure of nervous diseases.[328]

18. **Scarlet Fever and Measles.**—Bathe the child in warm water to bring out the rash, and put in about a dessertspoonful of mustard into each bath.

19. **Drinks.**—If a child is suffering with fevers, let it have all the water it wants. Toast-water will be found nourishing. When the stomach of the child is in an irritable condition, nourishments containing milk or any other fluid should be given very sparingly. Barley-water and rice-water are very soothing to an irritable stomach.

20. **Food.**—Mellin's Food and milk is very nourishing if the child will take it. Oatmeal gruel, white of eggs, etc. are excellent and nourishing articles. See "How to cook for the Sick."

21. **Eating Fruit.**—Let children who are recovering from sickness eat moderately of good fresh fruit. Never let a child, whether well or sick, eat the skins of any kind of fruit. The outer covering of fruit was not made to eat, and often has poisonous matter very injurious to health upon its surface. Contagious and infectious diseases are often communicated in that way.

22. **Sudden Startings** with the thumbs drawn into the palms, portend trouble with the brain, and often end in convulsions, which are far more serious in infants than in children. Convulsions in children often result from a suppression of urine. If you have occasion to believe that such is the case, get the patient to sweating as soon as possible. Give it a hot bath, after which cover it up in bed and put bags of hot salt over the lower part of the abdomen.

23. **Symptoms of Indigestion.**—If the baby shows symptoms of indigestion, do not begin giving it medicine. It is wiser to decrease the quantity and quality of the food and let the little one omit one meal entirely, that his stomach may rest. Avoid all starchy foods, as the organs of digestion are not sufficiently developed to receive them.

[329]

A Practical Rule for Feeding a Baby on Cow's Milk.

Cow's milk is steadily growing in favor as an artificial food. Country milk should be used instead of milk purchased in town or city.

RULE—Take the upper half of milk that has stood an hour of two, dilute, not hardly as much as a third, with sweetened water, and if there is a tendency to sour stomach, put in a teaspoonful of lime water to every quart. The milk and water should both be boiled separately. If the baby is constipated, it is best to heat the milk over boiling water and not allow it to boil.

INFANT FOOD FOR 24 HOURS.

Age of Child.	Milk.	Water.	Total.
2 to 10 days	1 ¼ gills	3 ¼ gills	4 ½ gills
10 to 20 days	1 ¾ gills	4 ¼ gills	6 gills
20 to 30 days	2	6	8

128

	½ gills	gills	½ gills
1 to 1½ months	3 gills	6 ¾ gills	9 ¾ gills
1½ to 2 months	3 ½ gills	7 gills	1 0½ gills
2 to 2½ months	4 gills	7 ½ gills	1 1½ gills
2½ to 3 months	4 ½ gills	7 ½ gills	1 2 gills
3 to 3½ months	5 gills	7 ½ gills	1 2½ gills
3½ to 4 months	5 ½ gills	7 ½ gills	1 3 gills
4 to 4½ months	6 gills	7 ½ gills	1 3½ gills
4½ to 5 months	6 ½ gills	7 ½ gills	1 4 gills
5 to 6 months	7 gills	7 gills	1 4 gills
6½ to 7 months	7 ½ gills	6 ½ gills	1 4 gills
7 to 8 months	8 gills	6 gills	1 4 gills
8 to 9 months	8 ¼ gills	6 gills	1 4¼ gills
9 to 10 months	8 ½ gills	6 gills	1 4½ gills
10 to 11 months	8 ¾ gills	6 gills	1 4¾ gills
11 to 12 months	9 gills	5 ½ gills	1 4½ gills
12 to 15 months	9 ¼ gills	5 ¼ gills	1 4½ gills
15 to 18 months	9 ½ gills	5 gills	1 4½ gills
18 and more months	1 0 gills	5 gills	1 5 gills

[330]

HOW TO KEEP A BABY WELL.

A delicate child should never be put into the bath, but bathed on the lap and kept warmly covered.

1. The mother's milk is the natural food, and nothing can fully take its place.

2. The infant's stomach does not readily accommodate itself to changes in diet; therefore, regularity in quality, quantity and temperature is extremely necessary.

3. Not until a child is a year old should it be allowed any food except that of milk, and possibly a little cracker or bread, thoroughly soaked and softened.

4. Meat should never be given to very young children. The best artificial food is cream, reduced and sweetened with sugar and milk. No rule can be given for its reduction.

Observation and experience must teach that, because every child's stomach is governed by a rule of its own.

5. A child can be safely weaned at one year of age, and sometimes less. It depends entirely upon the season, and upon the health of the child.

6. A child should never be weaned during the warm weather, in June, July or August.

7. When a child is weaned it may be given, in connection [331]with the milk diet, some such nourishment as broth, gruel, egg, or some prepared food.

8. A child should never be allowed to come to the table until two years of age.

9. A child should never eat much starchy food until four years old.

10. A child should have all the water it desires to drink, but it is decidedly the best to boil the water first, and allow it to cool. All the impurities and disease germs are thereby destroyed. This one thing alone will add greatly to the health and vigor of the child.

11. Where there is a tendency to bowel disorder, a little gum arabic, rice, or barley may be boiled with the drinking water.

12. If the child uses a bottle it should be kept absolutely clean. It is best to have two or three bottles, so that one will always be perfectly clean and fresh.

13. The nipple should be of black or pure rubber, and not of the white or vulcanized rubber; it should fit over the top of the bottle. No tubes should ever be used; it is impossible to keep them clean.

14. When the rubber becomes coated, a little coarse salt will clean it.

15. Babies should be fed at regular times. They should also be put to sleep at regular hours. Regularity is one of the best safeguards to health.

16. Milk for babies and children should be from healthy cows. Milk from different cows varies, and it is always better for a child to have milk from the same cow. A farrow cow's milk is preferable, especially if the child is not very strong.

17. Many of the prepared foods advertised for children are of little benefit. A few may be good, but what is good for one child may not be for another. So it must be simply a matter of experiment if any of the advertised foods are used.

18. It is a physiological fact that an infant is always healthier and better to sleep alone. It gets better air and is not liable to suffocation.

19. A healthy child should never be fed in less than two hours from the last time they finished before, gradually lengthening the time as it grows older. At 4 months 3½ or 4 hours; at 5 months a healthy child will be better if given nothing in the night except, perhaps, a little water.

20. Give an infant a little water several times a day.

21. A delicate child the first year should be oiled after each bath. The oiling may often take the place of the bath, in case of a cold.

22. In oiling a babe, use pure olive oil, and wipe off thoroughly after each application. For nourishing a weak child use also olive oil.

23. For colds, coughs, croup, etc., use goose oil externally and give a teaspoonful at bed-time.

[332]
HOW TO PRESERVE THE HEALTH AND LIFE OF YOUR INFANT DURING HOT WEATHER.
FOUND UPON THE DOOR STEP.
BATHING.

1. Bathe infants daily in tepid water and even twice a day in hot weather.

If delicate they should be sponged instead of immersing them in water, but cleanliness is absolutely necessary for the health of infants.

CLOTHING.

2. Put no bands in their clothing, but make all garments to hang loosely from the shoulders, and have all their clothing *scrupulously clean*; even the diaper should not be re-used without rinsing.[333]

SLEEP ALONE.

3. The child should in all cases sleep by itself on a cot or in a crib and retire at a regular hour. A child *always* early taught to go to sleep without rocking or nursing is the healthier and happier for it. Begin *at birth* and this will be easily accomplished.

CORDIALS AND SOOTHING SYRUPS.

4. Never give cordials, soothing syrups, sleeping drops, etc., without the advice of a physician. A child that frets and does not sleep is either hungry or ill. *If ill it needs a physician.* Never give candy or cake to quiet a small child, they are sure to produce disorders of the stomach, diarrhœa or some other trouble.

FRESH AIR.

5. Children should have plenty of fresh air summer as well as winter. Avoid the severe hot sun and the heated kitchen for infants in summer. Heat is the great destroyer of infants. In excessive hot weather feed them with chips of ice occasionally, if you have it.

CLEAN HOUSES.

6. Keep your house clean and cool and well aired night and day. Your cellars cleared of all rubbish and whitewashed every spring, your drains cleaned with strong solution of copperas or chloride of lime, poured down them once a week. Keep your gutters and yards clean and insist upon your neighbors doing the same.

EVACUATIONS OF A CHILD.

The healthy motion varies from light orange yellow to greenish yellow, in number, two to four times daily. Smell should never be offensive. Slimy mucous-like jelly passages indicate worms. Pale green, offensive, acrid motions indicate disordered stomach. Dark green indicate acid secretions and a more serious trouble.

Fetid dark brown stools are present in chronic diarrhœa. Putty-like pasty passages are due to acidity curdling the milk or to torpid liver.[334]

BREAST MILK.

7. Breast milk is the only proper food for infants, until after the second summer. If the supply is small keep what you have and feed the child in connection with it, for if the babe is ill this breast milk may be all that will save its life.

STERILIZED MILK.

8. Milk is the best food. Goat's milk best, cows milk next. If the child thrives on this *nothing else* should be given during the hot weather, until the front teeth are cut. Get fresh cow's milk twice a day if the child requires food in the night, pour it into a glass fruit jar with one-third pure water for a child under three months old, afterwards the proportion of water may be less and less, also a trifle of sugar may be added.

Then place the jar in a kettle or pan of cold water, like the bottom of an oatmeal kettle. Leave the cover of the jar loose. Place it on the stove and let the water come to a boil and boil ten minutes, screw down the cover tight and boil ten minutes more, then remove from the fire, and allow it to cool in the water slowly so as not to break the jar. When partly cool put on the ice or in a cool place, and keep tightly covered except when the milk is poured out for use. The glass jar must be kept perfectly clean and washed [335]and scalded carefully before use. A tablespoonful of lime water to a bottle of milk will aid indigestion. Discard the bottle as soon as possible and use a cup which you know is clean, whereas a bottle must be kept in water constantly when not in use, or the sour milk will make the child sick. Use no tube for it is exceedingly hard to keep it clean, and if pure milk cannot be had, condensed milk is admirable and does not need to be sterilized as the above.

DIET.

9. Never give babies under two years old such food as grown persons eat. Their chief diet should be milk, wheat bread and milk, oatmeal, possibly a little rare boiled egg, but always and chiefly milk. Germ wheat is also excellent.

EXERCISE.

10. Children should have exercise in the house as well as outdoors, but should not be jolted and jumped and jarred in rough play, not rudely rocked in the cradle, nor carelessly trundled over bumps in their carriages. They should not be held too much in the arms, but allowed to crawl and kick upon the floor and develop their limbs and muscles. A child should not be lifted by its arms, nor dragged along by one hand after it learns to take a few

feeble steps, but when they do learn to walk steadily it is the best of all exercise, especially in the open air.

Let the children as they grow older romp and play in the open air all they wish, girls as well as boys. Give the girls an even chance for health, while they are young at least, and don't mind about their complexion.

[336]

Infant Teething.

1. **Remarkable Instances.**—There are instances where babies have been born with teeth, and, on the other hand, there are cases of persons who have never had any teeth at all; and others that had double teeth all around in both upper and lower jaws, but these are rare instances, and may be termed as a sort of freaks of nature.

2. **Infant Teething.**—The first teeth generally make their appearance after the third month, and during the period of teething the child is fretful and restless, causing sometimes constitutional disturbances, such as diarrhœa, indigestion, etc. Usually, however, no serious results follow, and no unnecessary anxiety need be felt, unless the weather is extremely warm, then there is some danger of summer complaint setting in and seriously complicating matters.

3. **The Number of Teeth.**—Teeth are generally cut in pairs and make their appearance first in the front and going backwards until all are complete. It generally takes about [337]two years for a temporary set of children's teeth. A child two or three years old should have twenty teeth. After the age of seven they generally begin to loosen and fall out and permanent teeth take their place.

4. **Lancing the Gums.**—This is very rarely necessary. There are extreme cases when the condition of the mouth and health of the child demand a physician's lance but this should not be resorted to, unless it is absolutely necessary. When the gums are very much swollen and the tooth is nearly through, the pains may be relieved by the mother taking a thimble and pressing it down upon the tooth, the sharp edges of the tooth will cut through the swollen flesh, and instant relief will follow. A child in a few hours or a day will be perfectly happy after a very severe and trying time of sickness.

5. **Permanent Teeth.**—The teeth are firmly inserted in sockets of the upper and lower jaw. The permanent teeth which follow the temporary teeth, when complete, are sixteen in each jaw, or thirty-two in all.

6. **Names of Teeth.**—There are four incisors (front teeth), four cuspids (eye teeth), four bicuspids (grinders), and four molars (large grinders), in each jaw. Each tooth is divided into the crown, body, and root. The crown is the grinding surface; the body—the part projecting from the jaw—is the seat of sensation and nutrition; the root is that portion of the tooth which is inserted in the alveolus. The teeth are composed of dentine (ivory) and enamel. The ivory forms the greater portion of the body and root, while the enamel covers the exposed surface. The small white cords communicating with the teeth are the nerves.

[338]

HOME TREATMENT FOR THE DISEASES OF INFANTS AND CHILDREN.

1. Out of the 984,000 persons that died during the year of 1890, 227,264 did not reach one year of age, and 400,647 died under five years of age.

What a fearful responsibility therefore rests upon the parents who permit these hundreds of thousands of children to die annually. This terrible mortality among children is undoubtedly largely the result of ignorance as regarding to the proper care and treatment of sick children.

2. For very small children it is always best to use homœopathic remedies.

COLIC.

1. Babies often suffer severely with colic. It is not considered dangerous, but causes considerable suffering.

132

2. Severe colic is usually the result of derangement of the liver in the mother, or of her insufficient or improper nourishment, and it occurs more frequently when the child is from two to five months old.[339]

3. Let the mother eat chiefly barley, wheat and bread, rolled wheat, graham bread, fish, milk, eggs and fruit. The latter may be freely eaten, avoiding that which is very sour.

4. A rubber bag or bottle filled with hot water put into a crib, will keep the child, once quieted, asleep for hours. If a child is suffering from colic, it should be thoroughly warmed and kept warm.

5. Avoid giving opiates of any kind, such as cordials, Mrs. Winslow's Soothing Syrup, "Mother's Friend," and various other patent medicines. They injure the stomach and health of the child, instead of benefiting it.

6. REMEDIES.—A few tablespoonfuls of hot water will often allay a severe attack of the colic. Catnip tea is also a good remedy.

A drop of essence of peppermint in 6 or 7 teaspoonfuls of hot water will give relief.

If the stools are green and the child is very restless, give chamomilla.

If the child is suffering from constipation, and undigested curds of milk appear in its fæces, and the child starts suddenly in its sleep, give nux vomica.

An injection of a few spoonfuls of hot water into the rectum with a little asafœtida is an effective remedy, and will be good for an adult.

CONSTIPATION.

1. This is a very frequent ailment of infants. The first thing necessary is for the mother to regulate her diet.

2. If the child is nursed regularly and held out at the same time of each day, it will seldom be troubled with this complaint. Give plenty of *water*. Regularity of habit is the remedy. If this method fails, use a soap suppository. Make it by paring a piece of white castile soap round. It should be made about the size of a lead pencil, pointed at the end.

3. Avoid giving a baby drugs. Let the physician administer them if necessary.[340]

DIARRHŒA.

Great care should be exercised by parents in checking the diarrhœa of children. Many times serious diseases are brought on by parents being too hasty in checking this disorder of the bowels. It is an infant's first method of removing obstructions and overcoming derangements of the system.

SUMMER COMPLAINT.

1. Summer complaint is an irritation and inflammation of the lining membranes of the intestines. This may often be caused by teething, eating indigestible food, etc.

2. If the discharges are only frequent and yellow and not accompanied with pain, there is no cause for anxiety; but if the discharges are green, soon becoming gray, brown and sometimes frothy, having a mixture of phlegm, and sometimes containing food undigested, a physician had better be summoned.

3. For mild attacks the following treatment may be given:

1) Keep the child perfectly quiet and keep the room well aired.

2) Put a drop of tincture of camphor on a teaspoonful of sugar, mix thoroughly; then add 6 teaspoonfuls of hot water and give a teaspoonful of the mixture every ten minutes. This is indicated where the discharges are watery, and where there is vomiting and coldness of the feet and hands. Chamomilla is also an excellent remedy. Ipecac and nux vomica may also be given.

In giving homœopathic remedies, give 5 or 6 pellets every 2 or 3 hours.

3) The diet should be wholesome and nourishing.

FOR TEETHING.

If a child is suffering with swollen gums, is feverish, restless, and starts in its sleep, give nux vomica.[341]

WORMS.
PIN WORMS.

Pin worms and round worms are the most common in children. They are generally found in the lower bowels.

133

SYMPTOMS.—Restlessness, itching about the anus in the fore part of the evening, and worms in the fæces.

TREATMENT.—Give with a syringe an injection of a tablespoonful of linseed oil. Cleanliness is also very necessary.

ROUND WORMS.

A round worm is from six to sixteen inches in length, resembling the common earth worm. It inhabits generally the small intestines, but it sometimes enters the stomach and is thrown up by vomiting.

SYMPTOMS.—Distress, indigestion, swelling of the abdomen, grinding of the teeth, restlessness, and sometimes convulsions.

TREATMENT.—One teaspoonful of powdered wormseed mixed with a sufficient quantity of molasses, or spread on bread and butter.

Or, one grain of santonine every four hours for two or three days, followed by a brisk cathartic. Wormwood tea is also highly recommended.

SWAIM'S VERMIFUGE.

2 ounces wormseed,
1½ ounces valerian,
1½ ounces rhubarb,
1½ ounces pink-root,
1½ ounces white agaric.

Boil in sufficient water to yield 3 quarts of decoction, and add to it 30 drops of oil of tansy and 45 drops of oil of cloves, dissolved in a quart of rectified spirits. Dose, 1 teaspoonful at night.

ANOTHER EXCELLENT VERMIFUGE.

Oil of wormseed, 1 ounce,
Oil of anise, 1 ounce,
Castor oil, 1 ounce,
Tinct. of myrrh, 2 drops,
Oil of turpentine, 10 drops.

Mix thoroughly. Always shake well before using. Give 10 to 15 drops in cold coffee, once or twice a day.

[342]

HOW TO TREAT CROUP
SPASMODIC AND TRUE.
SPASMODIC CROUP.

DEFINITION.—A spasmodic closure of the glottis which interferes with respiration. Comes on suddenly and usually at night, without much warning. It is a purely nervous disease and may be caused by reflex nervous irritation from undigested food in the stomach or bowels, irritation of the gums in dentition, or from brain disorders.

SYMPTOMS.—Child awakens suddenly at night with suspended respiration or very difficult breathing. After a few respirations it cries out and then falls asleep quietly, or the attack may last an hour or so, when the face will become pale, veins in the neck become turgid and feet and hands contract spasmodically. In mild cases the attacks will only occur once during the night, but may recur on the following night.

HOME TREATMENT.—During the paroxysm dashing cold water in the face is a common remedy. To terminate the spasm and prevent its return give teaspoonful doses of[343]powdered alum. The syrup of squills is an old and tried remedy; give in 15 to 30 drop doses and repeat every 10 minutes till vomiting occurs. Seek out the cause if possible and remove it. It commonly lies in some derangement of the digestive organs.

TRUE CROUP.

DEFINITION.—This disease consists of an inflammation of the mucous membrane of the upper air passages, particularly of the larynx with the formation of a false membrane that obstructs the breathing. The disease is most common in children between the ages of two and seven years, but it may occur at any age.

SYMPTOMS.—Usually there are symptoms of a cold for three or four days previous to the attack. Marked hoarseness is observed in the evening with a ringing metallic cough and some difficulty in breathing, which increases and becomes somewhat paroxysmal till the face which was at first flushed becomes pallid and ashy in hue. The efforts at breathing become very great, and unless the child gets speedy relief it will die of suffocation.

HOME TREATMENT.—Patient should be kept in a moist warm atmosphere, and cold water applied to the neck early in the attack. As soon as the breathing seems difficult give a half to one teaspoonful of powdered alum in honey to produce vomiting and apply the remedies suggested in the treatment of diphtheria, as the two diseases are thought by many to be identical. When the breathing becomes labored and face becomes pallid, the condition is very serious and a physician should be called without delay.

SCARLET FEVER.

DEFINITION.—An eruptive contagious disease, brought about by direct exposure to those having the disease, or by contact with clothing, dishes, or other articles, used about the sick room.

The clothing may be disinfected by heating to a temperature of 230° Fahrenheit or by dipping in boiling water before washing.[344]

Dogs and cats will also carry the disease and should be kept from the house, and particularly from the sick room.

SYMPTOMS.—Chilly sensations or a decided chill, fever, headache, furred tongue, vomiting, sore throat, rapid pulse, hot dry skin and more or less stupor. In from 6 to 18 hours a fine red rash appears about the ears, neck and shoulders, which rapidly spreads to the entire surface of the body. After a few days, a scurf or branny scales will begin to form on the skin. These scales are the principal source of contagion.

HOME TREATMENT.

1. Isolate the patient from other members of the family to prevent the spread of the disease.

2. Keep the patient in bed and give a fluid diet of milk gruel, beef tea, etc., with plenty of cold water to drink.

3. Control the fever by sponging the body with tepid water, and relieve the pain in the throat by cold compresses, applied externally.

4. As soon as the skin shows a tendency to become scaly, apply goose grease or clean lard with a little boracic acid powder dusted in it, or better, perhaps, carbolized vaseline to relieve the itching and prevent the scales from being scattered about, and subjecting others to the contagion.

REGULAR TREATMENT.—A few drops of aconite every three hours to regulate the pulse, and if the skin be pale and circulation feeble, with tardy eruption, administer one to ten drops of tincture of belladonna, according to the age of the patient. At the end of third week, if eyes look puffy and feet swell, there is danger of Acute Bright's disease, and a physician should be consulted. If the case does not progress well under the home remedies suggested, a physician should be called at once.

WHOOPING COUGH.

DEFINITION.—This is a contagious disease which is known by a peculiar whooping sound in the cough. Considerable mucus is thrown off after each attack of spasmodic coughing.

SYMPTOMS.—It usually commences with the symptoms of a common cold in the head, some chilliness, feverishness, [345]restlessness, headache, a feeling of tightness across the chest, violent paroxysms of coughing, sometimes almost threatening suffocation, and accompanied with vomiting.

HOME TREATMENT.—Patient should eat plain food and avoid cold drafts and damp air, but keep in the open air as much as possible. A strong tea made of the tops of red clover is highly recommended. A strong tea made of chestnut leaves, sweetened with sugar, is also very good.

1 teaspoonful of powdered alum.
1 teaspoonful of syrup.

Mix in a tumbler of water, and give the child one teaspoonful every two or three hours. A kerosene lamp kept burning in the bed chamber at night is said to lessen the cough and shorten the course of the disease.

MUMPS.

DEFINITION.—This is a contagious disease causing the inflammation of the salivary glands, and is generally a disease of childhood and youth.

SYMPTOMS.—A slight fever, stiffness of the neck and lower jaw, swelling and soreness of the gland. It usually develops in four or five days and then begins to disappear.

HOME TREATMENT.—Apply to the swelling a hot poultice of cornmeal and bread and milk. A hop poultice is also excellent. Take a good dose of physic and rest carefully. A warm general bath, or mustard foot bath, is very good. Avoid exposure or cold drafts. If a bad cold is taken, serious results may follow.

MEASLES.

DEFINITION.—It is an eruptive, contagious disease, preceded by cough and other catarrhal symptoms for about four or five days. The eruption comes rapidly in small red spots, which are slightly raised.

SYMPTOMS.—A feeling of weakness, loss of appetite, some fever, cold in the head, frequent sneezing, watery eyes, dry cough and a hot skin. The disease takes effect nine or ten days after exposure.[346]

HOME TREATMENT.—Measles is not a dangerous disease in the child, but in an adult it is often very serious. In childhood very little medicine is necessary, but exposure must be carefully avoided, and the patient kept in bed, in a moderately warm room. The diet should be light and nourishing. Keep the room dark. If the eruption does not come out promptly, apply hot baths.

COMMON TREATMENT.—Two teaspoonfuls of spirits of nitre, one teaspoonful paregoric, one wineglassful of camphor water. Mix thoroughly, and give a teaspoonful in half a tea-cupful of water every two hours. To relieve the cough, if troublesome, flax seed tea, or infusion of slippery-elm bark, with a little lemon juice to render more palatable, will be of benefit.

CHICKEN POX.

DEFINITION.—This is a contagious, eruptive disease, which resembles to some extent small-pox. The pointed vesicles or pimples have a depression in the center in chicken-pox, and in small pox they do not.

SYMPTOMS.—Nine to seventeen days elapse after the exposure, before symptoms appear. Slight fever, a sense of sickness, the appearance of scattered pimples, some itching and heat. The pimples rapidly change into little blisters, filled with a watery fluid. After five or six days they disappear.

HOME TREATMENT.—Milk diet, and avoid all kinds of meat. Keep the bowels open, and avoid all exposure to cold. Large vesicles on the face should be punctured early, and irritation by rubbing should be avoided.

HOME TREATMENT OF DIPHTHERIA.

DEFINITION.—Acute, specific, constitutional disease, with local manifestations in the throat, mouth, nose, larynx, windpipe, and glands of the neck. The disease is infectious, but not very contagious under the proper precautions. It is a disease of childhood, though adults sometimes contract it. Many of the best physicians of the day consider true or membranous croup to be due to this diphtheritic membranous disease thus located in the larynx or trachea.[347]

SYMPTOMS.—Symptoms vary according to the severity of the attack. Chills, fever, headache, languor, loss of appetite, stiffness of neck, with tenderness about the angles of the jaw, soreness of the throat, pain in the ear, aching of the limbs, loss of strength, coated tongue, swelling of the neck, and offensive breath; lymphatic glands on side of neck enlarged and tender. The throat is first to be seen red and swollen, then covered with grayish white patches, which spread, and a false membrane is found on the mucous membrane. If the nose is attacked, there will be an offensive discharge, and the child will breathe through the mouth. If the larynx or throat are involved, the voice will become hoarse, and a croupy cough, with difficult breathing, shows that the air passage to the lungs is being obstructed by the false membrane.

HOME TREATMENT.—Isolate the patient, to prevent the spread of the disease. Diet should be of the most nutritious character, as milk, eggs, broths, and oysters. Give at intervals of every two or three hours. If patient refuses to swallow, from the pain caused by the effort, a nutrition injection must be resorted to. Inhalations of steam and hot water, and allowing the patient to suck pellets of ice, will give relief. Sponges dipped in hot water, and applied to the angles of the jaw, are beneficial. Inhalations of lime, made by slaking freshly burnt lime in a vessel, and directing the vapor to the child's mouth, by means of a newspaper, or similar contrivance. Flour of sulphur, blown into the back of the mouth and throat by means of a goose quill, has been highly recommended. Frequent gargling of the throat and mouth, with a solution of lactic acid, strong enough to taste sour, will help to keep the parts clean, and correct the foul breath. If there is great prostration, with the nasal passage affected, or hoarseness and difficult breathing, a physician should be called at once.

[348]

DISEASES OF WOMEN.
DISORDERS OF THE MENSES.
1. SUPPRESSION OF, OR SCANTY MENSES.

HOME TREATMENT.—Attention to the diet, and exercise in the open air to promote the general health. Some bitter tonic, taken with fifteen grains of dialyzed iron, well diluted, after meals, if patient is pale and debilitated. A hot foot bath is often all that is necessary.

2. PROFUSE MENSTRUATION.

HOME TREATMENT.—Avoid highly seasoned food, and the use of spirituous liquors; also excessive fatigue, either physical or mental. To check the flow, patient should be kept quiet, and allowed to sip cinnamon tea during the period.

3. PAINFUL MENSTRUATION.

HOME TREATMENT.—Often brought on by colds. Treat by warm hip baths, hot drinks (avoiding spirituous liquors), and heat applied to the back and extremities. A teaspoonful of the fluid extract of viburnum will sometimes act like a charm.

HOW TO CURE SWELLED AND SORE BREASTS.

Take and boil a quantity of chamomile, and apply the hot fomentations. This dissolves the knot, and reduce the swelling and soreness.[349]

LEUCORRHEA OR WHITES.

HOME TREATMENT.—This disorder, if not arising from some abnormal condition of the pelvic organs, can easily be cured by patient taking the proper amount of exercise and good nutritious food, avoiding tea and coffee. An injection every evening of one teaspoonful of Pond's Extract in a cup of hot water, after first cleansing the vagina well with a quart of warm water, is a simple but effective remedy.

INFLAMMATION OF THE WOMB.

HOME TREATMENT.—When in the acute form this disease is ushered in by a chill, followed by fever, and pain in the region of the womb. Patient should be placed in bed, and a brisk purgative given, hot poultices applied to the abdomen, and the feet and hands kept warm. If the symptoms do not subside, a physician should be consulted.

HYSTERIA.

DEFINITION.—A functional disorder of the nervous system of which it is impossible to speak definitely; characterized by disturbance of the reason, will, imagination, and emotions, with sometimes convulsive attacks that resemble epilepsy.

SYMPTOMS.—Fits of laughter, and tears without apparent cause; emotions easily excited; mind often melancholy and depressed; tenderness along the spine; disturbances of digestion, with hysterical convulsions, and other nervous phenomena.

HOME TREATMENT.—Some healthy and pleasant employment should be urged upon women afflicted with this disease. Men are also subject to it, though not so frequently. Avoid excessive fatigue and mental worry; also stimulants and opiates. Plenty of good food and fresh air will do more good than drugs.

137

Falling of the Womb.

Causes.—The displacement of the womb usually is the result of too much childbearing, miscarriages, abortions, or the taking of strong medicines to bring about menstruation. It may also be the result in getting up too quickly from the childbed. There are, however, other causes, such as a general breaking down of the health.

Symptoms.—If the womb has fallen forward it presses against the bladder, causing the patient to urinate frequently. If the womb has fallen back, it presses against the rectum, and constipation is the result with often severe pain at stool. If the womb descends into the vagina there is a feeling of heaviness. All forms of displacement produce pain in the back, with an irregular and scanty menstrual flow and a dull and exhausted feeling.

Home Treatment.—Improve the general health. Take some preparation of cod-liver oil, hot injections (of a teaspoonful of powdered alum with a pint of water), a daily sitz-bath, and a regular morning bath three times a week will be found very beneficial. There, however, can be no remedy unless the womb is first replaced to the proper position. This must be done by a competent physician who should frequently be consulted.

Menstruation.

1. **Its Importance.**—Menstruation plays a momentous part in the female economy; indeed, unless it be in every way properly and duly performed, it is neither possible that a lady can be well, nor is it at all probable that she will conceive. The large number of barren, of delicate, and of hysterical women there are in America arises mainly from menstruation not being duly and properly performed.

2. **The Boundary-Line.**—Menstruation—"the periods"—the appearance of the catamenia or the menses—is then one of the most important epochs in a girl's life. It is the boundary-line, the landmark between childhood and womanhood; it is the threshold, so to speak, of a woman's life. Her body now develops and expands, and her mental capacity enlarges and improves.

3. **The Commencement of Menstruation.**—A good beginning at this time is peculiarly necessary, or a girl's health is sure to suffer, and different organs of the body—her lungs, for instance, may become imperiled. A healthy continuation, at regular periods, is also much needed, or conception, when she is married, may not occur. Great attention and skillful management is required to ward off many formidable diseases, which at the close of menstruation—at "the change of life"—are more likely than at any time to be developed. If she marry when very young, marriage weakens her system, and prevents a full development of her body. Moreover, such an one is, during the progress of her labor, prone to convulsions—which is a very serious childbed complication.

4. **Early Marriages.**—Statistics prove that twenty per cent—20 in every 100—of females who marry are under age, and that such early marriages are often followed by serious, and sometimes even by fatal consequences to mother, to progeny, or to both. Parents ought, therefore, to persuade their daughters not to marry until they are of age—twenty-one; they should point out to them the risk and danger likely to ensue if their advice be not followed; they should impress upon their minds the old adage:

"Early wed,
Early dead."

5. **Time to Marry.**—Parents who have the real interest and happiness of their daughters at heart, ought, in consonance with the laws of physiology, to discountenance marriage before twenty; and the nearer the girls arrive at [352]the age of twenty-five before the consummation of this important rite, the greater the probability that, physically and morally, they will be protected against those risks which precocious marriages bring in their train.

6. **Feeble Parents.**—Feeble parents have generally feeble children; diseased parents, diseased children; nervous parents, nervous children;—"like begets like." It is sad to reflect, that the innocent have to suffer, not only for the guilty, but for the thoughtless and

inconsiderate. Disease and debility are thus propagated from one generation to another and the American race becomes woefully deteriorated.

7. **Time.**—Menstruation in this country usually commences at the ages of from thirteen to sixteen, sometimes earlier; occasionally as early as eleven or twelve; at other times later, and not until a girl be seventeen or eighteen years of age. Menstruation in large towns is supposed to commence at an earlier period than in the country, and earlier in luxurious than in simple life.

8. **Character.**—The menstrual fluid is not exactly blood, although, both in appearance and properties, it much resembles it; yet it never in the healthy state clots as blood does. It is a secretion of the womb, and, when healthy, ought to be of a bright red color, in appearance very much like the blood from a recently cut finger. The menstrual fluid ought not, as before observed, clot. If it does, a lady, during "her periods," suffers intense pain; moreover, she seldom conceives until the clotting has ceased.

9. **Menstruation during Nursing.**—Some ladies, though comparatively few, menstruate during nursing; when they do, it may be considered not as the rule, but as the exception. It is said in such instances, that they are more likely to conceive; and no doubt they are, as menstruation is an indication of a proneness to conception. Many persons have an idea that when a woman, during lactation, menstruates, her milk is both sweeter and purer. Such is an error. Menstruation during nursing is more likely to weaken the mother, and consequently to deteriorate her milk, and thus make it less sweet and less pure.

10. **Violent Exercise.**—During "the monthly periods" violent exercise is injurious; iced drinks and acid beverages are improper; and bathing in the sea, and bathing the feet in cold water, and cold baths are dangerous; indeed, at such times as these, no risks should be run, and no experiments should, for the moment, be permitted, otherwise serious consequences will, in all probability, ensue.[353]

11. **The Pale, Colorless-Complexioned.**—The pale, colorless-complexioned, helpless, listless, and almost lifeless young ladies who are so constantly seen in society, usually owe their miserable state of health to deficient, to absent, or to profuse menstruation. Their breathing is short—they are soon "out of breath," if they attempt to take exercise—to walk, for instance, either up stairs or up a hill, or even for half a mile on level ground, their breath is nearly exhausted—they pant as though they had been running quickly. They are ready, after the slightest exertion or fatigue, and after the least worry or excitement, to feel faint, and sometimes even to actually swoon away. Now such cases may, if judiciously treated, be generally soon cured. It therefore behooves mothers to seek medical aid early for their girls, and that before irreparable mischief has been done to the constitution.

12. **Poverty of Blood.**—In a pale, delicate girl or wife, who is laboring under what is popularly called poverty of blood, the menstrual fluid is sometimes very scant, at others very copious, but is, in either case, usually very pale—almost as colorless as water, the patient being very nervous and even hysterical. Now, these are signs of great debility; but, fortunately for such an one, a medical man is, in the majority of cases, in possession of remedies that will soon make her all right again.

13. **No Right to Marry.**—A delicate girl has no right until she be made strong, to marry. If she should marry, she will frequently, when in labor, not have strength, unless she has help, to bring a child into the world; which, provided she be healthy and well-formed, ought not to be. How graphically the Bible tells of delicate women not having strength to bring children into the world: "For the children are come to the birth, and there is not strength to bring forth."—2 Kings XIX, 3.

14. **Too Sparing.**—Menstruation at another time is too sparing; this is a frequent cause of sterility. Medical aid, in the majority of cases, will be able to remedy the defect, and, by doing so, will probably be the means of bringing the womb into a healthy state, and thus predispose to conception.

[354]
Celebrated Prescriptions for All Diseases and How to Use Them.

VINEGAR FOR HIVES.

After trying many remedies in a severe case of hives, Mr. Swain found vinegar lotion gave instant relief, and subsequent trials in other cases have been equally successful. One part of water to two parts of vinegar is the strength most suitable.

THROAT TROUBLE.

A teaspoonful of salt, in a cup of hot water, makes a safe and excellent gargle in most throat troubles.

FOR SWEATING FEET, WITH BAD ODOR.

Wash the feet in warm water with borax, and if this don't cure, use a solution of permanganate to destroy the fetor; about five grains to each ounce of water.[355]

AMENORRHŒA.

The following is recommended as a reliable emmenagogue in many cases of functional amenorrhœa:

Bichloride of mercury,
Arsenite of sodium, aa gr. iij.
Sulphate of strychnine, gr. iss.
Carbonate of potassium,
Sulphate of iron, aa gr. xlv.

Mix and divide into sixty pills. Sig. One pill after each meal.

SICK HEADACHE.

Take a spoonful of finely powdered charcoal in a small glass of warm water to relieve a sick headache.

It absorbs the gasses produced by the fermentation of undigested food.

AN EXCELLENT EYE WASH.

Acetate of zinc, 20 grains.
Acetate of morphia, 5 grains.
Rose water, 4 ounces. Mix.

FOR FILMS AND CATARACTS OF THE EYES.

Blood Root Pulverized, 1 ounce.
Hog's lard, 3 ounces.

Mix, simmer for 20 minutes, then strain; when cold put a little in the eyes twice or three times a day.

FOR BURNS AND SORES.

Pitch Burgundy, 2 pounds.
Bees' Wax, 1 pound.
Hog's lard, one pound.

Mix all together and simmer over a slow fire until the whole are well mixed together; then stir it until cold. Apply on muslin to the parts affected.

FOR CHAPPED HANDS.

Olive oil, 6 ounces.
Camphor beat fine, ½ ounce.

Mix, dissolve by gentle heat over slow fire and when cold apply to the hand freely.

INTOXICATION.

A man who is helplessly intoxicated may almost immediately restore the faculties and powers of locomotion by taking half a teaspoonful of chloride of ammonium in a goblet of water. A wineglassful of strong vinegar will have the same effect and is frequently resorted to by drunken soldiers.[356]

NERVOUS DISABILITY. HEADACHE. NEURALGIA. NERVOUSNESS.

Fluid extract of scullcap, 1 ounce.
Fluid extract American valerian, 1 ounce.
Fluid extract catnip, 1 ounce.

Mix all. Dose, from 15 to 30 drops every two hours, in water; most valuable.

A valuable tonic in all conditions of debility and want of appetite.

Comp. tincture of cinchona in teaspoonful doses in a little water, half hour before meals.

ANOTHER EXCELLENT TONIC.

Tincture of gentian, 1 ounce.

Tincture of Columba, 1 ounce.

Tincture of collinsonia, 1 ounce.

Mix all. Dose, one tablespoonful in one tablespoonful of water before meals.

REMEDY FOR CHAPPED HANDS.

When doing housework, if your hands become chapped or red, mix corn meal and vinegar into a stiff paste and apply to the hand two or three times a day, after washing them in hot water, then let dry without wiping, and rub with glycerine. At night use cold cream, and wear gloves.

BLEEDING.

Very hot water is a prompt checker of bleeding, besides, if it is clean, as it should be, it aids in sterilizing our wound.

TREATMENT FOR CRAMP.

Wherever friction can be conveniently applied, heat will be generated by it, and the muscle again reduced to a natural condition; but if the pains proceed from the contraction of some muscle located internally, burnt brandy is an excellent remedy.

A severe attack which will not yield to this simple treatment may be conquered by administering a small dose of laudanum or ether, best given under medical supervision.

TREATMENT FOR COLIC.

Castor oil, given as soon as the symptoms of colic manifest themselves, has frequently afforded relief. At any rate, the irritating substances may be expelled from the alimentary canal before the pains will subside. All local remedies will be ineffectual, and consequently the purgative should be given in large doses until a copious vacuation is produced.[357]

THE DOCTOR'S VISIT.
TREATMENT FOR HEARTBURN.

If soda, taken in small quantities after meals, does not relieve the distress, one may rest assured that the fluid is an alkali and requires an acid treatment. Proceed, after eating, to squeeze ten drops of lemon-juice into a small quantity of water, and swallow it. The habit of daily life should be made to conform to the laws of health, or local treatment will prove futile.

BILIOUSNESS.

For biliousness, squeeze the juice of a lime or small lemon into half a glass of cold water, then stir in a little baking soda and drink while it foams. This receipt will also relieve sick headache if taken at the beginning.

TURPENTINE APPLICATIONS.

Mix turpentine and lard in equal parts. Warmed and rubbed on the chest, it is a safe, reliable and mild counter irritant and revulsent in minor lung complications.[358]

TREATMENT FOR MUMPS.

It is very important that the face and neck be kept warm. Avoid catching cold, and regulate the stomach and bowels, because, when aggravated, this disease is communicated to other glands, and assumes there a serious form. Rest and quiet, with a good condition of the general health, will throw off this disease without further inconvenience.

TREATMENT FOR FELON.

All medication, such as poulticing, anointing, and the applications of lotions, is but useless waste of time. The surgeon's knife should be used as early as possible, for it will be required sooner or later, and the more promptly it can be applied, the less danger is there from the disease, and the more agony is spared to the unfortunate victim.

TREATMENT FOR STABS.

A wound made by thrusting a dagger or other oblong instrument into the flesh, is best treated, if no artery has been severed, by applying lint scraped from a linen cloth, which serves as an obstruction, allowing and assisting coagulation. Meanwhile cold water should be applied to the parts adjoining the wound.

TREATMENT FOR MASHED NAILS.

If the injured member be plunged into very hot water, the nail will become pliable and adapt itself to the new condition of things, thus alleviating agony to some extent. A small hole may be bored on the nail with a pointed instrument, so adroitly so as not to cause pain, yet so successfully as to relieve pressure on the sensitive tissues. Free applications of arnica or iodine will have an excellent effect.

TREATMENT FOR FOREIGN BODY IN THE EYE.

When any foreign body enters the eye, close it instantly, and keep it still until you have an opportunity to ask the assistance of some one; then have the upper lid folded over a pencil and the exposed surfaces closely searched; if the body be invisible, catch the everted lid by the lashes, and drawing it down over the lower lid, suddenly release it, and it will resume its natural position. Unsuccessful in this attempt, you may be pretty well assured that the object has become lodged in the tissues, and will require the assistance of a skilled operator to remove it.

CUTS.

A drop or two of creosote on a cut will stop its bleeding.[359]

Treatment for Poison Oak—Poison Ivy—Poison Sumach.—Mr. Charles Morris, of Philadelphia, who has studied the subject closely, uses, as a sovereign remedy, frequent bathing of the affected parts in water as hot as can be borne. If used immediately after exposure, it may prevent the eruption appearing. If later, it allays the itching, and gradually dries up the swellings, though, they are very stubborn after they have once appeared. But an application every few hours keeps down the intolerable itching, which is the most annoying feature of sumach poisoning. In addition to this, the ordinary astringent ointments are useful, as is also that sovereign lotion, "lead-water and laudanum." Mr. Morris adds to these a preventive prescription of "wide-open eyes."

Bites and Stings of Insects.—Wash with a solution of ammonia water.

Bites of Mad Dogs.—Apply caustic potash at once to the wound, and give enough whiskey to cause sleep.

Burns.—Make a paste of common baking soda and water, and apply it promptly to the burn. It will quickly check the pain and inflammation.

Cold on Chest.—A flannel rag wrung out in boiling water and sprinkled with turpentine, laid on the chest, gives the greatest relief.

Cough.—Boil one ounce of flaxseed in a pint of water, strain, and add a little honey, one ounce of rock candy, and the juice of three lemons. Mix and boil well. Drink as hot as possible.

Sprained Ankle or Wrist.—Wash the ankle very frequently with cold salt and water, which is far better than warm vinegar or decoction of herbs. Keep the foot as cool as possible to prevent inflammation, and sit with it elevated on a high cushion. Live on low diet, and take every morning some cooling medicine, such as Epsom salts. It cures in a few days.

Chilblains, Sprains, etc.—One raw egg well beaten, half a pint of vinegar, one ounce spirits of turpentine, a quarter of an ounce of spirits of wine, a quarter of an ounce of camphor. These ingredients to be beaten together, then put in a bottle and shaken for ten minutes, after which, to be corked down tightly to exclude the air. In half an hour it is fit for use. To be well rubbed in, two, three, or four times a day. For rheumatism in the head, to be rubbed at the back of the neck and behind the ears. In chilblains this remedy is to be used before they are broken.[360]

How To Remove Superfluous Hair.—Sulphuret of Arsenic, one ounce; Quicklime, one ounce; Prepared Lard, one ounce; White Wax, one ounce. Melt the Wax, add the Lard. When nearly cold, stir in the other ingredients. Apply to the superfluous hair, allowing it to remain on from five to ten minutes; use a table-knife to shave off the hair; then wash with soap and warm water.

Dyspepsia Cure.—Powdered Rhubarb, two drachms; Bicarbonate of Sodium, six drachms; Fluid Extract of Gentian, three drachms; Peppermint Water, seven and a half ounces. Mix them. Dose, a teaspoonful half an hour before meals.

For Neuralgia.—Tincture of Belladonna, one ounce; Tincture of Camphor, one ounce; Tincture of Arnica, one ounce; Tincture of Opium, one ounce. Mix them. Apply over the seat of the pain, and give ten to twenty drops in sweetened water every two hours.

For Coughs, Colds, etc.—Syrup of Morphia, three ounces; Syrup of Tar, three and a half ounces; Chloroform, one troy ounce; Glycerine, one troy ounce. Mix them. Dose, a teaspoonful three or four times a day.

To Cure Hives.—Compound syrup of Squill, U. S., three ounces; Syrup of Ipecac, U. S., one ounce. Mix them. Dose, a teaspoonful.

To Cure Sick Headache.—Gather sumach leaves in the summer, and spread them in the sun a few days to dry. Then powder them fine, and smoke, morning and evening for two weeks, also whenever there are symptoms of approaching headache. Use a new clay pipe. If these directions are adhered to, this medicine will surely effect a permanent cure.

Whooping Cough.—Dissolve a scruple of salt of tartar in a gill of water; add to it ten grains of cochineal; sweeten it with sugar. Give to an infant a quarter teaspoonful four times a day; two years old, one-half teaspoonful; from four years, a tablespoonful. Great care is required in the administration of medicines to infants. We can assure paternal inquirers that the foregoing may be depended upon.

Cut or Bruise.—Apply the moist surface of the inside coating or skin of the shell of a raw egg. It will adhere of itself, leave no scar, and heal without pain.

Disinfectant.—Chloride of lime should be scattered at least once a week under sinks and wherever sewer gas is likely to penetrate.

THE YOUNG DOCTOR.

[362]

Costiveness.—Common charcoal is highly recommended for costiveness. It may be taken in tea- or tablespoonful, or even larger doses, according to the exigencies of the case, mixed with molasses, repeating it as often as necessary. Bathe the bowels with pepper and vinegar. Or take two ounces of rhubarb, add one ounce of rust of iron, infuse in one quart of wine. Half a wineglassful every morning. Or take pulverized blood root, one drachm, pulverized rhubarb, one drachm, castile soap, two scruples. Mix. and roll into thirty-two pills. Take one, morning and night. By following these directions it may perhaps save you from a severe attack of the piles, or some other kindred disease.

To Cure Deafness.—Obtain pure pickerel oil, and apply four drops morning and evening to the ear. Great care should be taken to obtain oil that is perfectly pure.

Deafness.—Take three drops of sheep's gall, warm, and drop it into the ear on going to bed. The ear must be syringed with warm soap and water in the morning. The gall must be applied for three successive nights. It is only efficacious when the deafness is produced by cold. The most convenient way of warming the gall is by holding it in a silver spoon over the flame of a light. The above remedy has been frequently tried with perfect success.

Gout.—This is Col. Birch's recipe for rheumatic gout or acute rheumatism, commonly called in England the "Chelsea Pensioner." Half an ounce of nitre (saltpetre), half an ounce of sulphur, half an ounce of flour of mustard, half an ounce of Turkey rhubarb, quarter of an ounce of powdered guaicum. Mix, and take a teaspoonful every other night for three nights, and omit three nights, in a wine-glassful of cold water which has been previously well boiled.

Ringworm.—The head is to be washed twice a day with soft soap and warm soft water; when dried the places to be rubbed with a piece of linen rag dipped in ammonia from gas tar; the patient should take a little sulphur and molasses, or some other genuine aperient, every morning; brushes and combs should be washed every day, and the ammonia kept tightly corked.

Piles.—Hamamelis, both internally or as an injection in rectum. Bathe the parts with cold water or with astringent lotions, as alum water, especially in bleeding piles. Ointment of gallic acid and calomel is of repute. The best treatment of all is, suppositories of iodoform, ergotine, or tannic acid, which can be made at any drug store.[363]

Chicken Pox.—No medicine is usually needed, except a tea made from pleurisy root, to make the child sweat. Milk diet is the best; avoidance of animal food; careful attention to the bowels; keep cool and avoid exposure to cold.

Scarlet Fever.—Cold water compress on the throat. Fats and oils rubbed on hands and feet. The temperature of the room should be about 68 degrees Fahr., and all draughts avoided. Mustard baths for retrocession of the rash and to bring it out. Diet: ripe fruit, toast, gruel, beef tea and milk. Stimulants are useful to counteract depression of the vital forces.

False Measles or Rose Rash.—It requires no treatment except hygienic. Keep the bowels open. Nourishing diet, and if there is itching, moisten the skin with five per cent. solution of aconite or solution of starch and water.

Bilious Attacks.—Drop doses of muriatic acid in a wine glass of water every four hours, or the following prescription. Bicarbonate of soda, one drachm; Aromatic spirits of ammonia, two drachms; Peppermint water, four ounces. Dose: Take a teaspoonful every four hours.

Diarrhœa.—The following prescription is generally all that will be necessary: acetate of lead, eight grains; gum arabic, two drachms; acetate of morphia, one grain; and cinnamon water, eight ounces. Take a teaspoonful every three hours.

Be careful not to eat too much food. Some consider, the best treatment is to fast, and it is a good suggestion. Patients should keep quiet and have the room of a warm and even temperature.

Vomiting.—Ice dissolved in the mouth, often cures vomiting when all remedies fail. Much depends on the diet of persons liable to such attacks; this should be easily digestible food, taken often and in small quantities. Vomiting can often be arrested by applying a mustard paste over the region of the stomach. It is not necessary to allow it to remain until the parts are blistered, but it may be removed when the part becomes thoroughly red, and reapplied if required after the redness has disappeared. One of the secrets to relieve vomiting is to give the stomach perfect rest, not allowing the patient even a glass of water, as long as the tendency remains to throw it up again.

Nervous Headache.—Extract hyoscymus five grains, pulverized camphor five grains. Mix. Make four pills, one to be taken when the pain is most severe in nervous headache. Or three drops tincture nux vomica in a spoonful of water, two or three times a day.[364]

Bleeding from the Nose,—from whatever cause—may generally be stopped by putting a plug of lint into the nostril; if this does not do, apply a cold lotion to the forehead; raise the head and place both arms over the head, so that it will rest on both hands; dip the lint plug, slightly moistened, in some powdered gum arabic, and plug the nostrils again; or dip the plug into equal parts of gum arabic and alum. An easier and simpler method is to place a piece of writing paper on the gums of the upper jaw, under the upper lip, and let it remain there for a few minutes.

Boils.—These should be brought to a head by warm poultices of camomile flowers, or boiled white lily root, or onion root, by fermentation with hot water, or by stimulating plasters. When ripe they should be destroyed by a needle or lancet. But this should not be attempted until they are thoroughly proved.

Bunions may be checked in their early development by binding the joint with adhesive plaster, and keeping it on as long as any uneasiness is felt. The bandaging should be perfect, and it might be well to extend it round the foot. An inflamed bunion should be poulticed, and larger shoes be worn. Iodine 12 grains, lard or spermaceti ointment half an ounce, makes a capital ointment for bunions. It should be rubbed on gently twice or three times a day.

Felons.—One table-spoonful of red lead, and one table-spoonful of castile soap, and mix them with as much weak lye as will make it soft enough to spread like a salve, and apply it on the first appearance of the felon, and it will cure in ten or twelve days.

Cure for Warts.—The easiest way to get rid of warts, is to pare off the thickened skin which covers the prominent wart; cut it off by successive layers and shave it until you come to the surface of the skin, and till you draw blood in two or three places. Then rub the part thoroughly over with lunar caustic, and one effective operation of this kind will generally destroy the wart; if not, you cut off the black spot which has been occasioned by the caustic, and apply it again; or you may apply acetic acid, and thus you will get rid of it. Care must be taken in applying these acids, not to rub them on the skin around the wart.

144

Wens.—Take the yoke of some eggs, beat up, and add as much fine salt as will dissolve, and apply a plaster to the wen every ten hours. It cures without pain or any other inconvenience.

[365]

HOW TO CURE
Apoplexy, Bad Breath and Quinsy.

1. **Apoplexy.**—Apoplexy occurs only in the corpulent or obese, and those of gross or high living.

Treatment.—Raise the head to a nearly upright position; loosen all tight clothes, strings, etc., and apply cold water to the head and warm water and warm cloths to the feet. Have the apartment cool and well ventilated. Give nothing by the mouth until the breathing is relieved, and then only draughts of cold water.

2. **Bad Breath.**—Bad or foul breath will be removed by taking a teaspoonful of the following mixture after each meal: One ounce chloride of soda, one ounce liquor of potassa, one and one-half ounces phosphate of soda, and three ounces of water.

3. **Quinsy.**—This is an inflammation of the tonsils, or common inflammatory sore throat; commences with a slight feverish attack, with considerable pain and swelling of the tonsils, causing some difficulty in swallowing; as the attack advances, these symptoms become more intense, there is headache, thirst, a painful sense of tension, and acute darting pains in the ears. The attack is generally brought on by exposure to cold, and lasts from five to seven days, when it subsides naturally, or an abscess may form in tonsils and burst, or the tonsils may remain enlarged, the inflammation subsiding.

Home Treatment.—The patient should remain in a warm room, the diet chiefly milk and good broths, some cooling laxative and diaphoretic medicine may be given; but the greatest relief will be found in the frequent inhalation of the steam of hot water through an inhaler, or in the old-fashioned way through the spout of a teapot.

[366]

Sensible Rules for the Nurse.

"Remember to be extremely neat in dress; a few drops of hartshorn in the water used for *daily* bathing will remove the disagreeable odors of warmth and perspiration.

"Never speak of the symptoms of your patient in his presence, unless questioned by the doctor, whose orders you are always to obey *implicitly.*

"Remember never to be a gossip or tattler, and always to hold sacred the knowledge which, to a certain extent, you must obtain of the private affairs of your patient and the household in which you nurse.

"Never contradict your patient, nor argue with him, nor let him see that you are annoyed about anything.

"Never *whisper* in the sick room. If your patient be well enough, and wishes you to talk to him, speak in a low, distinct voice, on cheerful subjects. Don't relate painful hospital experiences, nor give details of the maladies of former patients, and remember never to startle him with accounts of dreadful crimes or accidents that you have read in the newspapers.

"*Write* down the orders that the physician gives you as to time for giving the medicines, food, etc.

"Keep the room bright (unless the doctor orders it darkened).

"Let the air of the room be as pure as possible, and keep everything in order, but without being fussy and bustling.

"The only way to remove dust in a sick room is to wipe everything with a damp cloth.

"Remember to carry out all vessels covered. Empty and wash them immediately, and keep some disinfectant in them.

"Remember that to leave the patient's untasted food by his side, from meal to meal, in hopes that he will eat it in the interval, is simply to prevent him from taking any food at all.

"Medicines, beef tea or stimulants, should never be kept where the patient can see them or smell them.

"Light-colored clothing should be worn by those who have the care of the sick, in preference to dark-colored apparel; particularly if the disease is of a contagious nature. Experiments have shown that black and other dark colors will absorb more readily the subtle effluvia that emanates from sick persons than white or light colors."

[367]

Longevity.

The following table exhibits very recent mortality statistics, showing the average duration of life among persons of various classes:

Employment	Years.
Judges	65
Farmers	64
Bank Officers	64
Coopers	58
Public Officers	57
Clergymen	56
Shipwrights	55
Hatters	54
Lawyers	54
Rope Makers	54
Blacksmiths	51
Merchants	51
Calico Printers	51
Physicians	51
Butchers	50
Carpenters	49
Masons	48
Traders	46
Tailors	44

Occupation	Age
Jewelers	44
Manufacturers	43
Bakers	43
Painters	43
Shoemakers	43
Mechanics	43
Editors	40
Musicians	39
Printers	38
Machinists	36
Teachers	34
Clerks	34
Operatives	32

"It will be easily seen, by these figures, how a quiet or tranquil life affects longevity. The phlegmatic man will live longer, all other things being equal, than the sanguine, nervous individual. Marriage is favorable to longevity, and it has also been ascertained that women live longer than men."[368]

HOT WATER THROAT BAG. HOT WATER BAG.

HOW TO APPLY AND USE HOT WATER IN ALL DISEASES.

1. THE HOT WATER THROAT BAG. The hot water throat bag is made from fine white rubber fastened to the head by a rubber band (see illustration), and is an unfailing remedy for catarrh, hay fever, cold, toothache, headache, earache, neuralgia, etc.

2. THE HOT WATER BOTTLE. No well regulated house should be without a hot water bottle. It is excellent in the application of hot water for inflammations, colic, headache, congestion, cold feet, rheumatism, sprains, etc., etc. It is an excellent warming pan and an excellent feet and hand warmer when riding. These hot water bags in any variety can be purchased at any drug store.

3. Boiling water may be used in the bags and the heat will be retained many hours. They are soft and pliable and pleasant to the touch, and can be adjusted to any part of the body.

4. Hot water is good for constipation, torpid liver, and relieves colic and flatulence, and is of special value.

5. *Caution.* When hot water bags or any hot fomentation [369]is removed, replace dry flannel and bathe parts in tepid water and rub till dry.

6. By inflammations it is best to use hot water and then cold water. It seems to give more immediate relief. Hot water is a much better remedy than drugs, paragoric, Dover's powder or morphine. Always avoid the use of strong poisonous drugs when possible.

147

7. Those who suffer from cold feet there is no better remedy than to bathe the feet in cold water before retiring and then place a hot water bottle in the bed at the feet. A few weeks of such treatment results in relief if not cure of the most obstinate case.

HOW TO USE COLD WATER.

Use a compress of cold water for acute or chronic inflammation, such as sore throat, bronchitis, croup, inflammation of the lungs, etc. If there is a hot and aching pain in the back apply a compress of cold water on the same, or it may simply be placed across the back or around the body. The most depends upon the condition of the patient.

[370]

Practical Rules for Bathing.

1. Bathe at least once a week all over, thoroughly. No one can preserve his health by neglecting personal cleanliness. Remember, "Cleanliness is akin to Godliness."

2. Only mild soap should be used in bathing the body.

3. Wipe quickly and dry the body thoroughly with a moderately coarse towel. Rub the skin vigorously.[371]

4. Many people have contracted severe and fatal diseases by neglecting to take proper care of the body after bathing.

5. If you get up a good reaction by thorough rubbing in a mild temperature, the effect is always good.

6. Never go into a cold room, or allow cold air to enter the room until you are dressed.

7. Bathing in cold rooms and in cold water is positively injurious, unless the person possesses a very strong and vigorous constitution, and then there is great danger of laying the foundation of some serious disease.

8. Never bathe within two hours after eating. It injures digestion.

9. Never bathe when the body or mind is much exhausted. It is liable to check the healthful circulation.

10. A good time for bathing is just before retiring. The morning hour is a good time also, if a warm room and warm water can be secured.

11. Never bathe a fresh wound or broken skin with cold water; the wound absorbs water, and causes swelling and irritation.

12. A person not robust should be very careful in bathing; great care should be exercised to avoid any chilling effects.

[372]

All the Different Kinds of Baths, and How to Prepare Them.
THE SULPHUR BATH.

For the itch, ringworm, itching, and for other slight skin irritations, bathe in water containing a little sulphur.

THE SALT BATH.

To open the pores of the skin, put a little common salt into the water. Borax, baking soda or lime used in the same way are excellent for cooling and cleansing the skin. A very small quantity in a bowl of water is sufficient.

THE VAPOR BATH.

1. For catarrh, bronchitis, pleurisy, inflammation of the lungs, rheumatism, fever, affections of the bowels and kidneys, and skin diseases, the vapor-bath is an excellent remedy.

2. APPARATUS.—Use a small alcohol lamp, and place over it a small dish containing water. Light the lamp and allow the water to boil. Place a cane-bottom chair over the lamp, and seat the patient on it. Wrap blankets or quilts around the chair and around the patient, closing it tightly about the neck. After free perspiration is produced the patient should be wrapped in warm blankets, and placed in bed, so as to continue the perspiration for some time.

3. A convenient alcohol lamp may be made by taking a tin box, placing a tube in it, and putting in a common lamp wick. Any tinner can make one in a few minutes, at a trifling cost.

THE HOT-AIR BATH.

1. Place the alcohol lamp under the chair, without the dish of water. Then place the patient on the chair, as in the vapor bath, and let him remain until a gentle and free perspiration is produced. This bath may be taken from time to time, as may be deemed necessary.

2. While remaining in the hot-air bath the patient may drink freely of cold or tepid water.

3. As soon as the bath is over the patient should be washed with hot water and soap.

4. The hot-air bath is excellent for colds, skin diseases, and the gout.[373]

THE SPONGE BATH.

1. Have a large basin of water of the temperature of 88 or 95 degrees. As soon as the patient rises rub the body over with a soft, dry towel until it becomes warm.

2. Now sponge the body with water and a little soap, at the same time keeping the body well covered, except such portions as are necessarily exposed. Then dry the skin carefully with a soft, warm towel. Rub the skin well for two or three minutes, until every part becomes red and perfectly dry.

3. Sulphur, lime or salt, and sometimes mustard, may be used in any of the sponge baths, according to the disease.

THE FOOT BATH.

1. The foot bath, in coughs, colds, asthma, headaches and fevers, is excellent. One or two tablespoonfuls of ground mustard added to a gallon of hot water, is very beneficial.

2. Heat the water as hot as the patient can endure it, and gradually increase the temperature by pouring in additional quantities of hot water during the bath.

THE SITZ BATH.

A tub is arranged so that the patient can sit down in it while bathing. Fill the tub about one-half full of water. This is an excellent remedy for piles, constipation, headache, gravel, and for acute and inflammatory affections generally.

THE ACID BATH.

Place a little vinegar in water, and heat to the usual temperature. This is an excellent remedy for the disorders of the liver.

A Sure Cure for Prickly Heat.

1. Prickly heat is caused by hot weather, by excess of flesh, by rough flannels, by sudden changes of temperature, or by over-fatigue.

2. TREATMENT—Bathe two or three times a day with warm water, in which a moderate quantity of bran and common soda has been stirred. After wiping the skin dry, dust the affected parts with common cornstarch.

[374]

Digestibility of Food.

Article of Food.	Condition.	Hours Required.	Article of Food.	Condition.	Hours Required.
Rice	Boiled	1.00	Soup, chicken	Boiled	3.00
Eggs, whipped	Raw	1.30	Apple dumpling	"	3.00
Trout, salmon, fresh	Boiled	1.30	Fresh oysters	Roasted	3.15
Apples, sweet and mellow	Raw	1.30	Pork steak	Broiled	3.15

149

Food	Preparation	Min.	Hr.	Food	Preparation	Min.	Hr.
Venison steak	Broiled	35	1.	Fresh mutton	Roasted	15	3.
Tapioca	Boiled	00	2.	Corn bread	Baked	15	3.
Barley	"	00	2.	Carrots	Boiled	15	3.
Milk	"	00	2.	Fresh sausage	Broiled	20	3.
Bullock's liver, fresh	Broiled	00	2.	Fresh flounder	Fried	30	3.
Fresh eggs	Raw	00	2.	Fresh catfish	"	30	3.
Codfish, cured and dry	Boiled	00	2.	Fresh oysters	Stewed	30	3.
Milk	Raw	15	2.	Butter	Melted	30	3.
Wild turkey	Roasted	15	2.	Old, strong cheese	Raw	30	3.
Domestic turkey	"	30	2.	Mutton soup	Boiled	30	3.
Goose	"	30	2.	Oyster soup	"	30	3.
Sucking pig	"	30	2.	Fresh wheat bread	Baked	30	3.
Fresh lamb	Broiled	30	2.	Flat turnips	Boiled	30	3.
Hash, meat and vegetables	Warmed	30	2.	Irish potatoes	"	30	3.
Beans and pod	Boiled	30	2.	Fresh eggs	Hard boiled	30	3.
Parsnips	"	30	2.	" "	Fried	30	3.
Irish potatoes	Roasted	30	2.	Green corn and beans	Boiled	45	3.
Chicken	Fricassee	45	2.	Beets	"	45	3.
Custard	Baked	45	2.	Fresh, lean beef	Fried	00	4.
Salt beef	Boiled	45	2.	Fresh veal	Broiled	00	4.
Sour and hard apples	Raw	50	2.	Domestic fowls	Roasted	00	4.
Fresh oysters	"	55	2.	Ducks	"	00	4.
Fresh eggs	Soft boiled	00	3.	Beef soup, vegetables and bread	Boiled	00	4.
Beef, fresh, lean and	Roasted	00	3.	Pork, recently salted	"	30	4.

rare Beef steak	Bro iled	3. 00	Fresh veal	Frie d	4. 30
Pork, recently salted	Ste wed	3. 00	Cabbage, with vinegar	Boil ed	4. 30
Fresh mutton	Boi led	3. 00	Pork, fat and lean	Roa sted	5. 30
Soup, beans	"	3. 00			

[375]

How to Cook for the Sick.
Useful Dietetic Recipes.

GRUELS.

1. **Oatmeal Gruel.**—Stir two tablespoonfuls of coarse oatmeal into a quart of boiling water, and let it simmer two hours. Strain, if preferred.

2. **Beef Tea and Oatmeal.**—Beat two tablespoonfuls of fine oatmeal, with two tablespoonfuls of cold water until very smooth, then add a pint of hot beef tea. Boil together six or eight minutes, stirring constantly. Strain through a fine sieve.

3. **Milk Gruel.**—Into a pint of scalding milk stir two tablespoonfuls of fine oatmeal. Add a pint of boiling water, and boil until the meal is thoroughly cooked.

4. **Milk Porridge.**—Place over the fire equal parts of milk and water. Just before it boils, add a small quantity (a tablespoonful to a pint of water) of graham flour or cornmeal, previously mixed with water, and boil three minutes.

5. **Sago Gruel.**—Take two tablespoonfuls of sago and place them in a small saucepan, moisten gradually with a little cold water. Set the preparation on a slow fire, and keep stirring till it becomes rather stiff and clear. Add a little grated nutmeg and sugar to taste; if preferred, half a pat of butter may also be added with the sugar.

6. **Cream Gruel.**—Put a pint and a half of water on the stove in a saucepan. Take one tablespoon of flour and the same of cornmeal; mix this with cold water, and as soon as the water in the saucepan boils, stir it in slowly. Let it boil slowly about twenty minutes, stirring constantly; then add a little salt and a gill of sweet cream. Do not let it boil after putting in the cream, but turn into a bowl and cover tightly. Serve in a pretty cup and saucer.[376]

DRINKS.

1. **Apple Water.**—Cut two large apples into slices and pour a quart of boiling water on them, or on roasted apples: strain in two or three hours and sweeten slightly.

2. **Orangeade.**—Take the thin peel of two oranges and of one lemon; add water and sugar the same as for hot lemonade. When cold add the juice of four or five oranges and one lemon and strain off.

3. **Hot Lemonade.**—Take two thin slices and the juice of one lemon; mix with two tablespoonfuls of granulated sugar, and add one-half pint of boiling water.

4. **Flaxseed Lemonade.**—Two tablespoonfuls of whole flaxseed to a pint of boiling water, let it steep three hours, strain when cool and add the juice of two lemons and two tablespoonfuls of honey. If too thick, put in cold water. Splendid for colds and suppression of urine.

5. **Jelly Water.**—Sour jellies dissolved in water make a pleasant drink for fever patients.

6. **Toast Water.**—Toast several thin pieces of bread a nice deep brown, but do not blacken or burn. Break into small pieces and put into a jar. Pour over the pieces a quart of boiling water; cover the jar and let it stand an hour before using. Strain if desired.

7. **White of Egg and Milk.**—The white of an egg beaten to a stiff froth, and stirred very quickly into a glass of milk, is a very nourishing food for persons whose digestion is weak, also for children who cannot digest milk alone.

151

8. **Egg Cocoa.**—One-half teaspoon cocoa with enough hot water to make a paste. Take one egg, beat white and yolk separately. Stir into a cup of milk heated to nearly boiling. Sweeten if desired. Very nourishing.

9. **Egg Lemonade.**—White of one egg, one tablespoonful pulverized sugar, juice of one lemon and one goblet of water. Beat together. Very grateful in inflammation of lungs, stomach or bowels.

10. **Beef Tea.**—For every quart of tea desired use one pound of fresh beef, from which all fat, bones and sinews have been carefully removed; cut the beef into pieces a quarter of an inch thick and mix with a pint of cold water. Let it stand an hour, then pour into a glass fruit can and place in a vessel of water; let it heat on the stove another hour, but do not let it boil. Strain before using.[377]

JELLIES.

1. **Sago Jelly.**—Simmer gently in a pint of water two tablespoonfuls of sago until it thickens, frequently stirring. A little sugar may be added if desired.

2. **Chicken Jelly.**—Take half a raw chicken, tie in a coarse cloth and pound, till well mashed, bones and meat together. Place the mass in a covered dish with water sufficient to cover it well. Allow it to simmer slowly till the liquor is reduced about one-half and the meat is thoroughly cooked. Press through a fine sieve or cloth, and salt to taste. Place on the stove to simmer about five minutes. When cold remove all particles of grease.

3. **Mulled Jelly.**—Take one tablespoonful of currant or grape jelly; beat it with the white of one egg and a little loaf sugar; pour on it one-half pint of boiling water and break in a slice of dry toast or two crackers.

4. **Bread Jelly.**—Pour boiling water over bread crumbs; place the mixture on the fire and let it boil until it is perfectly smooth. Take it off, and after pouring off the water, flavor with something agreeable, as a little raspberry or currant jelly water. Pour into a mold until required for use.

5. **Lemon Jelly.**—Moisten two tablespoonfuls of cornstarch, stir into one pint boiling water; add the juice of two lemons and one-half cup of sugar. Grate in a little of the rind. Put in molds to cool.

MISCELLANEOUS.

1. **To Cook Rice.**—Take two cups of rice and one and one-half pints of milk. Place in a covered dish and steam in a kettle of boiling water until it is cooked through, pour into cups and let it stand until cold. Serve with cream.

2. **Rice Omelet.**—Two cups boiled rice, one cup sweet milk, two eggs. Stir together with egg beater, and put into a hot buttered skillet. Cook slowly ten minutes, stirring frequently.

3. **Browned Rice.**—Parch or brown rice slowly. Steep in milk for two hours. The rice or the milk only is excellent in summer complaint.

4. **Stewed Oysters.**—Take one pint of milk, one cup of water, a teaspoon of salt: when boiling put in one pint of [378]bulk oysters. Stir occasionally and remove from the stove before it boils. An oyster should not be shriveled in cooking.

5. **Broiled Oysters.**—Put large oysters on a wire toaster. Hold over hot coals until heated through. Serve on toast moistened with cream. Very grateful in convalescence.

6. **Oyster Toast.**—Pour stewed oysters over graham gems or bread toasted. Excellent for breakfast.

7. **Graham Crisps.**—Mix graham flour and cold water into a very stiff dough. Knead, roll very thin, and bake quickly in a hot oven. Excellent food for dyspeptics.

8. **Apple Snow.**—Take seven apples, not very sweet ones, and bake till soft and brown. Then remove the skins and cores; when cool, beat them smooth and fine; add one-half cup of granulated sugar and the white of one egg. Beat till the mixture will hold on your spoon. Serve with soft custard.

9. **Eggs on Toast.**—Soften brown bread toast with hot water, put on a platter and cover with poached or scrambled eggs.

10. **Boiled Eggs.**—An egg should never be boiled. Place in boiling water and set back on the stove for from seven to ten minutes. A little experience will enable anyone to do it successfully.

11. **Cracked Wheat Pudding.**—In a deep two-quart pudding dish put layers of cold, cooked, cracked wheat, and tart apples sliced thin, with four tablespoonfuls of sugar. Raisins can be added if preferred. Fill the dish, having the wheat last, add a cup of cold water. Bake two hours.

12. **Pie for Dyspeptics.**—Four tablespoonfuls of oatmeal, one pint of water; let stand for a few hours, or until the meal is swelled. Then add two large apples, pared and sliced, a little salt, one cup of sugar, one tablespoonful of flour. Mix all well together and bake in a buttered dish; makes a most delicious pie, which can be eaten with safety by the sick or well.

13. **Apple Tapioca Pudding.**—Soak a teacup of tapioca in a quart of warm water three hours. Cut in thin slices six tart apples, stir them lightly with the tapioca, add half cup sugar. Bake three hours. To be eaten with whipped cream. Good either warm or cold.[379]

14. **Graham Muffins.**—Take one pint of new milk, one pint graham or entire wheat flour; stir together and add one beaten egg. Can be baked in any kind of gem pans or muffin rings. Salt must not be used with any bread that is made light with egg.

15. **Strawberry Dessert.**—Place alternate layers of hot cooked cracked wheat and strawberries in a deep dish; when cold, turn out on platter; cut in slices and serve with cream and sugar, or strawberry juice. Wet the molds with cold water before using. This, molded in small cups, makes a dainty dish for the sick. Wheatlet can be used in the same way.

16. **Fruit Blanc Mange.**—One quart of juice of strawberries, cherries, grapes or other juicy fruit; one cup water. When boiling, add two tablespoonfuls sugar and four tablespoonfuls cornstarch wet in cold water; let boil five or six minutes, then mold in small cups. Serve without sauce, or with cream or boiled custard. Lemon juice can be used the same, only requiring more water. This is a very valuable dish for convalescents and pregnant women, where the stomach rejects solid food.

[380]
Save the Girls.
GOOD ADVICE FROM GRANDPA.

1. **Public Balls.**—The church should turn its face like flint against the public ball. Its influence is evil, and nothing but evil. It is a well known fact that in all cities and large towns the ball room is the recruiting office for prostitution.

2. **Thoughtless Young Women.**—In cities public balls are given every night, and many thoughtless young women, [381]mostly the daughters of small tradesmen and mechanics, or clerks or laborers, are induced to attend "just for fun." Scarcely one in a hundred of the girls attending these balls preserve their purity. They meet the most desperate characters, professional gamblers, criminals and the lowest debauchees. Such an assembly and such influence cannot mean anything but ruin for an innocent girl.

3. **Vile Women.**—The public ball is always a resort of vile women who picture to innocent girls the ease and luxury of a harlot's life, and offer them all manner of temptations to abandon the paths of virtue. The public ball is the resort of the libertine and the adulterer, and whose object is to work the ruin of every innocent girl that may fall into their clutches.

4. **The Question.**—Why does society wonder at the increase of prostitution, when the public balls and promiscuous dancing is so largely endorsed and encouraged?

5. **Working Girls.**—Thousands of innocent working girls enter innocently and unsuspectingly into the paths which lead them to the house of evil, or who wander the streets as miserable outcasts all through the influence of the dance. The low theatre and dance halls and other places of unselected gatherings are the milestones which mark the working girl's downward path from virtue to vice, from modesty to shame.

6. **The Saleswoman**, the seamstress, the factory girl or any other virtuous girl had better, far better, die than take the first step in the path of impropriety and danger. Better, a thousand times better, better for this life, better for the life to come, an existence of humble, virtuous industry than a single departure from virtue, even though it were paid with a fortune.

7. **Temptations.**—There is not a young girl but what is more or less tempted by some unprincipled wretch who may have the reputation of a genteel society man. It

behooves parents to guard carefully the morals of their daughters, and be vigilant and cautious in permitting them to accept the society of young men. Parents who desire to save their daughters from a fate which is worse than death, should endeavor by every means in their power to keep them from falling into traps cunningly devised by some cunning lover. There are many good young men, but not all are safe friends to an innocent, confiding young girl.

8. **Prostitution.**—Some girls inherit their vicious tendency; others fall because of misplaced affections; many sin through a love of dress, which is fostered by society and[382]by the surroundings amidst which they may be placed; many, very many, embrace a life of shame to escape poverty. While each of these different phases of prostitution require a different remedy, we need better men, better women, better laws and better protection for the young girls.

A RUSSIAN SPINNING GIRL.

9. **A Startling Fact.**—Startling as it may seem to some, it is a fact in our large cities that there are many girls raised [383]by parents with no other aim than to make them harlots. At a tender age they are sold by fathers and mothers into an existence which is worse than slavery itself. It is not uncommon to see girls at the tender age of thirteen or fourteen—mere children—hardened courtesans, lost to all sense of shame and decency. They are reared in ignorance, surrounded by demoralizing influences, cut off from the blessings of church and Sabbath school, see nothing but licentiousness, intemperance and crime. These young girls are lost forever. They are beyond the reach of the moralist or preacher and have no comprehension of modesty and purity. Virtue to them is a stranger, and has been from the cradle.

10. **A Great Wrong.**—Parents too poor to clothe themselves bring children into the world, children for whom they have no bread, consequently the girl easily falls a victim in early womanhood to the heartless libertine. The boy with no other schooling but that of the streets soon masters all the qualifications for a professional criminal. If there could be a law forbidding people to marry who have no visible means of supporting a family, or if they should marry, if their children could be taken from them and properly educated by the State, it would cost the country less and be a great step in advancing our civilization.

11. **The First Step.**—Thousands of fallen women could have been saved from lives of degradation and deaths of shame had they received more toleration and loving forgiveness in their first steps of error. Many women naturally pure and virtuous have fallen to the lowest depths because discarded by friends, frowned upon by society, and sneered at by the world, after they had taken a single mis-step. Society forgives man, but woman never.

12. **In the beginning** of every girl's downward career there is necessarily a hesitation. She naturally ponders over what course to take, dreading to meet friends and looking into the future with horror. That moment is the vital turning point in her career; a kind word of forgiveness, a mother's embrace a father's welcome may save her. The bloodhounds, known as the seducer, the libertine, the procurer, are upon her track; she is trembling on the frightful brink of the abyss. Extend a helping hand and save her!

13. **Father**, if your daughter goes astray, do not drive her from your home. Mother, if your child errs, do not close your heart against her. Sisters and brothers and friends, do not force her into the pathway of shame, but rather strive to win her back into the Eden of virtue, and in nine cases out of ten you will succeed.[384]

14. **Society Evils.**—The dance, the theater, the wine-cup, the race-course, the idle frivolity and luxury of summer watering places, all have a tendency to demoralize the young.

15. **Bad Society.**—Much of our modern society admits libertines and seducers to the drawing-room, while it excludes their helpless and degraded victims, consequently it is not strange that there are skeletons in many closets, matrimonial infelicity and wayward girls.

16. **"'Know Thyself,'** says Dr. Saur, "is an important maxim for us all, and especially is it true for girls.

"All are born with the desire to become attractive—girls especially want to grow up, not only attractive, but beautiful. Some girls think that bright eyes, pretty hair and fine clothes alone make them beautiful. This is not so. Real beauty depends upon good health, good manners and a pure mind.

"As the happiness of our girls depends upon their health, it behoves us all to guide the girls in such a way as to bring forward the best of results.

17. **"There Is No One** who stands so near the girl as the mother. From early childhood she occupies the first place in the little one's confidence—she laughs, plays, and corrects, when necessary, the faults of her darling. She should be equally ready to guide in the important laws of life and health upon which rest her future. Teach your daughters that in all things the 'creative principle' has its source in life itself. It originates from Divine life, and when they know that it may be consecrated to wise and useful purposes, they are never apt to grow up with base thoughts or form bad habits. Their lives become a happiness to themselves and a blessing to humanity.

18. **Teach Wisely.**—"Teach your daughters that *all life* originates from a seed—a germ. Knowing this law, you need have no fears that base or unworthy thoughts of the reproductive function can ever enter their minds. The growth, development and ripening of human seed becomes a beautiful and sacred mystery. The tree, the rose and all plant life are equally as mysterious and beautiful in their reproductive life. Does not this alone prove to us, conclusively, that there is a Divinity in the background governing, controlling and influencing our lives? Nature has no secrets, and why should we? None at all. The only care we should experience is in teaching wisely.[385]

"Yes—lead them wisely—teach them that the seed, the germ of a new life, is maturing within them. Teach them that between the ages of eleven and fourteen this maturing process has certain physical signs. The breasts grow round and full, the whole body, even the voice, undergoes a change. It is right that they should be taught the natural law of life in reproduction and the physiological structure of their being. Again we repeat that these lessons should be taught by the mother, and in a tender, delicate and confidential way. Become, oh, mother, your daughter's companion, and she will not go elsewhere for this knowledge—which must come to all in time, but possibly too late and through sources that would prove more harm than good.

19. **The Organs of Creative Life** in women are: Ovaries, Fallopian tubes, uterus, vagina and mammary glands. The *ovaries* and *Fallopian tubes* have already been described under "The Female Generative Organs."

"The *uterus* is a pear-shaped muscular organ, situated in the lower portion of the pelvis, between the bladder and the rectum. It is less than three inches in length and two inches in width and one in thickness.

"The *vagina* is a membranous canal which joins the internal outlet with the womb, which projects slightly into it. The opening into the vagina is nearly oval, and in those who have never indulged in sexual intercourse or in handling the sexual organs is more or less closed by a membrane termed the *hymen*. The presence of this membrane was formerly considered as undoubted evidence of virginity; its absence, a lack of chastity.

"The *mammary glands* are accessory to the generative organs. They secrete milk, which the All-wise Father provided for the nourishment of the child after birth.

20. **"Menstruation**, which appears about the age of thirteen years, is the flow from the uterus that occurs every month as the seed-germ ripens in the ovaries. God made the sexual organs so that the race should not die out. He gave them to us so that we may reproduce life, and thus fill the highest position in the created universe. The purpose for which they are made is high and holy and honorable, and if they are used only for this purpose—and they must not be used at all until they are fully matured—they will be a source of greatest blessing to us all.

HOPEFUL YOUTH.

21. **"A Careful Study** of this organ, of its location, of its arteries and nerves, will convince the growing girl that [387]her body should never submit to corsets and tight lacing in response to the demands of fashion, even though nature has so bountifully provided for the safety of this important organ. By constant pressure the vagina and womb may be compressed into one-third their natural length or crowded into an unnatural position. We can readily see, then, the effect of lacing or tight clothing. Under these circumstances the ligaments lose their elasticity, and as a result we have prolapsus or falling of the womb.

22. **"I Am More Anxious** for growing girls than for any other earthly object. These girls are to be the mothers of future generations; upon them hangs the destiny of the world in coming time, and if they can be made to understand what is right and what is wrong with regard to their own bodies now, while they are young, the children they will give birth to and the men and women who shall call them mother will be of a higher type and belong to a nobler class than those of the present day.

23. **"All Women Cannot** have good features, but they can look well, and it is possible to a great extent to correct deformity and develop much of the figure. The first step to good looks is good health, and the first element of health is cleanliness. Keep clean— wash freely, bathe regularly. All the skin wants is leave to act, and it takes care of itself.

24. **"Girls Sometimes Get the Idea** that it is nice to be 'weak' and 'delicate,' but they cannot get a more false idea! God meant women to be strong and able-bodied, and only by being so can they be happy and capable of imparting happiness to others. It is only by being strong and healthy that they can be perfect in their sexual nature; and it is only by being perfect in this part of their being that you can become a noble, grand and beautiful woman.

25. **"Up to the Age** of puberty, if the girl has grown naturally, waist, hips and shoulders are about the same in width, the shoulders being, perhaps, a trifle the broadest. Up to this time the sexual organs have grown but little. Now they take a sudden start and need more room. Nature aids the girls; the tissues and muscles increase in size and the pelvis bones enlarge. The limbs grow plump, the girl stops growing tall and becomes round and full. Unsuspected strength comes to her; tasks that were once hard to perform are now easy; her voice becomes sweeter and stronger. The mind develops more rapidly even than the body; her brain is more active and quicker; subjects that once were [388]dull and dry have unwonted interest; lessons are more easily learned; the eyes sparkle with intelligence, indicating increased mental power; her manner denotes the consciousness of new power; toys of childhood are laid away; womanly thoughts and pursuits fill her mind; budding childhood has become blooming womanhood. Now, if ever, must be laid the foundation of physical vigor and of a healthy body. Girls should realize the significance of this fact. Do not get the idea that men admire a weakly, puny, delicate, small-waisted, languid, doll-like creature, a libel on true womanhood. Girls admire men with broad chests, square shoulders, erect form, keen bright eyes, hard muscles and undoubted vigor. Men also turn naturally to healthy, robust, well-developed girls, and to win their admiration girls must meet their ideals. A good form, a sound mind and a healthy body are within the reach of nine out of ten of our girls by proper care and training. Physical bankruptcy may claim the same proportion if care and training are neglected.

26. **"A Woman Five Feet Tall** should measure two feet around the waist and thirty-three inches around the hips. A waist less than this proportion indicates compression either by lacing or tight clothing. Exercise in the open air, take long walks and vigorous exercise, using care not to overdo it. Housework will prove a panacea for many of the ills which flesh is heir to. One hour's exercise at the wash-*tub is of far more value, from a physical standpoint, than hours at the piano. Boating is most excellent exercise and within the reach of many. Care in dressing is also important, and, fortunately, fashion is coming to the rescue here. It is essential that no garments be suspended from the waist. Let the shoulders bear the weight of all the clothing, so that the organs of the body may be left free and unimpeded.

27. **"Sleep Should be Had** regularly and abundantly. Avoid late hours, undue excitement, evil associations; partake of plain, nutritious food, and health will be your reward. There is one way of destroying health, which, fortunately, is not as common among girls as boys, and which must be mentioned ere this chapter closes. Self-abuse is practised among growing girls to such an extent as to arouse serious alarm. Many a girl has been led to handle and play with her sexual organs through the advice of some girl who has obtained temporary pleasure in that [389]way; or, perchance, chafing has been followed by rubbing until the organs have become congested with blood, and in this accidental manner the girl discovered what seems to her a source of pleasure, but which, alas, is a source of misery, and even death.

28. **"As In the Boy, So In the Girl**, self-abuse causes an undue amount of blood to flow to those organs, thus depriving other parts of the body of its nourishment, the weakest

part first showing the effect of want of sustenance. All that has been said upon this loathsome subject in the preceding chapter for boys might well be repeated here, but space forbids. Read that chapter again, and know that the same signs that betray the boy will make known the girl addicted to the vice. The bloodless lips, the dull, heavy eye surrounded with dark rings, the nerveless hand, the blanched cheek, the short breath, the old, faded look, the weakened memory and silly irritability tell the story all too plainly. The same evil result follows, ending perhaps in death, or worse, in insanity. Aside from the injury the girl does herself by yielding to this habit, there is one other reason which appeals to the conscience, and that is, self-abuse is an offence against moral law—it is putting to a vile, selfish use the organs which were given for a high, sacred purpose.

29. **"Let Them Alone**, except to care for them when care is needed, and they may prove the greatest blessing you have ever known. They were given you that you might become a mother, the highest office to which God has ever called one of His creatures. Do not debase yourself and become lower than the beasts of the field. If this habit has fastened itself upon any one of our readers, stop it now. Do not allow yourself to think about it, give up all evil associations, seek pure companions, and go to your mother, older sister, or physician for advice.

30. **"And You, Mother**, knowing the danger that besets your daughters at this critical period, are you justified in keeping silent? Can you be held guiltless if your daughter ruins body and mind because you were *too modest* to tell her the laws of her being? There is no love that is dearer to your daughter than *yours*, no advice that is more respected than *yours*, no one whose warning would be more potent. Fail not in your duty. As motherhood has been your sweetest joy, so help your daughter to make it hers."

[390]

Save the Boys.
PLAIN WORDS TO PARENTS.
YOUNG GARFIELD DRIVING TEAM ON THE CANAL.

1. With a shy look, approaching his mother when she was alone, the boy of fifteen said, "There are some things I want to ask you. I hear the boys speak of them at school, and I don't understand, and a fellow doesn't like to ask any one but his mother."

2. Drawing him down to her, in the darkness that was closing about them, the mother spoke to her son and the son to his mother freely of things which everybody must know sooner or later, and which no boy should learn from "anyone but his mother" or father.

3. If you do not answer such a natural question, your boy will turn for answer to others, and learn things, perhaps, which your cheeks may well blush to have him know.

4. Our boys and girls are growing faster than we think. The world moves; we can no longer put off our children [391]with the old nurses' tales; even MacDonald's beautiful statement,

"Out of the everywhere into the there",

does not satisfy them when they reverse his question and ask, "Where did I come from?"

5. They must be answered. If we put them off, they may be tempted to go elsewhere for information, and hear half-truths, or whole truths so distorted, so mingled with what is low and impure that, struggle against it as they may in later years, their minds will always retain these early impressions.

6. It is not so hard if you begin early. The very flowers are object lessons. The wonderful mystery of life is wrapped in one flower, with its stamens, pistils and ovaries. Every child knows how an egg came in the nest, and takes it as a matter of course; why not go one step farther with them and teach the wonder, the beauty, the holiness that surrounds maternity anywhere? Why, centuries ago the Romans honored, and taught their boys to honor, the women in whose safety was bound up the future of their existence as a nation! Why should we do less?

7. Your sons and mine, your daughters and mine, need to be wisely taught and guarded just along these lines, if your sons and mine, your daughters and mine, are to grow up into a pure, healthy, Christian manhood and womanhood.

157

8. ⊔"How grand is the boy who has kept himself undefiled! His complexion clear, his muscles firm, his movements vigorous, his manner frank, his courage undaunted, his brain active, his will firm, his self-control perfect, his body and mind unfolding day by day. His life should be one song of praise and thanksgiving. If you want your boy to be such a one, train him, my dear woman, *to-day,* and his *to-morrow* will take care of itself.

9. "Think you that good seed sown will bring forth bitter fruit? A thousand times, No! As we sow, so shall we reap. Train your boys in morality, temperance and virtue. Teach them to embrace good and shun evil. Teach them the true from the false; the light from the dark. Teach them that when they take a thing that is not their own, they commit a sin. Teach them that *sin means disobedience of God's laws of every kind.*

10. "God made every organ of our body with the intention that it should perform a certain work. If we wish to see, we use our eyes; if we want to hear, our ears are called into use. In fact, nature teaches us the proper use of *all our organs.* I say to you, mother, and oh, so earnestly: 'Go teach your boy that which you may never be ashamed to do, about these organs that make him *specially a boy.'*

11. "Teach him they are called *sexual organs;* that they are not impure, but of special importance, and made by God for a definite purpose. Teach him that there are impurities taken from the system in fluid form called urine, and that it passes through the sexual organs, but that nature takes care of that. Teach him that these organs are given as a sacred trust, that in maturer years he may be the means of giving life to those who shall live forever.

12. "Impress upon him that if these organs are abused, or if they are put to any use besides that for which God made them—and He did not intend they should be used at all until man is fully grown—they will bring disease and ruin upon those who abuse and disobey the laws which God has made to govern them. If he has ever learned to handle his *sexual organs,* or to touch them in any way except to keep them clean, not to do it again. If he does he will not grow up happy, healthy and strong.

13. "Teach him that when he handles or excites the [393]sexual organs all parts of the body suffer, because they are connected by nerves that run throughout the system; this is why it is called 'self-abuse.' The whole body is abused when this part of the body is handled or excited in any manner whatever. Teach them to shun all children who indulge in this loathsome habit, or all children who talk about these things. The sin is terrible, and is, in fact, worse than lying or stealing. For, although these are wicked and will ruin their souls, yet this habit of self-abuse will ruin both soul and body.

14. "If the sexual organs are handled, it brings too much blood to these parts, and this produces a diseased condition; it also causes disease in other organs of the body, because they are left with a less amount of blood than they ought to have. The sexual organs, too, are very closely connected with the spine and the brain by means of the nerves, and if they are handled, or if you keep thinking about them, these nerves get excited and become exhausted, and this makes the back ache, the brain heavy and the whole body weak.

15. "It lays the foundation for consumption, paralysis and heart disease. It weakens the memory, makes a boy careless, negligent and listless. It even makes many lose their minds; others, when grown, commit suicide. How often mothers see their little boys handling themselves, and let it pass, because they think the boy will outgrow the habit, and do not realize the strong hold it has upon them. I say to you who love your boys—'Watch!'

16. "Don't think it does no harm to your boy because he does not suffer now, for the effects of this vice come on so slowly that the victim is often very near death before you realize that he has done himself harm. The boy with no knowledge of the consequences, and with no one to warn him, finds momentary pleasure in its practice, and so contracts a habit which grows upon him, undermining his health, poisoning his mind, arresting his development, and laying the foundation for future misery.

17. "Do not read this book and forget it, for it contains earnest and living truths. Do not let false modesty stand in your way, but from this time on keep this thought in mind—'the saving of your boy.' Follow its teachings and you will bless God as long as you live. Read

it to your neighbors, who, like yourself, have growing boys, and urge them for the sake of humanity to heed its advice.[394]

18. "Right here we want to emphasize the importance of *cleanliness*. We verily believe that oftentimes these habits originate in a burning and irritating sensation about the organs, caused by a want of thorough washing.

19. "It is worthy of note that many eminent physicians now advocate the custom of circumcision, claiming that the removal of a little of the foreskin induces cleanliness, thus preventing the irritation and excitement which come from the gathering of the whiteish matter under the foreskin at the beginning of the glands. This irritation being removed, the boy is less apt to tamper with his sexual organs. The argument seems a good one, especially when we call to mind the high physical state of those people who have practiced the custom.

20. "Happy is the mother who can feel she has done her duty, in this direction, while her boy is still a child. For those mothers, though, whose little boys have now grown to boyhood with the evil still upon them, and *you*, through ignorance, permitted it, we would say, 'Begin at once; it is never too late.' If he has not lost all will power, he can be saved. Let him go in confidence to a reputable physician and follow his advice. Simple diet, plentiful exercise in open air and congenial employment will do much. Do not let the mind dwell upon evil thoughts, shun evil companions, avoid vulgar stories, sensational novels, and keep the thoughts pure.

21. "Let him interest himself in social and benevolent affairs, participate in Sunday-school work, farmers' clubs, or any organizations which tend to elevate and inspire noble sentiment. Let us remember that 'a perfect man is the noblest work of God.' God has given us a life which is to last forever, and the little time we spend on earth is as nothing to the ages which we are to spend in the world beyond; so our earthly life is a very important part of our existence, for it is here that the foundation is laid for either happiness or misery in the future. It is here that we decide our destiny, and our efforts to know and obey God's laws in our bodies as well as in our souls will not only bring blessings to us in this life, but never-ending happiness throughout eternity."

22. **A Question.**—How can a father chew and smoke tobacco, drink and swear, use vulgar language, tell obscene stories, and raise a family of pure, clean-minded children?LET THE ECHO ANSWER.

[396]
The Inhumanities of Parents.
AN OLD ADAGE: "HE WHO LOVES CHILDREN WILL DO YOU NO HARM."

1. Not long ago a Presbyterian minister in Western New York whipped his three-year-old boy to death for refusing to say his prayers. The little fingers were broken; the tender flesh was bruised and actually mangled; strong men wept when they looked on the lifeless body. Think of a strong man from one hundred and fifty to two hundred pounds in weight, pouncing upon a little child, like a Tiger upon a Lamb, and with his strong arm inflicting physical blows on the delicate tissues of a child's body. See its frail and trembling flesh quiver and its tender nervous organization shaking with terror and fear.

2. How often is this the case in the punishment of children all over this broad land! Death is not often the immediate consequence of this brutality as in the above stated case, but the punishment is often as unjust, and the physical constitution of children is often ruined and the mind by fright seriously injured.

3. Everyone knows the sudden sense of pain, and sometimes dizziness and nausea follow, as the results of an accidental hitting of the ankle, knee or elbow against a hard substance, and involuntary tears are brought to the eyes; but what is such a pain as this compared with the pains of a dozen or more quick blows on the body of a little helpless child from the strong arm of a parent in a passion? Add to this overwhelming terror of fright, the strangulating effects of sighing and shrieking, and you have a complete picture of child-torture.

4. Who has not often seen a child receive, within an hour or two of the first whipping, a second one, for some small ebullition of nervous irritability, which was simply inevitable from its spent and worn condition?

5. Would not all mankind cry out at the inhumanity of one who, as things are to-day, should propose the substitution of pricking or cutting or burning for whipping? It would, however, be easy to show that small jabs or pricks or cuts are more human than the blows many children receive. Why may not lying be as legitimately cured by blisters made with hot coals as by black and blue spots made with a ruler or whip? The principle is the same; and if the principle is right, why not multiply methods?

6. How many loving mothers will, without any thought of cruelty, inflict half a dozen quick blows on the little hand of her child, and when she could no more take a pin and make [397]the same number of thrusts into the tender flesh, than she could bind the baby on a rack. Yet the pin-thrust would hurt far less, and would probably make a deeper impression on the child's mind.

7. We do not intend to be understood that a child must have everything that it desires and every whim and wish to receive special recognition by the parents. Children can soon be made to understand the necessity of obedience, and punishment can easily be brought about by teaching them self-denial. Deny them the use of a certain plaything, deny [398]them the privilege of visiting certain of their little friends, deny them the privilege of the table, etc., and these self-denials can be applied according to the age and condition of the child, with firmness and without any yielding. Children will soon learn obedience if they see the parents are sincere. Lessons of home government can be learned by the children at home as well as they can learn lessons at school.

8. The trouble is, many parents need more government, more training and more discipline than the little ones under their control.

9. Scores of times during the day a child is told in a short, authoritative way to do or not to do certain little things, which we ask at the hands of elder persons as favors. When we speak to an elder person, we say, would you be so kind as to close the door, when the same person making the request of a child will say, "*Shut the door.*" "*Bring me the chair.*" "*Stop that noise.*" "*Sit down there.*" Whereas, if the same kindness was used towards the child it would soon learn to imitate the example.

10. On the other hand, let a child ask for anything without saying "please," receive anything without saying "thank you," it suffers a rebuke and a look of scorn at once. Often a child insists on having a book, chair or apple to the inconveniencing of an elder, and what an outcry is raised: "Such rudeness;" "Such an ill-mannered child;" "His parents must have neglected him strangely." Not at all: The parents may have been steadily telling him a great many times every day not to do these precise things which you dislike. But they themselves have been all the time doing those very things before him, and there is no proverb that strikes a truer balance between two things than the old one which weighs example over against precept.

11. It is a bad policy to be rude to children. A child will win and be won, and in a long run the chances are that the child will have better manners than its parents. Give them a good example and take pains in teaching them lessons of obedience and propriety, and there will be little difficulty in raising a family of beautiful and well-behaved children.

12. Never correct a child in the presence of others; it is a rudeness to the child that will soon destroy its self-respect. It is the way criminals are made and should always and everywhere be condemned.

13. But there are no words to say what we are or what we deserve, if we do this to the little children whom we [399]have dared for our own pleasure to bring into the perils of this life, and whose whole future may be blighted by the mistakes of our careless hands. There are thousands of young men and women to-day groaning under the penalties and burdens of life, who owe their misfortunes, their shipwreck and ruin to the ignorance or indifference of parents.

14. Parents of course love their children, but with that love there is a responsibility that cannot be shirked. The government and training of children is a study that demands a parent's time and attention often much more than the claims of business.

15. Parents, study the problems that come up every day in your home. Remember, your future happiness, and the future welfare of your children, depend upon it.

16. **Criminals and Heredity.**—Wm. M. F. Round was for many years in charge of the House of Refuge on Randall's Island, New York, and his opportunities for observation in the work among criminals surely make him a competent judge, and he says in his letter to the New York Observer: "Among this large number of young offenders I can state with entire confidence that not one per cent. were children born of criminal parents; and with equal confidence I am able to say that the common cause of their delinquency was found in bad parental training, in bad companionship, and in lack of wholesome restraint from evil associations and influences. It was this knowledge that led to the establishing of the House of Refuge nearly three-quarters of a century ago."

17. **Bad Training.**—Thus it is seen from one of the best authorities in the United States that criminals are made either by the indifference or the neglect of parents, or both, or by too much training without proper judgment and knowledge. Give your children a good example, and never tell a child to do something and then become indifferent as to whether they do it or not. A child should never be told twice to do the same thing. Teach the child in childhood obedience and never vary from that rule. Do it kindly but firmly.

18. **If Your Children Do Not Obey or Respect You** in their childhood and youth, how can you expect to govern them when older and shape their character for future usefulness and good citizenship?

19. **The Fundamental Rule.**—Never tell a child twice to do the same thing. Command the respect of your children, and there will be no question as to obedience.

[400]
Chastity and Purity of Character.

1. **Chastity** is the purest and brightest jewel in human character. Dr. Pierce in his widely known *Medical Adviser* says: For the full and perfect development of mankind, both mental and physical, chastity is necessary. The health demands abstinence from unlawful intercourse. Therefore children should be instructed to avoid all impure works of fiction, which tend to inflame the mind and excite the passions. Only in total abstinence from illicit pleasures is there safety, morals, and health, while integrity, peace and happiness are the conscious rewards of virtue. Impurity travels downward with intemperance, obscenity and corrupting diseases, to degradation and death. A dissolute, licentious, free-and-easy life is filled with the dregs of human suffering, iniquity and despair. The penalties which follow a violation of the law of chastity are found to be severe and swiftly retributive.

2. **The Union** of the sexes in holy Matrimony is a law of nature, finding sanction in both morals and legislation. Even some of the lower animals unite in this union for life and instinctively observe the law of conjugal fidelity with a consistency which might put to blush other animals more highly endowed. It seems important to discuss this subject and understand our social evils, as well as the intense passional desires of the sexes, which must be controlled, or they lead to ruin.

3. **Sexual Propensities** are possessed by all, and these must be held in abeyance, until they are needed for legitimate purposes. Hence parents ought to understand the value to their children of mental and physical labor, to elevate and strengthen the intellectual and moral faculties, to develop the muscular system and direct the energies of the blood into healthful channels. Vigorous employment of mind and body engrosses the vital energies and diverts them from undue excitement of the sexual desires.

Give your young people plenty of outdoor amusement; less of dancing and more of croquet and lawn tennis. Stimulate the methods of pure thoughts in innocent amusement, and your sons and daughters will mature to manhood and womanhood pure and chaste in character.[401]

4. **Ignorance Does Not Mean Innocence.**—It is a current idea, especially among our good common people, that the child should be kept in ignorance regarding the mystery

of his own body and how he was created or came into the world. This is a great mistake. Parents must know that the sources of social impurity are great, and the child is a hundred times more liable to have his young mind poisoned if entirely ignorant of the functions of his nature than if judiciously enlightened on these important truths by the parent. The parent must give him weapons of defense against the putrid corruption he is sure to meet outside the parental roof. The child cannot get through the A, B, C period of school without it.

5. **Conflicting Views.**—There is a great difference of opinion regarding the age at which the child should be taught the mysteries of nature: some maintain that he cannot comprehend the subject before the age of puberty; others say "they will find it out soon enough, it is not best to have them over-wise while they are so young. Wait a while." That is just the point (*they will find it out*), and we ask in all candor, is it not better that they learn it from the pure loving mother, untarnished from any insinuating remark, than that they should learn it from some foul-mouthed libertine on the street, or some giddy girl at school? Mothers! fathers! which think you is the most sensible and fraught with the least danger to your darling boy or girl?

6. **Delay is Fraught With Danger.**—Knowledge on a subject so vitally connected with moral health must not be deferred. It is safe to say that no child, no boy at least in these days of excitement and unrest, reaches the age of ten years without getting some idea of nature's laws regarding parenthood. And ninety-nine chances to one, those ideas will be vile and pernicious unless they come from a wise, loving and pure parent. Now, we entreat you, parents, mothers! do not wait; begin before a false notion has had chance to find lodgment in the childish mind. But remember this is a lesson of life, it cannot be told in one chapter; it is as important as the lessons of love and duty.

7. **The First Lessons.**—Should you be asked by your four or five-year old, "Mamma, where did you get me?" Instead of saying, "The doctor brought you," or "God made you and a stork brought you from Babyland on his back," tell him the truth as you would about any ordinary question. One mother's explanation was something like this: "My dear, you were not made any more than apples are made, or the little chickens are made. Your dolly was [402]made, but it has no life like you have. God has provided that all living things such as plants, trees, little chickens, little kittens, little babies, etc., should grow from seeds or little tiny eggs. Apples grow, little chickens grow, little babies grow. Apple and peach trees grow from seeds that are planted in the ground, and the apples and peaches grow on the trees. Baby chickens grow inside the eggs that are kept warm by the mother hen for a certain time. Baby boys and girls do not grow inside an egg, but they start to grow inside of a snug warm nest, from an egg that is so small you cannot see it with just your eye." This was not given at once, but from time to time as the child asked questions and in the simplest language, with many illustrations from plant and animal life. It may have occupied months, but in time the lesson was fully understood.

8. **The Second Lesson.**—The second lesson came with the question, "But *where* is the nest?" The ice is now broken, as it were; it was an easy matter for the mother to say, "The nest in which you grew, dear, was close to your mother's heart inside her body. All things that do not grow inside the egg itself, and which are kept warm by the mother's body, begin to grow from the egg in a nest inside the mother's body." It may be that this mother had access to illustrations of the babe in the womb which were shown and explained to the child, a boy. He was pleased and satisfied with the explanations. It meant nothing out of the ordinary any more than a primary lesson on the circulatory system did, it was knowledge on nature in its purity and simplicity taught by mother, and hence caused no surprise. The subject of the male and female generative organs came later; the greatest pains and care was taken to make it clear, the little boy was taught that the *sexual organs* were made for a high and holy purpose, that their office at present is only to carry off impurities from the system in the fluid form called urine, and that he must never handle his *sexual organs* nor touch them in any way except to keep them clean, and if he does this, he will grow up a bright, happy and healthy boy. But if he excites or *abuses* them, he will become puny, sickly and unhappy. All this was explained in language pure and simple. There is now in the boy a sturdy base of character building along the line of virtue and purity through knowledge.

9. Silly Dirty Trash.—But I hear some mother say "Such silly dirty trash to tell a child!" It is not dirty nor silly; it is nature's untarnished truth. God has ordained that children should thus be brought into the world, do you call the works of God silly? Remember, kind mother, and [403]don't forget it, if you fail to teach your children, boys or girls, these important lessons early in life, they will learn them from other sources, perhaps long ere you dream of it, and ninety-nine times out of one hundred they will get improper, perverted, impure and vile ideas of these important truths; besides you have lost their confidence and you will never regain it in these matters. They will never come to mamma for information on these subjects. And, think you, that your son and daughter, later in life will make you their confidant as they ought? Will your beautiful daughter hand the first letters she receives from her lover to mamma to read, and seek her counsel and advice when she replies to them? Will she ask mamma whether it is ever proper to sit in her lover's lap? I think not; you have blighted her confidence and alienated her affections. You have kept knowledge from her that she had a right to know; you even failed to teach her the important truths of menstruation. Troubled and excited at the first menstrual flow, she dashed her feet in cold water hoping to stop the flow. You know the results—she is now twenty-five but is suffering from it to this day. You, her mother, over fastidious, *so very nice* you would never mention "*such silly trash*," but by your consummate foolishness and mock modesty you have ruined your daughter's health, and though in later years she may forgive you, yet she can never love and respect you as she ought.

10. "Knowledge the Preserver of Purity."—Laura E. Scammon, writing on this subject, in the *Arena* of November, 1893, says: "When questions arise that can not be answered by observation, reply to each as simply and directly as you answer questions upon other subjects, giving scientific names and facts, and such explanations as are suited to the comprehension of the child. Treat nature and her laws always with serious, respectful attention. Treat the holy mysteries of parenthood reverently, never losing sight of the great law upon which are founded all others—the law of love. Say it and sing it, play it and pray it into the soul of your child, that *love is lord of all*."

11. Conclusion of the Whole Matter.—Observation and common sense should teach every parent that lack of knowledge on these subjects and proper counsel and advice in later years is the main cause of so many charming girls being seduced and led astray, and so many bright promising boys wrecked by *self-abuse* or *social impurity*. Make your children your confidants early in life, especially in these things, have frequent talks with them on nature, and you will never, other things being equal, mourn over a ruined daughter or a wreckless, debased son.

[404]
Exciting the Passions in Children.

1. Conversation before Children.—The conduct and conversation of adults before children and youth, how often have I blushed with shame, and kindled with indignation at the conversation of parents, and especially of mothers, to their children: "John, go and kiss Harriet, for she is your sweet-heart." Well may shame make him hesitate and hang his head. "Why, John, I did not think you so great a coward. Afraid of the girls, are you? That will never do. Come, go along, and hug and kiss her. There, that's a man. I guess you will love the girls yet." Continually is he teased about the girls and being in love, till he really selects a sweet-heart.

2. The Loss of Maiden Purity and Natural Delicacy.—I will not lift the veil, nor expose the conduct of children among themselves. And all this because adults have filled their heads with those impurities which surfeit their own. What could more effectually wear off that natural delicacy, that maiden purity and bashfulness, which form the main barriers against the influx of vitiated Amativeness? How often do those whose modesty has been worn smooth, even take pleasure in thus saying and doing things to raise the blush on the cheek of youth and innocence, merely to witness the effect of this improper illusion upon them; little realizing that they are thereby breaking down the barriers of their virtue, and prematurely kindling the fires of animal passion!

163

3. **Balls, Parties and Amusements.**—The entire machinery of balls and parties, of dances and other amusements of young people, tend to excite and inflame this passion. Thinking it a fine thing to get in love, they court and form attachments long before either their mental or physical powers are matured. Of course, these young loves, these greenhouse exotics, must be broken off, and their miserable subjects left burning up with the fierce fires of a flaming passion, which, if left alone, would have slumbered on for years, till they were prepared for its proper management and exercise.

4. **Sowing the Seeds for Future Ruin.**—Nor is it merely the conversation of adults that does all this mischief; their manners also increase it. Young men take the hands of girls from six to thirteen years old, kiss them, press them, and play with them so as, in a great variety of ways, to excite their innocent passions, combined, I grant, with friendship and refinement—for all this is genteely done. They [405]intend no harm, and parents dream of none: and yet their embryo love is awakened, to be again still more easily excited. Maiden ladies, and even married women, often express similar feelings towards lads, not perhaps positively improper in themselves, yet injurious in their ultimate effects.

5. **Reading Novels.**—How often have I seen girls not twelve years old, as hungry for a story or novel as they should be for their dinners! A sickly sentimentalism is thus formed, and their minds are sullied with impure desires. Every fashionable young lady must of course read every new novel, though nearly all of them contain exceptionable allusions, perhaps delicately covered over with a thin gauze of fashionable refinement; yet, on that very account, the more objectionable. If this work contained one improper allusion to their ten, many of those fastidious ladies who now eagerly devour the vulgarities of Dumas, and the double-entendres of Bulwer, and even converse with gentlemen about their contents, would discountenance or condemn it as improper. *Shame on novel-reading women;* for they cannot have pure minds or unsullied feelings but Cupid and the beaux, and waking of dreams of love, are fast consuming their health and virtue.

6. **Theater-going.**—Theaters and theatrical dancing, also inflame the passions, and are "the wide gate" of "the broad road" of moral impurity. Fashionable music is another, especially the verses set to it, being mostly love-sick ditties, or sentimental odes, breathing this tender passion in its most melting and bewitching strains. Improper prints often do immense injury in this respect, as do also balls, parties, annuals, newspaper articles, exceptional works, etc.

7. **The Conclusion of the Whole Matter.**—Stop for one moment and think for yourself and you will be convinced that the sentiment herein announced is for your good and the benefit of all mankind.

[406]

Puberty, Virility and Hygienic Laws.

1. **What is Puberty?**—The definition is explained in another portion of this book, but it should be understood that it is not a prompt or immediate change; it is a slow extending growth and may extend for many years. The ripening of physical powers do not take place when the first signs of puberty appear.

2. **Proper Age.**—The proper age for puberty should vary from twelve to eighteen years. As a general rule, in the more vigorous and the more addicted to athletic exercise or out-door life, this change is slower in making its approach.

3. **Hygienic Attention.**—Youths at this period should receive special private attention. They should be taught the purpose of the sexual organs and the proper hygienic laws that govern them, and they should also be taught to rise in the morning and not to lie in bed after waking up, because it is largely owing to this habit that the secret vice is contracted. One of the common causes of premature excitement in many boys is a tight foreskin. It may cause much evil and ought always to be remedied. Ill-fitting garments often cause much irritation in children and produce unnatural passions. It is best to have boys sleep in separate beds and not have them sleep together if it can be avoided.[407]

4. **Proper Influence.**—Every boy and girl should be carefully trained to look with disgust on everything that is indecent in word or action. Let them be taught a sense of shame

in doing shameful things, and teach them that modesty is honorable, and that immodesty is indecent and dishonorable. Careful training at the proper age may save many a boy or girl from ruin.

5. **Sexual Passions.**—The sexual passions may be a fire from heaven, or a subtle flame from hell. It depends upon the government and proper control. The noblest and most unselfish emotions take their rise in the passion of sex. Its sweet influence, its elevating ties, its vibrations and harmony, all combine to make up the noble and courageous traits of man.

6. **When Passions Begin.**—It is thought by some that passions begin at the age of puberty, but the passions may be produced as early as five or ten years. All depends upon the training or the want of it. Self-abuse is not an uncommon evil at the age of eight or ten. A company of bad boys often teach an innocent child that which will develop his ruin. A boy may feel a sense of pleasure at eight and produce a slight discharge, but not of semen. Thus it is seen that parents may by neglect do their child the greatest injury.

7. **False Modesty.**—Let there be no false modesty on part of the parents. Give the child the necessary advice and instructions as soon as necessary.

8. **The Man Unsexed**, by Mutilation or Masturbation. Eunuchs are proverbial for their cruelty and crafty and unsympathizing dispositions. Their mental powers are feeble and their physical strength is inferior. They lack courage and physical endurance. When a child is operated upon before the age of puberty, the voice retains its childish treble, the limbs their soft and rounded outlines, and the neck acquires a feminine fulness; no beard makes its appearance. In ancient times and up to this time in Oriental nations eunuchs are found. They are generally slaves who have suffered mutilation at a tender age. It is a scientific fact that where boys have been taught the practice of masturbation in their early years, say from eight to fourteen years of age, if they survive at all they often have their powers reduced to a similar condition of a eunuch. They generally however suffer a greater disadvantage. Their health will be more or less injured. In the eunuch the power of sexual intercourse is not entirely lost but of course there is sterility and little if any satisfaction, and the same thing may be true of the victim of self-abuse.[408]

9. **Signs of Virility.**—As the young man develops in strength and years the sexual appetite will manifest itself. The secretion of the male known as the seed or semen depends for the life-transmitting power upon little minute bodies called spermatozoa. These are very active and numerous in a healthy secretion, being many hundreds in a single drop and a single one of them is capable to bring about conception in a female. Dr. Napheys in his "Transmission of Life," says: "The secreted fluid has been frozen and kept at a temperature of zero for four days, yet when it was thawed these animalcules, as they are supposed to be, were as active as ever. They are not, however, always present, and when present may be of variable activity. In young men, just past puberty, and in aged men, they are often scarce and languid in motion." At the proper age the secretion is supposed to be the most active, generally at the age of twenty-five, and decreases as age increases.

10. **Hygienic Rule.**—The man at mid-life should guard carefully his passions and the husband his virile powers, and as the years progress, steadily wean himself more from his desire, for his passions will become weaker with age and any excitement in middle life may soon debilitate and destroy his virile powers.

11. **Follies of Youth.**—Dr. Napheys says: "Not many men can fritter away a decade or two of years in dissipation and excess, and ever hope to make up their losses by rigid surveillance in later years." "The sins of youth are expiated in age," is a proverb which daily examples illustrate. In proportion as puberty is precocious, will decadence be premature; the excesses of middle life draw heavily on the fortune of later years. "The mill of the gods grinds slow, but it grinds exceedingly fine," and though nature may be a tardy creditor, she is found at last to be an inexorable one.

[409]

Our Secret Sins.

1. **Passions.**—Every healthful man has sexual desires, and he might as well refuse to satisfy his hunger as to deny their existence. The Creator has given us various appetites, intended they should be indulged, and has provided the means.

2. **Reason.**—While it is true that a healthy man has strongly developed sexual passions, yet, God has crowned man with reason, and with a proper exercise of this wonderful faculty of the human mind no lascivious thoughts need to control the passions. A pure heart will develop pure thoughts and bring out a good life.

3. **Rioting in Visions.**—Dr. Lewis says: "Rioting in visions of nude women may exhaust one as much as an excess in actual intercourse. There are multitudes who would never spend the night with an abandoned female, but who rarely meet a young girl that their imaginations are not busy with her person. This species of indulgence is well-nigh universal; and it is the source of all other forms—the fountain from which the external vices spring, and the nursery of masturbation."

4. **Committing Adultery in the Heart.**—A young man who allows his mind to dwell upon the vision of nude women will soon become a victim of ruinous passion, and either fall under the influence of lewd women or resort to self-abuse. The man who has no control over his mind and allows impure thoughts to be associated with the name of every female that may be suggested to his mind, is but committing adultery in his heart, just as guilty at heart as though he had committed the deed.

5. **Unchastity.**—So far as the record is preserved, unchastity has contributed above all other causes, more to the ruin and exhaustion and demoralization of the race than all other wickedness. And we shall not be likely to vanquish the monster, even in ourselves, unless we make the thoughts our point of attack. So long as they are sensual we are indulging in sexual abuse, and are almost sure, when temptation is presented, to commit the overt acts of sin. If we cannot succeed within, we may pray in vain for help to resist the tempter outwardly. A young man who will indulge in obscene language will be guilty of a worse deed if opportunity is offered.

6. **Bad Dressing.**—If women knew how much mischief they do men they would change some of their habits of [410]dress. The dress of their busts, the padding in different parts, are so contrived as to call away attention from the soul and fix it on the bosom and hips. And then, many, even educated women, are careful to avoid serious subjects in our presence—one minute before a gentleman enters the room they may be engaged in thoughtful discussion, but the moment he appears their whole style changes; they assume light fascinating ways, laugh sweet little bits of laughs, and turn their heads this way and that, all which forbids serious thinking and gives men over to imagination.

7. **The Lustful Eye.**—How many men there are who lecherously stare at every woman in whose presence they happen to be. These monsters stare at women as though they were naked in a cage on exhibition. A man whose whole manner is full of animal passion is not worthy of the respect of refined women. They have no thoughts, no ideas, no sentiments, nothing to interest them but the bodies of women whom they behold. The moral character of young women has no significance or weight in their eyes. This kind of men are a curse to society and a danger to the community. No young lady is safe in their company.

8. **Rebuking Sensualism.**—If the young women would exercise an honorable independence and heap contempt upon the young men that allow their imagination to take such liberties, a different state of things would soon follow. Men of that type of character should have no recognition in the presence of ladies.

9. **Early Marriages.**—There can be no doubt that early marriages are bad for both parties. For children of such a marriage always lack vitality. The ancient Germans did not marry until the twenty-fourth or twenty-fifth year, previous to which they observed the most rigid chastity, and in consequence they acquired a size and strength that excited the astonishment of Europe. The present incomparable vigor of that race, both physically and mentally, is due in a great measure to their long established aversion to marrying young. The results of too early marriages are in brief, stunted growth and impaired strength on the part of the male; delicate if not utterly bad health in the female; the premature old age or death of one or both, and a puny, sickly offspring.

10. **Signs of Excesses.**—Dr. Dio Lewis says: "Some of the most common effects of sexual excess are backache, lassitude, giddiness, dimness of sight, noises in the ears, numbness of the fingers, and paralysis. The drain is universal, but the more sensitive organs

and tissues suffer [411]most. So the nervous system gives way and continues the principal sufferer throughout. A large part of the premature loss of sight and hearing, dizziness, numbness and pricking in the hands and feet, and other kindred developments, are justly chargeable to unbridled venery. Not unfrequently you see men whose head or back or nerve testifies of such reckless expenditure."

11. **Non-Completed Intercourse.**—Withdrawal before the emission occurs is injurious to both parties. The soiling of the conjugal bed by the shameful manœuvres is to be deplored.

12. **The Extent of the Practice.**—One cannot tell to what extent this vice is practiced, except by observing its consequences, even among people who fear to commit the slightest sin, to such a degree is the public conscience perverted upon this point. Still, many husbands know that nature often renders nugatory the most subtle calculations, and reconquers the rights which they have striven to frustrate. No matter; they persevere none the less, and by the force of habit they poison the most blissful moments of life, with no surety of averting the result that they fear. So who knows if the too often feeble and weakened infants are not the fruit of these in themselves incomplete procreations, and disturbed by preoccupations foreign to the natural act.

13. **Health of Women.**—Furthermore, the moral relations existing between the married couple undergo unfortunate changes; this affection, founded upon reciprocal esteem, is little by little effaced by the repetition of an act which pollutes the marriage bed. If the good harmony of families and the reciprocal relations are seriously menaced by the invasion of these detestable practices, the health of women, as we have already intimated, is fearfully injured.

14. **The Practice of Abortion.**—Then we have the practice of abortion reduced in modern times to a science, and almost to a distinct profession. A large part of the business is carried on by the means of medicines advertised in obscure but intelligible terms as embryo-destroyers or preventives of conception. Every large city has its professional abortionist. Many ordinary physicians destroy embryos to order, and the skill to do this terrible deed has even descended among the common people.

15. **Sexual Exhaustion.**—Every sexual excitement is exhaustive in proportion to its intensity and continuance. If a man sits by the side of a woman, fondles and kisses her three or four hours, and allows his imagination to run riot with sexual visions, he will be five times as much exhausted [412]as he would by the act culminating in emission. It is the sexual excitement more than the emission which exhausts. As shown in another part of this work, thoughts of sexual intimacies, long continued, lead to the worst effects. To a man, whose imagination is filled with erotic fancies the emission comes as a merciful interruption to the burning, harassing and wearing excitement which so constantly goads him.

16. **The Desire of Good.**—The desire of good for its own sake—this is Love. The desire of good for bodily pleasure—this is Lust. Man is a moral being, and as such should always act in the animal sphere according to the spiritual law. Hence, to break the law of the highest creative action for the mere gratification of animal instinct is to perform the act of sin and to produce the corruption of nature.

17. **Cause Of Prostitution.**—Dr. Dio Lewis says: "Occasionally we meet a diseased female with excessive animal passion, but such a case is very rare. The average woman has so little sexual desire that if licentiousness depended upon her, uninfluenced by her desire to please man or secure his support, there would be very little sexual excess. Man is strong—he has all the money and all the facilities for business and pleasure; and woman is not long in learning the road to his favor. Many prostitutes who take no pleasure in their unclean intimacies not only endure a disgusting life for the favor and means thus gained, but affect intense passion in their sexual contacts because they have learned that such exhibitions gratify men."

18. **Husband's Brutality.**—Husbands! It is your licentiousness that drives your wives to a deed so abhorrent to their every wifely, womanly and maternal instinct—a deed which ruins the health of their bodies, prostitutes their souls, and makes marriage, maternity and womanhood itself degrading and loathsome. No terms can sufficiently characterize the cruelty, meanness and disgusting selfishness of your conduct when you impose on them a

maternity so detested as to drive them to the desperation of killing their unborn children and often themselves.

19. **What Drunkards Bequeath to Their Offspring.**—Organic imperfections unfit the brain for sane action, and habit confirms the insane condition; the man's brain has become unsound. Then comes in the law of hereditary descent, by which the brain of a man's children is fashioned after his own—not as it was originally, but as it has become, in consequence of frequent functional disturbance. Hence, of all appetites, the inherited appetite for drunkenness is [413]the most direful. Natural laws contemplate no exceptions, and sins against them are never pardoned.

20. **The Reports of Hospitals.**—The reports of hospitals for lunatics almost universally assign intemperance as one of the causes which predispose a man's offspring to insanity. This is even more strikingly manifested in the case of congenital idiocy. They come generally from a class of families which seem to have degenerated physically to a low degree. They are puny and sickly.

21. **Secret Diseases.**—See the weakly, sickly and diseased children who are born only to suffer and die, all because of the private disease of the father before his marriage. Oh, let the truth be told that the young men of our land may learn the lessons of purity of life. Let them learn that in morality there is perfect protection and happiness.

GETTING A DIVORCE

[414]

Physical and Moral Degeneracy.

THE DEGENERATE TURK.

1. **Moral Principle.**—"Edgar Allen Poe, Lord Byron, and Robert Burns," says Dr. Geo. F. Hall, "were men of marvelous strength intellectually. But measured by the true rule of high moral principle, they were very weak. Superior endowment in a single direction—physical, mental, or spiritual—is not of itself sufficient to make one strong in all that that heroic word means.

2. **Insane Asylum.**—Many a good man spiritually has gone to an untimely grave because of impaired physical powers. Many a good man spiritually has gone to the insane asylum because of bodily and mental weaknesses. Many a good man spiritually has fallen from virtue in an evil moment because of a weakened will, or, a too demanding fleshly passion, or, worse than either, too lax views on the subject of personal chastity."

3. **Boys Learning Vices.**—Some ignorant and timid people argue that boys and young men in reading a work of this character will learn vices concerning which they had [415]never so much as dreamed of before. This is, however, certain, that vices cannot be condemned unless they are mentioned; and if the condemnation is strong enough it surely will be a source of strength and of security. If light and education, on these important subjects, does injury, then all knowledge likewise must do more wrong than good. Knowledge is power, and the only hope of the race is enlightenment on all subjects pertaining to their being.

4. **Moral Manhood.**—It is clearly visible that the American manhood is rotting down—decaying at the center. The present generation shows many men of a small body and weak principles, and men and women of this kind are becoming more and more prevalent. Dissipation and indiscretions of all kind are working ruin. Purity of life and temperate habits are being too generally disregarded.

5. **Young Women.**—The vast majority of graduates from the schools and colleges of our land to-day, and two-thirds of the membership of our churches, and three-fourths of the charitable workers, are females. Everywhere girls are carrying off most of the prizes in competitive examinations, because women, as a sex, naturally maintain a better character, take better care of their bodies, and are less addicted to bad and injurious habits. While all this is true in reference to females, you will find that the male sex furnishes almost the entire number of criminals. The saloons, gambling dens, the brothels, and bad literature are drawing down all that the public schools can build up. Seventy per cent. of the young men of this land do not darken the church door. They are not interested in moral improvement or moral education. Eighty-five per cent. leave school under 15 years of age; prefer the loafer's honors to the benefit of school.

6. **Promotion.**—The world is full of good places for good young men, and all the positions of trust now occupied by the present generation will soon be filled by the competent young men of the coming generation; and he that keeps his record clean, lives a pure life, and avoids excesses or dissipations of all kinds, and fortifies his life with good habits, is the young man who will be heard from, and a thousand places will be open for his services.

7. **Personal Purity.**—Dr. George F. Hall says: "Why not pay careful attention to man in all his elements of strength, physical, mental, and moral? Why not make personal purity a fixed principle in the manhood of the present and coming generations, and thus insure the best men the world has ever seen? It can be done. Let every reader of these lines resolve that he will be one to help do it."

[416]
Immorality, Disease and Death.
Charles Dickens' Chair and Desk.

1. **The Policy of Silence.**—There is no greater delusion than to suppose that vast number of boys know nothing about practices of sin. Some parents are afraid that unclean thoughts may be suggested by these very defences. The danger is slight. Such cases are barely possible, but when the untold thousands are thought of on the other side, who have been demoralized from childhood through ignorance, and who are to-day suffering the result of these vicious practices, the policy of silence stands condemned, and intelligent knowledge abundantly justified. The emphatic words of Scripture are true in this respect also, "The people are destroyed for lack of knowledge."

2. **Living Illustrations.**—Without fear of truthful contradiction we affirm that the homes, public assemblies, and streets of all our large cities abound to-day with living illustrations and proofs of the widespread existence of this physical and moral scourge. An enervated and stunted manhood, a badly developed physique, a marked absence of manly and womanly strength and beauty, are painfully common everywhere. Boys and girls, young men and women, exist by thousands, of whom it may be said, they were badly born and ill-developed. Many of these are, to some extent, bearing the penalty of the sins and excesses of their parents, especially their fathers, whilst the great majority are reaping the fruits of their own immorality in a dwarfed and ill-formed body, and effeminate appearance, weak and enervated mind.[417]

3. **Effeminate and Sickly Young Men.**—The purposeless and aimless life of any number of effeminate and sickly young men, is to be distinctly attributed to these sins. The large class of mentally impotent "ne'er-do-wells" are being constantly recruited and added to by those who practice what the celebrated Erichson calls "that hideous sin engendered by vice, and practiced in solitude"—the sin, be it observed, which is the common cause of physical and mental weakness, and of the fearfully impoverishing night-emissions, or as they are commonly called, "wet-dreams."

4. **Weakness, Disease, Deformity, and Death.**—Through self-pollution and fornication the land is being corrupted with weakness, disease, deformity, and death. We regret to say that we cannot speak with confidence concerning the moral character of the Jew; but we have people amongst us who have deservedly a high character for the tone of their moral life—we refer to the members of the Society of Friends. The average of life amongst these reaches no less than fifty-six years; and, whilst some allowance must be made for the fact that amongst the Friends the poor have not a large representation, these figures show conclusively the soundness of this position,

5. **Sowing Their Wild Oats.**—It is monstrous to suppose that healthy children should die just as they are coming to manhood. The fact that thousands of young people do reach the age of sixteen or eighteen, and then decline and die, should arouse parents to ask the question: Why? Certainly it would not be difficult to tell the reason in thousands of instances, and yet the habit and practice of the deadly sin of self-pollution is actually ignored; it is even spoken of as a boyish folly not to be mentioned, and young men literally burning up with lust are mildly spoken of as "sowing their wild oats." Thus the cemetery is being filled with masses of the youth of America who, as in Egypt of old, fill up the graves of

uncleanness and lust. Some time since a prominent Christian man was taking exception to my addressing men on this subject; observe this! one of his own sons was at that very time near the lunatic asylum through these disgusting sins. What folly and madness this is!

6. **Death to True Manhood.**—The question for each one is, "In what way are you going to divert the courses of the streams of energy which pertain to youthful vigor and manhood?" To be destitute of that which may be described as raw material in the human frame, means that no really vigorous manhood can have place; to burn up the juices of the system in the fires of lust is madness and wanton folly, [418]but it can be done. To divert the currents of life and energy from blood and brain, from memory and muscle, in order to secrete it for the shambles of prostitution, is death to true manhood; but remember, it can be done! The generous liquid life may inspire the brain and blood with noble impulse and vital force, or it may be sinned away and drained out of the system until the jaded brain, the faded cheek, the enervated young manhood, the gray hair, narrow chest, weak voice, and the enfeebled mind show another victim in the long catalogue of the degraded through lust.

7. **The Sisterhood of Shame and Death.**—Whenever we pass the sisterhood of death, and hear the undertone of song, which is one of the harlot's methods of advertising, let us recall the words, that these represent the "pestilence which walketh in darkness, the destruction that wasteth at noonday." The allusion, of course, is to the fact that the great majority of these harlots are full of loathsome physical and moral disease; with the face and form of an angel, these women "bite like a serpent and sting like an adder;" their traffic is not for life, but inevitably for shame, disease, and death. Betrayed and seduced themselves, they in their turn betray and curse others.

8. **Warning Others.**—Have you never been struck with the argument of the Apostle, who, warning others from the corrupt example of the fleshy Esau, said, "Lest there be any fornicator or profane person as Esau, who for one mess of meat sold his own birthright. For ye know that even afterward, when he desired to inherit the blessing, he was rejected, he found no place for repentance, though he sought it diligently with tears." Terrible and striking words are these. His birthright sold for a mess of meat. The fearful costs of sin— yes, that is the thought, particularly the sin of fornication! Engrave that word upon your memories and hearts—"One mess of meat."

9. **The Harlot's Mess of Meat.**—Remember it, young men, when you are tempted to this sin. For a few minutes' sensual pleasure, for a mess of harlot's meat, young men are paying out the love of the son and brother; they are deceiving, lying, and cheating for a mess of meat; for a mess, not seldom of putrid flesh, men have paid down purity and prayer, manliness and godliness; for a mess of meat some perhaps have donned their best attire, and assumed the manners of the gentleman, and then, like an infernal hypocrite, dogged the steps of maiden or harlot to satisfy their degrading lust; for a mess of meat young men have deceived father and mother, and shrunk from the embrace of [419]love of the pure-minded sister. For the harlot's mess of meat some listening to me have spent scores of hours of invaluable time. They have wearied the body, diseased and demoralized the mind. The pocket has been emptied, theft committed, lies unnumbered told, to play the part of the harlot's mate—perchance a six-foot fool, dragged into the filth and mire of the harlot's house. You called her your friend, when, but for her mess of meat, you would have passed her like dirt in the street.

10. **Seeing life.**—You consorted with her for your mutual shame and death, and then called it "seeing life." Had your mother met you, you would have shrunk away like a craven cur. Had your sister interviewed you, she had blushed to bear your name; or had she been seen by you in company with some other whoremaster, for similar commerce, you would have wished that she had been dead. Now what think you of this "seeing life?" And it is for this that tens of thousands of strong men in our large cities are selling their birthright.

11. **The Devil's Decoys.**—Some may be ready to affirm that physical and moral penalties do not appear to overtake all men; that many men known to be given to intemperance and sensuality are strong, well, and live to a good age. Let us not make any mistake concerning these; they are exceptions to the rule; the appearance of health in them is but the grossness of sensuality. You have only carefully to look into the faces of these men

to see that their countenances, eyes, and speech betray them. They are simply the devil's decoys.

12. **Grossness of Sensuality.**—The poor degraded harlot draws in the victims like a heavily charged lodestone; these men are found in large numbers throughout the entire community; they would make fine men were they not weighted with the grossness of sensuality; as it is, they frequent the race-course, the card-table, the drinking-saloon, the music-hall, and the low theaters, which abound in our cities and towns; the great majority of these are men of means and leisure. Idleness is their curse, their opportunity for sin; you may know them as the loungers over refreshment-bars, as the retailers of the latest filthy joke, or as the vendors of some disgusting scandal; indeed, it is appalling the number of these lepers found both in our business and social circles.

[421]

Poisonous Literature and Bad Pictures.
PALESTINE WATER CARRIERS.

1. **Obscene Literature.**—No other source contributes so much to sexual immorality as obscene literature. The mass of stories published in the great weeklies and the cheap novels are mischievous. When the devil determines to take charge of a young soul, he often employs a very ingenious method. He slyly hands a little novel filled with "voluptuous forms," "reclining on bosoms," "languishing eyes," etc.

2. **Moral Forces.**—The world is full of such literature. It is easily accessible, for it is cheap, and the young will procure it, and therefore become easy prey to its baneful influence and effects. It weakens the moral forces of the young, and they thereby fall an easy prey before the subtle schemes of the libertine.

3. **Bad Books.**—Bad books play not a small part in the corruption of the youth. A bad book is as bad as an evil companion. In some respects it is even worse than a living teacher of vice, since it may cling to an individual at all times. It will follow him and poison his mind with the venom of evil. The influence of bad books in making bad boys and men is little appreciated. Few are aware how much evil seed is being sown among the young everywhere through the medium of vile books.

4. **Sensational Story Books.**—Much of the evil literature which is sold in nickel and dime novels, and which constitutes the principal part of the contents of such papers as the "Police Gazette," the "Police News," and a large proportion of the sensational story books which flood the land. You might better place a coal of fire or a live viper in your bosom, than allow yourself to read such a book. The thoughts that are implanted in the mind in youth will often stick there through life, in spite of all efforts to dislodge them.

5. **Papers and Magazines.**—Many of the papers and magazines sold at our news stands, and eagerly sought after by young men and boys, are better suited for the parlors of a house of ill-fame than for the eyes of pure-minded youth. A newsdealer who will distribute such vile sheets ought to be dealt with as an educator in vice and crime, an agent of evil, and a recruiting officer of hell and perdition.

6. **Sentimental Literature of Low Fiction.**—Sentimental literature, whether impure in its subject matter or not, has [422]a direct tendency in the direction of impurity. The stimulation of the emotional nature, the instilling of sentimental ideas into the minds of the young, has a tendency to turn the thoughts into a channel which leads in the direction of the formation of vicious habits.

7. **Impressions Left by Reading Questionable Literature.**—It is painful to see strong intelligent men and youths reading bad books, or feasting their eyes on filthy pictures, for the practice is sure to affect their personal purity. Impressions will be left which cannot fail to breed a legion of impure thoughts, and in many instances criminal deeds. Thousands of elevator boys, clerks, students, traveling men, and others, patronize the questionable literature counter to an alarming extent.

8. **The Nude in Art.**—For years there has been a great craze after the nude in art, and the realistic in literature. Many art galleries abound in pictures and statuary which cannot fail to fan the fires of sensualism, unless the thoughts of the visitor are trained to the strictest purity. Why should artists and sculptors persist in shocking the finer sensibilities of old and

young of both sexes by crowding upon their view representations of naked human forms in attitudes of luxurious abandon? Public taste may demand it. But let those who have the power endeavor to reform public taste.

9. **Widely Diffused.**—Good men have ever lamented the pernicious influence of a depraved and perverted literature. But such literature has never been so systematically and widely diffused as at the present time. This is owing to two causes, its cheapness and the facility of conveyance.

10. **Inflame the Passions.**—A very large proportion of the works thus put in circulation are of the worst character, tending to corrupt the principles, to inflame the passions, to excite impure desire, and spread a blight over all the powers of the soul. Brothels are recruited from this more than any other source. Those who search the trunks of convicted criminals are almost sure to find in them one or more of these works; and few prisoners who can read at all fail to enumerate among the causes which led them into crime the unhealthy stimulus of this depraved and poisonous literature.

[423]

Startling Sins.

1. **Nameless Crimes.**—The nameless crimes identified with the hushed-up Sodomite cases; the revolting condition of the school of Sodomy; the revelations of the Divorce Court concerning the condition of what is called national nobility, and upper classes, as well as the unclean spirit which attaches to "society papers," has revealed a condition which is perfectly disgusting.

2. **Unfaithfulness.**—Unfaithfulness amongst husbands and wives in the upper classes is common and adultery rife everywhere; mistresses are kept in all directions; thousands of these rich men have at least two, and not seldom three establishments.

3. **A Frightful Increase.**—Facts which have come to light during the past ten years show a frightful increase in every form of licentiousness; the widely extended area over which whoredom and degrading lust have thrown the glamor of their fascinating toils is simply appalling.[424]

4. **Moral Carnage.**—We speak against the fearful moral carnage; would to God that some unmistakable manifestation of the wrath of God should come in and put a stop to this huge seed-plot of national demoralization! We are reaping in this disgusting centre the harvest of corruption which has come from the toleration and encouragements given by the legislature, the police, and the magistrates to immorality, vice, and sin; the awful fact is, that we are in the midst of the foul and foetid harvest of lust. Aided by some of the most exalted personages in the land, assisted by thousands of educated and wealthy whoremongers and adulterers, we are reaping also, in individual physical ugliness and deformity, that which has been sown; the puny, ill-formed and mentally weak youths and maidens, men and women, to be seen in large numbers in our principal towns and cities, represent the widespread nature of the curse which has, in a marked manner, impaired the physique, the morality, and the intelligence of the nation.

5. **Daily Press.**—The daily press has not had the moral courage to say one word; the quality of demoralizing novels such as have been produced from the impure brain and unclean imaginations; the subtle, clever, and fascinating undermining of the white-winged angel of purity by modern sophists, whose prurient and vicious volumes were written to throw a halo of charm and beauty about the brilliant courtesan and the splendid adulteress; the mixing up of lust and love; the making of corrupt passion to stand in the garb of a deep, lasting, and holy affection—these are some of the hideous seedlings which, hidden amid the glamor and fascination of the seeming "angel of light," have to so large an extent corrupted the morality of the country.

6. **Nightly Exhibitions.**—Some of you know what the nightly exhibitions in these garlanded temples of whorish incentive are. There is the variety theatre, with its disgusting ballet dancing, and its shamelessly indecent photographs exhibited in every direction. What a clear gain to morality it would be if the accursed houses were burnt down, and forbidden by

172

law ever to be re-built or re-opened; the whole scene is designed to act upon and stimulate the lusts and evil passions of corrupt men and women.

7. **Confidence and Exposure.**—I hear some of you say, cannot some influence be brought to bear upon this plague-spot? Will the legislature or congress do nothing? Is the law and moral right to continue to be trodden under foot? Are the magistrates and the police powerless? The truth is the harlots and whoremongers are master of the situation; the moral sense of the legislators, the magistrates, and the [425]police is so low that anything like confidence is at present out of the question.

8. **The Sisterhood of Shame and Death.**—It is enough to make angels weep to see a great mass of America's wealthy and better-class sons full of zeal and on fire with interest in the surging hundreds of the sisterhood of shame and death. Many of these men act as if they were—if they do not believe they are—dogs. No poor hunted dog in the streets was ever tracked by a yelping crowd of curs more than is the fresh girl or chance of a maid in the accursed streets of our large cities. Price is no object, nor parentage, nor home; it is the truth to affirm that hundreds and thousands of well-dressed and educated men come in order to the gratification of their lusts, and to this end they frequent this whole district; they have reached this stage, they are being burned up in this fire of lust; men of whom God says, "Having eyes full of adultery and that cannot cease sin."

9. **Law Makers.**—Now should any member of the legislature rise up and testify against this "earthly hell," and speak in defence of the moral manhood and womanhood of the nation, he would be greeted as a fanatic, and laughed down amid derisive cheers; such has been the experience again and again. Therefore attack this great stronghold which for the past thirty years has warred and is warring against our social manhood and womanhood, and constantly undermining the moral life of the nation; against this citadel of licentiousness, this metropolitan centre of crime, and vice, and sin, direct your full blast of righteous and manly indignation.

10. **Temples of Lust.**—Here stand the foul and splendid temples of lust, intemperance, and passion, into whose vortex tens of thousands of our sons and daughters are constantly being drawn. Let it be remembered that this whole area represents the most costly conditions, and proves beyond question that an enormous proportion of the wealthy manhood of the nation, and we as citizens sustain, partake, and share in this carnival of death. Is it any wonder that the robust type of godly manhood which used to be found in the legislature, is sadly wanting now, or that the wretched caricatures of manhood which find form and place in such papers as "Truth" and the "World" are accepted as representing "modern society?"

11. **Puritanic Manhood.**—It is a melancholy fact that by reason of uncleanness, we have almost lost regard for the type of puritanic manhood which in the past held aloft the standard of a chaste and holy life; such men in this day are spoken of as "too slow" as "weak-kneed," and [426]"goody-goody" men. Let me recall that word, the fast and indecently-dressed "things," the animals of easy virtue, the "respectable" courtesans that flirt, chaff, gamble, and waltz with well-known high-class licentious lepers—such is the ideal of womanhood which a large proportion of our large city society accepts, fawns upon, and favors.

12. **Shameful Conditions.**—Perhaps one of the most inhuman and shameful conditions of modern fashionable society, both in England and America, is that which wealthy men and women who are married destroy their own children in the embryo stage of being, and become murderers thereby. This is done to prevent what should be one of our chief glories, viz., large and well-developed home and family life.

[427]

The Prostitution of Men.
CAUSE AND REMEDY.

1. **Exposed Youth.**—Generally even in the beginning of the period when sexual uneasiness begins to show itself in the boy, he is exposed in schools, institutes, and elsewhere to the temptations of secret vice, which is transmitted from youth to youth, like a

contagious corruption, and which in thousands destroys the first germs of virility. Countless numbers of boys are addicted to these vices for years. That they do not in the beginning of nascent puberty proceed to sexual intercourse with women, is generally due to youthful timidity, which dares not reveal its desire, or from want of experience for finding opportunities. The desire is there, for the heart is already corrupted.

2. **Boyhood Timidity Overcome.**—Too often a common boy's timidity is overcome by chance or by seduction, which is rarely lacking in great cities where prostitution is flourishing, and thus numbers of boys immediately after the transition period of youth, in accordance with the previous secret practice, accustom themselves to the association with prostitute women, and there young manhood and morals are soon lost forever.

3. **Marriage-bed Resolutions.**—Most men of the educated classes enter the marriage-bed with the consciousness of leaving behind them a whole army of prostitutes or seduced women, in whose arms they cooled their passions and spent the vigor of their youth. But with such a past the married man does not at the same time leave behind him its influence on his inclinations. The habit of having a feminine being at his disposal for every rising appetite, and the desire for change inordinately indulged for years, generally make themselves felt again as soon as the honeymoon is over. Marriage will not make a morally corrupt man all at once a good man and a model husband.

4. **The Injustice of Man.**—Now, although many men are in a certain sense "not worthy to unloose the latchet of the shoes" of the commonest woman, much less to "unfasten her girdle," yet they make the most extravagant demands on the feminine sex. Even the greatest debauchee, who has spent his vigor in the arms of a hundred courtesans, will cry out fraud and treachery if he does not receive his newly married bride as an untouched virgin. Even the most dissolute husband will look on his wife as deserving of death if his daily infidelity is only once reciprocated.[428]

5. **Unjust Demands.**—The greater the injustice a husband does to his wife, the less he is willing to submit from her; the oftener he becomes unfaithful to her, the stricter he is in demanding faithfulness from her. We see that despotism nowhere denies its own nature: the more a despot deceives and abuses his people, the more submissiveness and faithfulness he demands of them.

6. **Suffering Women.**—Who can be astonished at the many unhappy marriages, if he knows how unworthy most men are of their wives? Their virtues they rarely can appreciate, and their vices they generally call out by their own. Thousands of women suffer from the results of a mode of life of which they, having remained pure in their thought, have no conception whatever; and many an unsuspecting wife nurses her husband with tenderest care in sicknesses which are nothing more than the consequences of his amours with other women.

7. **An Inhuman Criminal.**—When at last, after long years of delusion and endurance, the scales drop from the eyes of the wife, and revenge or despair drives her into a hostile position towards her lord and master, she is an inhuman criminal, and the hue and cry against the fickleness of women and the falsity of their nature is endless. Oh, the injustice of society and the injustice of cruel man. Is there no relief for helpless women that are bound by the ties of marriage to men who are nothing but rotten corruption?

8. **Vulgar Desire.**—The habit of regarding the end and aim of woman only from the most vulgar side—not to respect in her the noble human being, but to see in her only the instrument of sensual desire—is carried so far among men that they will allow it to force into the background considerations among themselves, which they otherwise pretend to rank very high.

9. **The Only Remedy.**—But when the feeling of women has once been driven to indignation with respect to the position which they occupy, it is to be hoped that they will compel men to be pure before marriage, and they will remain loyal after marriage.

10. **Worse than Savages.**—With all our civilization we are put to shame even by the savages. The savages know of no fastidiousness of the sexual instinct and of no brothels. We are, indeed, likewise savages, but in quite a different sense. Proof of this is especially furnished by our youth. But that our students, and young men in general, usually pass

through the school of corruption and drag the filth of the road which they have traversed before marriage along [429]with them throughout life, is not their fault so much as the fault of prejudices and of our political and social conditions that prohibits a proper education, and the placing of the right kind of literature on these subjects into the hands of young people.

11. **Reason and Remedy.**—Keep the youth pure by a thorough system of plain unrestricted training. The seeds of immorality are sown in youth, and the secret vice eats out their young manhood often before the age of puberty. They develop a bad character as they grow older. Young girls are ruined, and licentiousness and prostitution flourish. Keep the boys pure and the harlot would soon lose her vocation. Elevate the morals of the boys, and you will have pure men and moral husbands.

[430]

The Road to Shame.
SUICIDE LAKE.

1. **Insult to Mother or Sister.**—Young men, it can never under any circumstances be right for you to do to a woman that, which, if another man did to your mother or sister, you could never forgive! The very thought is revolting. Let us suppose a man guilty of this shameful sin, and I apprehend that each of us would feel ready to shoot the villain. We are not justifying the shooting, but appealing to your instinctive sense of right, in order to show the enormity of this fearful crime, and to fasten strong conviction in your mind against this sin.[431]

2. **A Ruined Sister.**—What would you think of a man, no matter what his wealth, culture, or gentlemanly bearing, who should lay himself out for the seduction and shame of your beloved sister? Her very name now reminds you of the purest affection: think of her, if you can bear it, ruined in character, and soon to become an unhappy mother. To whom can you introduce her? What can you say concerning her? How can her own brothers and sisters associate with her? and, mark! all this personal and relative misery caused by this genteel villain's degrading passion.

3. **Young Man Lost.**—Another terrible result of this sin is the practical overthrow of natural affection which it effects. A young man comes from his father's house to Chicago. Either through his own lust or through the corrupt companions that he finds in the house of business where he resides, he becomes the companion of lewd women. The immediate result is a bad conscience, a sense of shame, and a breach in the affections of home. Letters are less frequent, careless, and brief. He cannot manifest true love now. He begins to shrink from his sister and mother, and well he may.

4. **The Harlot's Influence.**—He has spent the strength of his affection and love for home. In their stead the wretched harlot has filled him with unholy lust. His brain and heart refuse to yield him the love of the son and brother. His hand can not write as aforetime, or at best, his expressions become a hypocritical pretence. Fallen into the degradation of the fornicator, he has changed a mother's love and sister's affection for the cursed fellowship of the woman "whose house is the way to hell." (Prov. VII. 27.)

5. **The Way of Death.**—Observe, that directly the law of God is broken, and wherever promiscuous intercourse between the sexes takes place, gonorrhœa, syphilis, and every other form of venereal disease is seen in hideous variety. It is only true to say that thousands of both sexes are slain annually by these horrible diseases. What must be the moral enormity of a sin, which, when committed, produces in vast numbers of cases such frightful physical and moral destruction as that which is here portrayed?

6. **A Harlot's Woes.**—Would to God that something might be done to rescue fallen women from their low estate. We speak of them as "fallen women". Fallen, indeed, they are, but surely not more deserving of the application of that term than the "fallen men" who are their partners and paramours. It is easy to use the words, "a fallen woman", but who can apprehend all that is involved in the [432]expression, seeing that every purpose for which God created woman is prostituted and destroyed? She is now neither maiden, wife, nor

175

mother; the sweet names of sister and betrothed can have no legitimate application in her case.

7. **The Penalties for Lost Virtue.**—Can the harlot be welcomed where either children, brothers, sisters, wife, or husband are found? Surely, no. Home is a sphere alien to the harlot's estate. See such an one wherever you may—she is a fallen outcast from woman's high estate. Her existence—for she does not live—now culminates in one dread issue, viz., prostitution. She sleeps, but awakes a harlot. She rises in the late morning hours, but her object is prostitution; she washes, dresses, and braids her hair, but it is with one foul purpose before her. To this end she eats, drinks, and is clothed. To this end her house is hidden and the blinds are drawn.

8. **Lost Forever.**—To this end she applies the unnatural cosmetique, and covers herself with sweet perfumes, which vainly try to hide her disease and shame. To this end she decks herself with dashing finery and tawdry trappings, and with bold, unwomanly mien essays the streets of the great city. To this end she is loud and coarse and impudent. To this end she is the prostituted "lady," with simpering words, and smiles, and glamour of refined deceit. To this end an angel face, a devil in disguise. There is one foul and ghastly purpose towards which all her energies now tend. So low has she fallen, so lost is she to all the design of woman, that she exists for one foul purpose only, viz., to excite, stimulate, and gratify the lusts of degraded, ungodly men. Verily, the word "prostitute" has an awful meaning. What plummet can sound the depths of a woman's fall who has become a harlot?

9. **Sound the Alarm.**—Remember, young man, you can never rise above the degradation of the companionship of lewd women. Your virtue once lost is lost forever. Remember, young woman, your wealth or riches is your good name and good character— you have nothing else. Give a man your virtue and he will forsake you, and you will be forsaken by all the world. Remember that purity of purpose brings nobility of character, and an honorable life is the joy and security of mankind.

[433]
The Curse of Manhood.

THE GREAT PHILANTHROPIST.

1. **Moral Lepers.**—We cannot but denounce in the strongest terms, the profligacy of many married men. Not content with the moderation permitted in the divine appointed relationship of marriage, they become adulterers, in order to gratify their accursed lust. The man in them is trodden down by the sensual beast which reigns supreme. These are the moral outlaws that make light of this scandalous social iniquity, and by their damnable example encourage young men to sin.

2. **A Sad Condition.**—It is constantly affirmed by prostitutes, that amongst married men are found their chief supporters. Evidence from such a quarter must be received with considerable caution. Nevertheless, we believe that there is much truth in this statement. Here, again, we lay [434]the ax to the root of the tree; the married man who dares affirm that there is a particle of physical necessity for this sin, is a liar, and the truth is not in him. Whether these men be princes, peers, legislators, professional men, mechanics, or workmen, they are moral pests, a scandal to the social state, and a curse to the nation.

3. **Excesses.**—Many married men exhaust themselves by these excesses; they become irritable, liable to cold, to rheumatic affections, and nervous depression. They find themselves weary when they rise in the morning. Unfitted for close application to business, they become dilatory and careless, often lapsing into entire lack of energy, and not seldom into the love of intoxicating stimulants. Numbers of husbands and wives entering upon these experiences lose the charm of health, the cheerfulness of life and converse. Home duties become irksome to the wife; the brightness, vivacity, and bloom natural to her earlier years, decline; she is spoken of as highly nervous, poorly, and weak, when the whole truth is that she is suffering from physical exhaustion which she cannot bear. Her features become angular, her hair prematurely gray, she rapidly settles down into the nervous invalid, constantly needing medical aid, and, if possible, change of air.

176

4. **Ignorance.**—These conditions are brought about in many cases through ignorance on the part of those who are married. Multitudes of men have neither read, heard, nor known the truth of this question. We sympathize with our fellow-men in this, that we have been left in practical ignorance concerning the exceeding value and legitimate uses of these functions of our being. Some know, that, had they known these things in the early days of their married life, it would have proved to them knowledge of exceeding value. If this counsel is followed, thousands of homes will scarcely know the need of the physician's presence.

5. **Animal Passion.**—Common-sense teaches that children who are begotten in the heat of animal passion, are likely to be licentious when they grow up. Many parents through excesses of eating and drinking, become inflamed with wine and strong drink., They are sensualists, and consequently, morally diseased. Now, if in such conditions men beget their children, who can affect surprise if they develop licentious tendencies? Are not such parents largely to blame? Are they not criminals in a high degree? Have they not fouled their own nest, and transmitted to their children predisposition to moral evil?

6. **Fast Young Men.**—Many of our "fast young men" have been thus corrupted, even as the children of the [435]intemperate are proved to have been. Certainly no one can deny that many of our "well-bred" young men are little better than "high-class dogs" so lawless are they, and ready for the arena of licentiousness.

7. **The Pure-Minded Wife.**—Happily, as tens of thousands of husbands can testify, the pure-minded wife and mother is not carried away, as men are liable to be, with the force of animal passion. Were it not so, the tendencies to licentiousness in many sons would be stronger than they are. In the vast majority of cases suggestion is never made except by the husband, and it is a matter of deepest gratitude and consideration, that the true wife may become a real helpmeet in restraining this desire in the husband.

8. **Young Wife and Children.**—We often hear it stated that a young wife has her children quickly. This cannot happen to the majority of women without injury to health and jeopardy to life. The law which rendered it imperative for the land to lie fallow in order to rest and gain renewed strength, is only another illustration of the unity which pervades physical conditions everywhere. It should be known that if a mother nurses her own babe, and the child is not weaned until it is nine or ten months old, the mother, except in rare cases, will not become enceinte again, though cohabitation with the husband takes place.

9. **Selfish and Unnatural Conduct.**—It is natural and rational that a mother should feed her own children; in the selfish and unnatural conduct of many mothers, who, to avoid the self-denial and patience which are required, hand the little one over to the wet-nurse, or to be brought up by hand, is found in many cases the cause and reason of the unnatural haste of child-bearing. Mothers need to be taught that the laws of nature cannot be broken without penalty. For every woman whose health has been weakened through nursing her child, a hundred have lost strength and health through marital excesses. The haste of having children is the costly penalty which women pay for shirking the mother's duty to the child.

10. **Law of God.**—So graciously has the law of God been arranged in regard to the mother's strength, that, if it be obeyed, there will be, as a rule, an interval of at least from eighteen months to two years between the birth of one child and that of another. Every married man should abstain during certain natural seasons. In this periodical recurrence God has instituted to every husband the law of restraint, and insisted upon self-control.

11. **To Young People Who Are Married.**—Be exceedingly careful of license and excess in your intercourse with [436]one another. Do not needlessly expose, by undress, the body. Let not the purity of love degenerate into unholy lust. See to it that you walk according to the divine Word, "Dwelling together as being heirs of the grace of life, that your prayers be not hindered."

12. **Lost Powers.**—Many young men after their union showed a marked difference. They lost much of their natural vivacity, energy, and strength of voice. Their powers of application, as business men, students, and ministers, had declined, as also their enterprise, fervor, and kindliness. They had become irritable, dull, pale, and complaining. Many cases of rheumatic fever have been induced through impoverishment, caused by excesses on the part of young married men.

177

13. **Middle Age.**—After middle age the sap of a man's life declines in quantity. A man who intends close application to the ministry, to scientific or literary pursuits, where great demands are made upon the brain, must restrain this passion. The supplies for the brain and nervous system are absorbed, and the seed diverted through sexual excesses in the marriage relationship, by fornication, or by any other form of immorality, the man's power must decline: that to this very cause may be attributed the failure and breakdown of so many men of middle age.

14. **Intoxicating Drinks.**—By all means avoid intoxicating drinks. Immorality and alcoholic stimulants, as we have shown, are intimately related to one another. Wine and strong drink inflame the blood, and heat the passions. Attacking the brain, they warp the judgment, and weaken the power of restraint. Avoid what is called good living; it is madness to allow the pleasures of the table to corrupt and corrode the human body. We are not designed for gourmands, much less for educated pigs. Cold water bathing, water as a beverage, simple and wholesome food, regularity of sleep, plenty of exercise; games such as cricket, football, tennis, boating, or bicycling, are among the best possible preventives against lust and animal passion.

15. **Beware of Idleness.**—Indolent leisure means an unoccupied mind. When young men lounge along the streets, in this condition they become an easy prey to the sisterhood of shame and death. Bear in mind that evil thoughts precede evil actions. The hand of the worst thief will not steal until the thief within operates upon the hand without. The members of the body which are capable of becoming instruments of sin, are not involuntary actors. Lustful desires must proceed from brain and heart, ere the fire that consumes burns in the member.

[437]

A Private Talk to Young Men.
Young Lincoln Starting to School.

1. The most valuable and useful organs of the body are those which are capable of the greatest dishonor, abuse and corruption. What a snare the wonderful organism of the eye may become when used to read corrupt books or look upon licentious scenes at the theatre, or when used to meet the fascinating gaze of the harlot! What an instrument for depraving the whole man may be found in the matchless powers of the brain, the hand, the ear, the mouth, or the tongue! What potent instruments may these become in accomplishing the ruin of the whole being for time and eternity!

2. In like manner the organ concerning the uses of which I am to speak, has been, and continues to be, made one of the chief instruments of man's immorality, shame, disease, and death. How important to know what the legitimate uses of this member of the body are, and how great the [438]dignity conferred upon us in the possession of this gift. On the human side this gift may be truly said to bring men nearer to the high and solemn relationship of the Creator than any other which they possess.

3. I first deal with the destructive sin of self-abuse. There can be little doubt that vast numbers of boys are guilty of this practice. In many cases the degrading habit has been taught by others, e.g., by elder boys at school, where association largely results in mutual corruption. With others, the means of sensual gratification is found out by personal action; whilst in other cases fallen and depraved men have not hesitated to debauch the minds of mere children by teaching them this debasing practice.

4. Thousands of youths and young men have only to use the looking-glass to see the portrait of one guilty of this loathsome sin. The effects are plainly discernible in the boy's appearance. The face and hands become pale and bloodless. The eye is destitute of its natural fire and lustre. The flesh is soft and flabby, the muscles limp and lacking healthy firmness. In cases where the habit has become confirmed, and where the system has been drained of this vital force, it is seen in positive ugliness, in a pale and cadaverous appearance, slovenly gait, slouching walk, and an impaired memory.

5. It is obvious that if the most vital physical force of a boy's life is being spent through this degrading habit—a habit, be it observed, of rapid growth, great strength, and difficult to break—he must develop badly. In thousands of cases the result is seen in a low

stature, contracted chest, weak lungs, and liability to sore throat. Tendency to cold, indigestion, depression, drowsiness, and idleness, are results distinctly traceable to this deadly practice. Pallor of countenance, nervous and rheumatic affections, loss of memory, epilepsy, paralysis, and insanity find their principal predisposing cause in the same shameful waste of life. The want of moral force and strength of mind often observable is youths and young men is largely induced by this destructive and deadly sin.

6. Large numbers of youths pass from an exhausted boyhood into the weakness, intermittent fevers, and consumption, which are said to carry off so many. If the deaths were attributed primarily to loss of strength occasioned by self-pollution, it would be much nearer the truth. It is monstrous to suppose that a boy who comes from healthy parents should decline and die. Without a shade of doubt the chief cause of decay and death amongst youths and young men, is to be traced to this baneful habit.[439]

7. It is a well-known fact that any man who desires to excel and retain his excellence as an accurate shot, an oarsman, a pedestrian, a pugilist, a first-class cricketer, bicyclist, student, artist, or literary man, must abstain from self-pollution and fornication. Thousands of school boys and students lose their positions in the class, and are plucked at the time of their examination by reason of failure of memory, through lack of nerve and vital force, caused mainly by draining the physical frame of the seed which is the vigor of the life.

8. It is only true to say that thousands of young men in the early stages of a licentious career would rather lose a right hand than have their mothers or sisters know what manner of men they are. From the side of the mothers and sisters it may also be affirmed that, were they aware of the real character of those brothers and sons, they would wish that they had never been born.

9. Let it be remembered that sexual desire is not in itself dishonorable or sinful, any more than hunger, thirst, or any other lawful and natural desire is. It is the gratification by unlawful means of this appetite which renders it so corrupting and iniquitous.

10. Leisure means the opportunity to commit sin. Unclean pictures are sought after and feasted upon, paragraphs relating to cases of divorce and seduction are eagerly read, papers and books of an immoral character and tendency greedily devoured, low and disgusting conversation indulged in and repeated.

11. The practical and manly counsel to every youth and young man is, entire abstinence from indulgence of the sexual faculty until such time as the marriage relationship is entered upon. Neither is there, nor can there be, any exception to this rule.

12. No man can affirm that self-denial ever injured him. On the contrary, self-restraint has been liberty, strength and blessing. Beware of the deceitful streams of temporary gratification, whose eddying current drifts towards license, shame, disease and death. Remember, how quickly moral power declines, how rapidly the edge of the fatal maelstrom is reached, how near the vortex, how terrible the penalty, how fearful the sentence of everlasting punishment.

13. Be a young man of principle, honor, and preserve your powers. How can you look an innocent girl in the face when you are degrading your manhood with the vilest practice? Keep your mind and life pure, and nobility will be your crown.

[440]
Remedies for the Social Evil.
1. **Man Responsible.**—Every great social reform must begin with the male sex. They must either lead, or give it its support. Prostitution is a sin wholly of their own making. All the misery, all the lust, as well as all the blighting consequences, are chargeable wholly to the uncontrolled sexual passion of the male. To reform sinful women, *reform the men.* Teach them that the physiological truth means permanent moral, physical and mental benefit, while seductive indulgence blights and ruins.

2. **Contagious Diseases.**—A man or woman cannot long live an impure life without sooner or later contracting disease which brings to every sufferer not only moral degradation, but often serious and vital injuries and many times death itself becomes the only relief.

179

3. **Should It Be Regulated by Law?**—Dr. G. J. Ziegler, of Philadelphia, in several medical articles says that the act of sexual connection should be made in itself the solemnization of marriage, and that when any such single act can be proven against an unmarried man, by an unmarried woman, the latter be at once invested with all the legal privileges of a wife. By bestowing this power on women very few men would risk the dangers of the society of a dissolute and scheming woman who might exercise the right to force him to a marriage and ruin his reputation and life. The strongest objection of this would be that it would increase the temptation to destroy the purity of married women, for they could be approached without danger of being forced into another marriage. But this objection could easily be harmonized with a good system of well regulated laws. Many means have been tried to mitigate the social evils, but with little encouragement. In the city of Paris a system of registration has been inaugurated and houses of prostitution are under the supervision of the police, yet prostitution has not been in any degree diminished. Similar methods have been tried in other European towns, but without satisfactory results.

4. **Moral Influence.**—Let it be an imperative to every clergyman, to every educator, to every statesman and to every philanthropist, to every father and to every mother, to impart that moral influence which may guide and direct the youth of the land into the natural channels of morality, chastity and health. Then, and not till then, shall we see righteous laws and rightly enforced for the mitigation and extermination of the modern house of prostitution.

[441]
The Selfish Slaves of Doses of Disease and Death.
A TURKISH CIGARETTE GIRL.

1. **Most Devilish Intoxication.**—What is the most devilish, subtle alluring, unconquerable, hopeless and deadly form of intoxication, with which science struggles and to which it often succumbs; which eludes the restrictive grasp of legislation; lurks behind lace curtains, hides in luxurious boudoirs, haunts the solitude of the study, and with waxen [442]face, furtive eyes and palsied step totters to the secret recesses of its self-indulgence? It is the drunkenness of drugs, and woe be unto him that crosseth the threshold of its dream-curtained portal, for though gifted with the strength of Samson, the courage of Richard and the genius of Archimedes, he shall never return, and of him it is written that forever he leaves hope behind.

2. **The Material Satan.**—The material Satan in this sensuous syndicate of soul and body-destroying drugs is opium, and next in order of hellish potency come cocaine and chloral.

3. **Gum Opium.**—Gum opium, from which the sulphate of morphine is made, is the dried juice of the poppy, and is obtained principally in the orient. Taken in moderate doses it acts specially upon the nervous system, deadens sensibility, and the mind becomes inactive. When used habitually and excessively it becomes a tonic, which stimulates the whole nervous system, producing intense mental exaltation and delusive visions. When the effects wear off, proportionate lassitude follows, which begets an insatiate and insane craving for the drug. Under the repeated strain of the continually increasing doses, which have to be taken to renew the desired effect, the nervous system finally becomes exhausted, and mind and body are utterly and hopelessly wrecked.

4. **Cocaine.**—Cocaine is extracted from the leaves of the Peruvian cocoa tree, and exerts a decided influence upon the nervous system, somewhat akin to that of coffee. It increases the heart action and is said to be such an exhilarant that the natives of the Andes are enabled to make extraordinary forced marches by chewing the leaves containing it. Its after effects are more depressing even than those of opium, and insanity more frequently results from its use.

5. **Chloral.**—The name which is derived from the first two syllables of chlorine and alcohol, is made by passing dry chlorine gas in a continuous stream through absolute alcohol for six or eight weeks. It is a hypnotic or sleep-producing drug, and in moderate doses acts on the caliber of the blood vessels of the brain, producing a soothing effect, especially in cases of passive congestion. Some patent medicines contain chloral, bromide

180

and hyoscymus, and they have a large sale, being bought by persons of wealth, who do not know what they are composed of and recklessly take them for the effect they produce.

6. **Victims Rapidly Increasing.**—"From my experience," said a leading and conservative druggist, "I infer that the [443]number of what are termed opium, cocaine, and chloral "fiends" is rapidly increasing, and is greater by two or three hundred per cent than a year ago, with twice as many women as men represented. I should say that one person out of every fifty is a victim of this frightful habit, which claims its doomed votaries from the extremes of social life, those who have the most and the least to live for, the upper classes and the cyprian, professional men of the finest intelligence, fifty per cent of whom are doctors and walk into the pit with eyes wide open. And lawyers and other professional men must be added to this fated vice."

7. **Destroys the Moral Fiber.**—"It is a habit which utterly destroys the moral fiber of its slaves, and makes unmitigated liars and thieves and forgers of them, and even murder might be added to the list of crimes, were no other road left open to the gratification of its insatiate and insane appetite. I do not know of a single case in which it has been mastered, but I do know of many where the end has been unspeakable misery, disgrace, suffering, insanity and death."

8. **Shameful Death.**—To particularize further would be profitless so far as the beginners are concerned, but would to heaven that those not within the shadow of this shameful death would take warning from those who are. There are no social or periodical drunkards in this sort of intoxication. The vice is not only solitary, unsocial and utterly selfish, but incessant and increasing in its demands.

9. **Appetite Stronger than for Liquor.**—This appetite is far stronger and more uncontrollable than that for liquor, and we can spot its victim as readily as though he were an ordinary bummer. He has a pallid complexion, a shifting, shuffling manner and can't look you in the face. If you manage to catch his eye for an instant you will observe that its pupil is contracted to an almost invisible point. It is no exaggeration to say that he would barter his very soul for that which indulgence has made him too poor to purchase, and where artifice fails he will grovel in abject agony of supplication for a few grains. At the same time he resorts to all kinds of miserable and transparent shifts, to conceal his degradation. He never buys for himself, but always for some fictitious person, and often resorts to purchasing from distant points.

10. **Opium Smoking.**—"Opium smoking," said another representative druggist, "is almost entirely confined to the Chinese and they seem to thrive on it. Very few others hit the pipe that we know of."

[444]

11. **Malt and Alcoholic Drunkenness.**—Alcoholic stimulants have a record of woe second to nothing. Its victims are annually marching to drunkards' graves by the thousands. Drunkards may be divided into three classes: First, the accidental or social drunkard; second, the periodical or spasmodic drunkard; and third, the sot.

12. **The Accidental or Social Drunkard** is yet on safe ground. He has not acquired the dangerous craving for liquor. It is only on special occasions that he yields to excessive indulgence; sometimes in meeting a friend, or at some political blow-out. On extreme occasions he will indulge until he becomes a helpless victim, and usually as he grows older occasions will increase, and step by step he will be lead nearer to the precipice of ruin.

13. **The Periodical or Spasmodic Drunkard**, with whom it is always the unexpected which occurs, and who at intervals exacts from his accumulated capital the usury of as prolonged a spree as his nerves and stomach will stand. Science is inclined to charitably label this specimen of man a sort of a physiologic puzzle, to be as much pitied as blamed. Given the benefit of every doubt, when he starts off on one of his hilarious tangents, he becomes a howling nuisance; if he has a family, keeps them continually on the ragged edge of apprehension, and is unanimously pronounced a "holy terror" by his friends. His life and future is an uncertainty. He is unreliable and cannot be long trusted. Total reformation is the only hope, but it rarely is accomplished.

14. **The Sot.**—A blunt term that needs no defining, for even the children comprehend the hopeless degradation it implies. Laws to restrain and punish him are

framed; societies to protect and reform him are organized, and mostly in vain. He is prone in life's very gutter; bloated, reeking and polluted with the doggery's slops and filth. He can fall but a few feet lower, and not until he stumbles into an unmarked, unhonored grave, where kind mother earth and the merciful mantle of oblivion will cover and conceal the awful wreck he made of God's own image. To the casual observer, the large majority of the community, these three phases, at whose vagaries many laugh, and over whose consequences millions mourn, comprehend intoxication and its results, from the filling of the cup to its shattering fall from the nerveless hand, and this is the end of the matter. Would to God that it were! for at that it would be bad enough. But it is not, for wife, children and friends must suffer and drink the cup of trouble and sorrow to its dregs.

[445]

OBJECT LESSONS OF THE EFFECTS OF ALCOHOL AND CIGARETTE SMOKING.

By PROF. GEORGE HENKLE, who personally made the postmortem examinations and drew the following illustrations from the diseased organs just as they appeared when first taken from the bodies of the unfortunate victims.

THE STOMACH of an habitual drinker of alcoholic stimulants, showing the ulcerated condition of the mucous membrane, incapacitating this important organ for digestive functions.

THE STOMACH (interior view) of a healthy person with the first section of the small intestines.

[446]

The Liver of a drunkard who died of Cirrhosis of the liver, also called granular liver, or "gin drinker's liver." The organ is much shrunken and presents rough, uneven edges, with carbuncular non-suppurative sores. In this self-inflicted disease the tissues of the liver undergo a cicatrical retraction which strangulates and partly destroys the parenchyma of the liver.

THE LIVER IN HEALTH.

[447]

THE KIDNEY of a man who died a drunkard, showing in upper portion the

THE KIDNEY in health, with the lower section

182

sores so often found on kidneys of hard drinkers, and in the lower portion, the obstruction formed in the internal arrangement of this organ. Alcohol is a great enemy to the kidneys, and after this poison has once set in on its destructive course in these organs no remedial agents are known to exist to stop the already established disease.

[448]

| The Lungs and Heart of a boy who died from the effects of cigarette smoking, showing the nicotine sediments in lungs and shrunken condition of the heart. | THE LUNGS AND HEART IN HEALTH. | A section of the diseased Lung of a cigarette smoker, highly magnified. |

removed, to show the filtering apparatus (Malphigian pyramids). Natural size.

THE DESTRUCTIVE EFFECTS OF CIGARETTE SMOKING.

Illustrating the shrunken condition of one of the Lungs of an excessive smoker

[449]

Cigarettes have been analyzed, and the most physicians and chemists were surprised to find how much opium is put into them. A tobacconist himself says that "the extent to which drugs are used in cigarettes is appalling." "Havana flavoring" for this same purpose is sold everywhere by the thousand barrels. This flavoring is made from the tonka-bean, which contains a deadly poison. The wrappers, warranted to be rice paper, are sometimes made of common paper, and sometimes of the filthy scrapings of ragpickers bleached white with arsenic. What a thing for human lungs.

The habit burns up good health, good resolutions, good manners, good memories, good faculties, and often honesty and truthfulness as well.

Cases of epilepsy, insanity and death are frequently reported as the result of smoking cigarettes, while such physicians as Dr. Lewis Sayre, Dr. Hammond, and Sir Morell Mackenzie of England, name heart trouble, blindness, cancer and other diseases as occasioned by it.

Leading physicians of America unanimously condemn [450]cigarette smoking as "one of the vilest and most destructive evils that ever befell the youth of any country," declaring that "its direct tendency is a deterioration of the race."

Look at the pale, wilted complexion of a boy who indulges in excessive cigarette smoking. It takes no physician to diagnose his case, and death will surely mark for his own every boy and young man who will follow up the habit. It is no longer a matter of guess. It is a scientific fact which the microscope in every case verifies.

[451]

The Dangerous Vices.

183

INNOCENT YOUTH.

Few persons are aware of the extent to which masturbation or self-pollution is practiced by the young of both sexes in civilized society.

SYMPTOMS.

The hollow, sunken eye, the blanched cheek, the withered hands, and emaciated frame, and the listless life, have other sources than the ordinary illnesses of all large communities.

When a child, after having given proofs of memory and intelligence, experiences daily more and more difficulty in retaining and understanding what is taught him, it is not only from unwillingness and idleness, as is commonly supposed, but from a disease eating out life itself, brought on by a self-abuse of the private organs. Besides the slow and progressive derangement of his or her health, the diminished energy of application, the languid movement, the stooping gait, the desertion of social games, the solitary walk, late rising, livid and sunken eye, and many other symptoms, will fix the attention of every intelligent and competent guardian of youth that something is wrong.

[453]

MARRIED PEOPLE.

Nor are many persons sufficiently aware of the ruinous extent to which the amative propensity is indulged by married persons. The matrimonial ceremony does, indeed, sanctify the act of sexual intercourse, but it can by no means atone for nor obviate the consequences of its abuse. Excessive indulgence in the married relation is, perhaps, as much owing to the force of habit, as to the force of the sexual appetite.

GUARD WELL THE CRADLE.
EDUCATION CANNOT BEGIN TOO YOUNG.

EXTREME YOUTH.

More lamentable still is the effect of inordinate sexual excitement of the young and unmarried. It is not very uncommon to find a confirmed onanist, or, rather, masturbator, who has not yet arrived at the period of puberty. Many cases are related in which young boys and girls, from eight to ten years of age, were taught the method of self-pollution by their older playmates, and had made serious encroachments on the fund of constitutional vitality even before any considerable degree of sexual appetite was developed.

FORCE OF HABIT.

Here, again, the fault was not in the power of passion, but in the force of habit. Parents and guardians of youth can not be too mindful of the character and habits of those with whom they allow young persons and children under their charge to associate intimately, and especially careful should they be with whom they allow them to sleep.

SIN OF IGNORANCE.

It is customary to designate self-pollution as among the "vices." I think misfortune is the more appropriate term. It is true, that in the physiological sense, it is one of the very worst "transgressions of the law." But in the moral sense it is generally the sin of ignorance in the commencement, and in the end the passive submission to a morbid and almost resistless impulse.

QUACKS.

The time has come when the rising generation must be thoroughly instructed in this matter. That quack specific "ignorance" has been experimented with quite too long already. The true method of insuring all persons, young or old, against the abuses of any part, organ, function, or faculty of the wondrous machinery of life, is to teach them its use. "Train a child in the way it should go" or be sure it [454]will, amid the ten thousand surrounding temptations, find out a way in which it should not go. Keeping a child in ignorant innocence is, I aver, no part of the "training" which has been taught by a wiser than Solomon. Boys and girls do know, will know, and must know, that between them are important anatomical differences and interesting physiological relations. Teach them, I repeat, their use, or expect their abuse. Hardly a young person in the world would ever become addicted to self-pollution if he or she understood clearly the consequences; if he or she knew at the outset that the practice was directly destroying the bodily stamina, vitiating the moral tone, and enfeebling the intellect. No one would pursue the disgusting habit if he or she was fully aware that it was blasting all prospects of health and happiness in the approaching period of manhood and womanhood.

GENERAL SYMPTOMS OF THE SECRET HABIT.

The effects of either self-pollution or excessive sexual indulgence, appear in many forms. It would seem as if God had written an instinctive law of remonstrance, in the innate moral sense, against this filthy vice.

All who give themselves up to the excesses of this debasing indulgence, carry about with them, continually, a consciousness of their defilement, and cherish a secret suspicion that others look upon them as debased beings. They feel none of that manly confidence and gallant spirit, and chaste delight in the presence of virtuous females, which stimulate young men to pursue the course of ennobling refinement, and mature them for the social relations and enjoyments of life.

This shamefacedness, or unhappy quailing of the countenance, on meeting the look of others, often follows them through life, in some instances even after they have entirely abandoned the habit, and became married men and respectable members of society.

In some cases, the only complaint the patient will make on consulting you, is that he is suffering under a kind of continued fever. He will probably present a hot, dry skin, with something of a hectic appearance. Though all the ordinary means of arresting such symptoms have been tried, he is none the better.

The sleep seems to be irregular and unrefreshing—restlessness during the early part of the night, and in the advanced stages of the disease, profuse sweats before morning. There is also frequent starting in the sleep, from [455]disturbing dreams. The characteristic feature is, that your patient almost always dreams of sexual intercourse. This is one of the earliest, as well as most constant symptoms. When it occurs most frequently, it is apt to be accompanied with pain. A gleety discharge from the urethra may also be frequently discovered, especially if the patient examine when at stool or after urinating. Other common symptoms are nervous headache, giddiness, ringing in the ears, and a dull pain in the back part of the head. It is frequently the case that the patient suffers a stiffness in the neck, darting pains in the forehead, and also weak eyes are among the common symptoms.

One very frequent, and perhaps early symptom (especially in young females) is solitariness—a disposition to seclude themselves from society. Although they may be tolerably cheerful when in company, they prefer rather to be alone.

The countenance has often a gloomy and worn-down expression. The patient's friends frequently notice a great change. Large livid spots under the eyes is a common feature. Sudden flashes of heat may be noticed passing over the patient's face. He is liable also to palpitations. The pulse is very variable, generally too slow. Extreme emaciation, without any other assignable cause for it, may be set down as another very common symptom.

If the evil has gone on for several years, there will be a general unhealthy appearance, of a character so marked as to enable an experienced observer at once to detect the cause. In the case of onanists especially there is a peculiar rank odor emitted from the body, by which they may be readily distinguished. One striking peculiarity of all these patients is, that they cannot look a man in the face! Cowardice is constitutional with them.

HOME TREATMENT OF THE SECRET HABIT.

1. The first condition of recovery is a prompt and permanent abandonment of the ruinous habit. Without a faithful adherence to this prohibitory law on the part of the patient all medication on the part of the physician will assuredly fail. The patient must plainly understand that future prospects, character, health, and life itself, depend on an unfaltering resistance to the morbid solicitation; with the assurance, however, that a due perseverance will eventually render what now seems like a resistless and overwhelming[456]propensity, not only controllable but perfectly loathsome and undesirable.

2. Keep the mind employed by interesting the patient in the various topics of the day, and social features of the community.

3. Plenty of bodily out of door exercise, hoeing in the garden, walking, or working on the farm; of course not too heavy work must be indulged in.

185

4. If the patient is weak and very much emaciated, cod liver oil is an excellent remedy.

5. **Diet.** The patient should live principally on brown bread, oat meal, graham crackers, wheat meal, cracked or boiled wheat, or hominy, and food of that character. No meats should be indulged in whatever; milk diet if used by the patient is an excellent remedy. Plenty of fruit should be indulged in; dried toast and baked apples make an excellent supper. The patient should eat early in the evening, never late at night.

6. Avoid all tea, coffee, or alcoholic stimulants of any kind.

7. "Early to bed and early to rise," should be the motto of every victim of this vice. A patient should take a cold bath every morning after rising. A cold water injection in moderate quantities before retiring has cured many patients.

8. If the above remedies are not sufficient, a family physician should be consulted.

9. Never let children sleep together, if possible, to avoid it. Discourage the children of neighbors and friends from sleeping with your children.

10. Have your children rise early. It is the lying in bed in the morning that plays the mischief.

(l) Healthy Semen, Greatly Magnified. (r) The Semen of a Victim of Masturbation.
[457]

NOCTURNAL EMISSIONS

Involuntary emissions of semen during amorous dreams at night is not at all uncommon among healthy men. When this occurs from one to three or four times a month, no anxiety or concern need be felt.

When the emissions take place without dreams, manifested only by stained spots in the morning on the linen, or take place at stool and are entirely beyond control, then the patient should at once seek for remedies or consult a competent physician. When blood stains are produced, then medical aid must be sought at once.

HOME TREATMENT FOR NOCTURNAL EMISSIONS.

Sleep in a hard bed, and rise early and take a sponge bath in cold water every morning. Eat light suppers and refrain from eating late in the evening. Empty the bladder thoroughly before retiring, bathe the spine and hips with a sponge dipped in cold water.

Never sleep lying on the back.

Avoid all highly seasoned food and read good books, and keep the mind well employed. Take regular and vigorous outdoor exercise every day.

A Testicle wasted by Masturbation.

Healthy Testicle.

Avoid all coffee, tea, wine, beer and all alcoholic liquors. Don't use tobacco, and keep the bowels free.

Prescription.—Ask your druggist to put you up a good Iron Tonic and take it regularly according to his directions.

BEWARE OF ADVERTISING QUACKS.

Beware of these advertising schemes that advertise a speedy cure for "Loss of Youth," "Lost Vitality," "A Cure for Impotency," "Renewing of Old Age," etc. Do not allow these circulating pamphlets and circulars to concern you the least. If you have a few *Nocturnal Emissions*, remember it is only a mark of vitality and health, and not a sign of a deathly disease, as many of these advertising quacks would lead you to believe.

Use your private organs only for what your Creator intended they should be used, and there will be no occasion for you to be frightened by the deception of quacks.

[458]

THE TWO PATHS: WHAT WILL THE BOY BECOME?

[459]

Lost Manhood Restored.

1. **Resolute Desistence.**—The first step towards the restoration of lost manhood is a resolute desistence from these terrible sins. Each time the temptation is overcome, the power to resist becomes stronger, and the fierce fire declines. Each time the sin is

committed, its hateful power strengthens, and the fire of lust is increased. Remember, that you cannot commit these sins, and maintain health and strength.

2. **Avoid Being Alone.**—Avoid being alone when the temptation comes upon you to commit self-abuse. Change your thoughts at once; "keep the heart diligently, for out of it are the issues of life."

3. **Avoid Evil Companions.**—Avoid evil companions, lewd conversation, bad pictures, corrupt and vicious novels, books, and papers. Abstain from all intoxicating drinks. These inflame the blood, excite the passions, and stimulate sensuality; weakening the power of the brain, they always impair the power of self-restraint. Smoking is very undesirable. Keep away from the moral pesthouses. Remember that these houses are the great resort of fallen and depraved men and women. The music, singing, and dancing are simply a blind to cover the intemperance and lust, which hold high carnival in these guilded hells. This, be it remembered, is equally true of the great majority of the theatres.

4. **Avoid Strong Tea, or Coffee.**—Take freely of cocoa, milk, and bread and milk, or oatmeal porridge. Meats, such as beef and mutton, use moderately. We would strongly recommend to young men of full habit, vegetarian diet. Fruits in their season, partake liberally; also fresh vegetables. Brown bread and toast, as also rice, and similar puddings, are always suitable. Avoid rich pastry and new bread.

5. **Three Meals a Day Are Abundant.**—Avoid suppers, and be careful, if troubled with nightly emissions, not to take any liquid, not even water, after seven o'clock in the evening, at latest. This will diminish the secretions of the body, when asleep, and the consequent emissions, which in the early hours or the morning usually follow the taking of any kind of drink. Do not be anxious or troubled by an occasional emission, say, for example, once a fortnight.

6. **Rest on a Hard Mattress.**—Keep the body cool when asleep; heat arising from a load of bed-clothes is most [460]undesirable. Turn down the counterpane, and let the air have free course through the blankets.

7. **Relieve the System.**—As much as possible relieve the system of urine before going to sleep. On rising, bathe if practicable. If you cannot bear cold water, take the least possible chill off the water (cold water, however, is best). If bathing is not practicable, wash the body with cold water, and keep scrupulously clean. The reaction caused by cold water, is most desirable. Rub the body dry with a rough towel. Drink a good draught of cold water.

8. **Exercise.**—Get fifteen minutes' brisk walk, if possible before breakfast. If any sense of faintness exists, eat a crust of bread, or biscuit. Be regular in your meals, and do not fear to make a hearty breakfast. This lays a good foundation for the day. Take daily good, but not violent exercise. Walk until you can distinctly feel the tendency to perspiration. This will keep the pores of the skin open and in healthy condition.

9. **Medicines.**—Take the medicines, if used, regularly and carefully. Bromide of Potassium is a most valuable remedy in allaying lustful and heated passions and appetites. Unless there is actual venereal disease, medicine should be very little resorted to.

10. **Avoid the Streets at Night.**—Beware of corrupt companions. Fast young men and women should be shunned everywhere. Cultivate a taste for good reading and evening studies. Home life with its gentle restraints, pure friendships, and healthful discipline, should be highly valued. There is no liberty like that of a well-regulated home. To large numbers of young men in business houses, home life is impracticable.

11. **Be of Good Cheer and Courage.**—Recovery will be gradual, and not sudden; vital force is developed slowly from within. The object aimed at by medicine and counsel is to aid and increase nervous and physical vigor, and give tone to the demoralized system. Do not pay the slightest heed to the exaggerated statements of the wretched quack doctors, who advertise everywhere. Avoid them as you would a pestilence. Their great object is, through exciting your fears, to get you into their clutches, in order to oppress you with heavy and unjust payments. Be careful, not to indulge in fancies, or morbid thoughts and feelings. Be hopeful, and play the part of a man determined to overcome.

[461]

Manhood Wrecked and Rescued.

1. **The Noblest Functions of Manhood.**—The noblest functions of manhood are brought into action in the office of the parent. It is here that man assumes the prerogative of a God and becomes a creator. How essential that every function of his physical system should be perfect, and every faculty of his mind free from that which would degrade; yet how many drag their purity through the filth of masturbation, revel in the orgies of the debauchee, and worship at the shrine of the prostitute, until, like a tree blighted by the livid lightning, they stand with all their outward form of men, but without life.

2. **Threshold of Honor.**—Think of a man like that; in whom the passions and vices have burned themselves out, putting on the airs of a saint and claiming to have reformed! Aye, reformed, when there is no longer sweetness in the indulgence of lust. Think of such loathsome bestiality, dragging its slimy body across the threshold of honor and nobility and asking a pure woman, with the love-light of heaven in her eyes, to pass her days with him; to accept him as her lord; to be satisfied with the burnt-out, shriveled forces of manhood left; to sacrifice her purity that he may be redeemed, and to respect in a husband what she would despise in the brute.

3. **Stop.**—If you are, then, on the highway to this state of degradation, stop. If already you have sounded the depths of lost manhood, then turn, and from the fountain of life regain your power, before you perpetrate the terrible crime of marriage, thus wrecking a woman's life and perhaps bringing into the world children who will live only to suffer and curse the day on which they were born and the father who begat them.

4. **Sexual Impotency.**—Sexual impotency means sexual starvation, and drives many wives to ruin, while a similar lack among wives drives husbands to libertinism. Nothing so enhances the happiness of married couples as this full, life-abounding, sexual vigor in the husband, thoroughly reciprocated by the wife, yet completely controlled by both.

5. **Two Classes of Sufferers.**—There are two classes of sufferers. First, those who have only practiced self-abuse and are suffering from emissions. Second, those who by overindulgence in marital relations, or by dissipation with women, have ruined their forces.

6. **The Remedy.**—For self-abuse: When the young man has practiced self-abuse for some time, he finds, upon [462]quitting the habit, that he has nightly emissions. He becomes alarmed, reads every sensational advertisement in the papers, and at once comes to the conclusion that he must take something. *Drugs are not necessary.*

7. **Stop the Cause.**—The one thing needful, above all others, is to stop the cause. I have found that young men are invariably mistaken as to what is the cause. When asked as to the first cause of their trouble, they invariably say it was self-abuse, etc., but it is not. *It is the thought.* This precedes the handling, and, like every other cause, must be removed in order to have right results.

8. **Stop the Thought.**—But remember, *stop the thought!* You must not look after every woman with lustful thoughts, nor go courting girls who will allow you to hug, caress and kiss them, thus rousing your passions almost to a climax. Do not keep the company of those whose only conversation is of a lewd and depraved character, but keep the company of those ladies who awaken your higher sentiments and nobler impulses, who appeal to the intellect and rouse your aspiration, in whose presence you would no more feel your passions aroused than in the presence of your own mother.

9. **You Will Get Well.**—Remember you will get well. Don't fear. Fear destroys strength and therefore increases the trouble. Many get downhearted, discouraged, despairing—the very worst thing that can happen, doing as much harm, and in many cases more, than their former dissipation. Brooding kills; hope enlivens. Then sing with joy that the savior of knowledge has vanquished the death-dealing ignorance of the past; that the glorious strength of manhood has awakened and cast from you forever the grinning skeleton of vice. Be your better self, proud that your thoughts in the day-time are as pure as you could wish your dreams to be at night.

10. **Helps.**—Do not use tobacco or liquor. They inflame the passions and irritate the nervous system; they only gratify base appetites and never rouse the higher feelings. Highly spiced food should be eschewed, not chewed. Meat should be eaten sparingly, and never at the last meal.

11. **Don't Eat too Much.**—If not engaged in hard physical labor, try eating two meals a day. Never neglect the calls of nature, and if possible have a passage from the bowels every night before retiring. When this is not done the feces often drop into the rectum during sleep, producing heat which extends to the sexual organs, causing the lascivious dreams and emission. This will be noticed especially in the morning, when the feces usually distend [463]the rectum and the person nearly always awakes with sexual passions aroused. If necessary, use injections into the rectum of from one to two quarts of water, blood heat, two or three times a week. Be sure to keep clean and see to it that no matter collects under the foreskin. Wash off the organ every night and take a quick, cold hand-bath every morning. Have something to do. Never be idle. Idleness always worships at the shrine of passion.

12. **The Worst Time of All.**—Many are ruined by allowing their thoughts to run riot in the morning. Owing to the passions being roused as stated above, the young man lies half awake and half dozing, rousing his passions and reveling in lascivious thought for hours perhaps, thus completely sapping the fountains of purity, establishing habits of vice that will bind him with iron bands, and doing his physical system more injury than if he had practiced self-abuse, and had the emission in a few minutes. Jump out of bed at once on waking, and never allow the thought to master you.

13. **A Hand Bath.**—A hand bath in cold water every morning will diminish those rampant sexual cravings, that crazy, burning, lustful desire so sensualizing to men by millions; lessen prostitution by toning down that passion which alone patronizes it, and relieve wives by the millions of those excessive conjugal demands which ruin their sexual health; besides souring their tempers, and then demanding millions of money for resultant doctor bills.

14. **Will Get Well.**—Feel no more concern about your self. Say to yourself, "I shall and will get well under this treatment," as you certainly will. Pluck is half the battle. Mind acts and reads directly on the sexual organs. Determining to get well gets you well; whilst all fear that you will become worse makes you worse. All worrying over your case as if it were hopeless, all moody and despondent feelings, tear the life right out of these organs whilst hopefulness puts new life into them.

[464]
The Curse and Consequence of Secret Diseases.
INNOCENT CHILDHOOD.

1. **The Sins of the Fathers Are Visited on the Children.**—If persons who contract secret diseases were the only sufferers, there would be less pity and less concern manifested by the public and medical profession.

2. There are many secret diseases which leave an hereditary taint, and innocent children and grandchildren are compelled to suffer as well as those who committed the immoral act.

3. **Gonorrhœa** (Clap) is liable to leave the parts sensitive and irritable, and the miseries of spermatorrhœa, impotence, chronic rheumatism, stricture and other serious ailments may follow.

4. **Syphilis** (Pox).—Statistics prove that over 30 per cent. of the children born alive perish within the first year. Outside of this frightful mortality, how many children are born, inheriting eruptions of the skin, foul ulcerations, [465]swelling of the bones, weak eyes or blindness, scrofula, idiocy, stunted growth, and finally insanity, all on account of the father's early vices. The weaknesses and afflictions of parents are by natural laws visited upon their children.

5. The mother often takes the disease from her husband, and she becomes an innocent sufferer to the dreaded disease. However, some other name generally is applied to the disease, and with perfect confidence in her husband she suffers pain all her life, ignorant of the true cause. Her children have diseases of the eyes, skin, glands and bones, and the doctor will apply the term scrofula, when the result is nothing more or less than inherited syphilis. Let every man remember, the vengeance to a vital law knows only justice, not mercy, and a single moment of illicit pleasure will bring many curses upon him, and drain

out the life of his innocent children, and bring a double burden of disease and sorrow to his wife.

6. If any man who has been once diseased is determined to marry, he should have his constitution tested thoroughly and see that every seed of the malady in the system has been destroyed. He should bathe daily in natural sulphur waters, as, for instance, the hot springs in Arkansas, or the sulphur springs in Florida, or those springs known as specific remedies for syphilic diseases. As long as the eruptions on the skin appear by bathing in sulphur water there is danger, and if the eruptions cease and do not appear, it is very fair evidence that the disease has left the system, yet it is not an infallible test.

7. How many bright and intelligent young men have met their doom and blighted the innocent lives of others, all on account of the secret follies and vices of men.

8. **Protection.**—Girls, you, who are too poor and too honest to disguise aught in your character, with your sweet soul shining through every act of your lives, beware of the men who smile upon you. Study human nature, and try and select a virtuous companion.

Transcriber's note: there is no 9. in the original.

10. **Syphilitic Poison Ineradicable.**—Many of our best and ablest physicians assert that syphilitic poison, once infected, there can be no total disinfection during life; some of the virus remains in the system, though it may seem latent. Boards of State Charities in discussing the causes of the existence of whole classes of defectives hold to the opinion given above. The Massachusetts board in its report has these strong words on the subject:

"The worst is that, though years may have passed since its active stage, it permeates the very seed of life and [466]causes strange affections or abnormalities in the offspring, or it tends to lessen their vital force, to disturb or to repress their growth, to lower their standard of mental and bodily vigor, and to render life puny and short.

11. **A Serpent's Tooth.**—"*The direct blood-poisoning, caused by the absorption into the system of the virus (syphilis) is more hideous and terrible in its effect than that of a serpent's tooth.* This may kill outright, and there's an end; but that, stingless and painless, slowly and surely permeates and vitiates the whole system of which it becomes part and parcel, like myriads of trichinæ, and can never be utterly cast out, even by salivation.

"Woe to the family and to the people in whose veins the poison courses!

"It would seem that nothing could end the curse except utter extermination. That, however, would imply a purpose of eternal vengeance, involving the innocent with the guilty."

This disease compared with small-pox is as an ulcer upon a finger to an ulcer in the vitals. Small-pox does not vitiate the blood of a people; this disease does. Its existence in a primary form implies moral turpitude.

12. **Cases Cited.**—Many cases might be cited. We give but one. A man who had contracted the disease reformed his ways and was apparently cured. He married, and although living a moral life was compelled to witness in his little girl's eye-balls, her gums, and her breath the result of his past sins. No suffering, no expense, no effort would have been too great could he but be assured that his offspring might be freed from these results.

13. **Prevention Better than Cure.**—Here is a case where the old adage, "An ounce of prevention is worth a pound of cure," may be aptly applied. Our desire would be to herald to all young men in stentorian tones the advice, "Avoid as a deadly enemy any approaches or probable pitfalls of the disease. Let prevention be your motto and then you need not look for a cure."

14. **Help Proffered.**—Realizing the sad fact that many are afflicted with this disease we would put forth our utmost powers to help even these, and hence give on the following pages some of the best methods of cure.

HOW TO CURE GONORRHŒA (Clap).
Causes, Impure Connections, etc.

Symptoms.—As the disease first commences to manifest itself, the patient notices a slight itching at the point of the the [467]male organ, which is shortly followed by a tingling or smarting sensation, especially on making water. This is on account of the inflammation, which now gradually extends backward, until the whole canal is involved. The orifice of the urethra is now noticed to be swollen and reddened, and on inspection a slight discharge will be found to be present. And if the penis is pressed between the finger and thumb, matter or pus exudes. As the inflammatory stage commences, the formation of pus is increased, which changes from a thin to a thick yellow color, accompanied by a severe scalding on making water. The inflammation increases up to the fifth day, often causing such pain, on urinating, that the patient is tortured severely. When the disease reaches its height, the erections become somewhat painful, when the discharge may be streaked with blood.

Home Treatment.

First, see that the bowels are loose—if not, a cathartic should be given. If the digestive powers are impaired, they should be corrected and the general health looked after. If the system is in a good condition, give internally five drops of gelseminum every two hours. The first thing to be thought of is to pluck the disease in its bud, which is best done by injections. The best of these are: tinct. hydrastis, one drachm; pure water, four ounces; to be used three times a day after urinating. Zinc, sulphate, ten grains; pure water, eight ounces; to be used after urinating every morning and night. Equal parts of red wine and pure water are often used, and are of high repute, as also one grain of permanganate of potash to four ounces of water.

If the above remedies are ineffectual, a competent physician should be consulted.

General Treatment.—One of the best injections for a speedy cure is:

Hydrastis, 1 oz.

Water, 5 oz.

Mix and with a small syringe inject into the penis four or five times a day after urinating, until relieved, and diminish the number of injections as the disease disappears. No medicine per mouth need be given, unless the patient is in poor health.

SYPHILIS (Pox).

1. This is the worst of all diseases except cancer—no tissue of the body escapes the ravages of this dreadful [468]disease—bone, muscle, teeth, skin and every part of the body are destroyed by its deforming and corroding influence.

2. **Symptoms.**—About eight days after the exposure a little redness and then a pimple, which soon becomes an open sore, makes its appearance, on or about the end of the penis in males or on the external or inner parts of the uterus of females. Pimples and sores soon multiply, and after a time little hard lumps appear in the groin, which soon develop into a blue tumor called *bubo*. Copper colored spots may appear in the face, hair fall out, etc. Canker and ulcerations in the mouth and various parts of the body soon develop.

3. **Treatment.**—Secure the very best physician your means will allow without delay.

4. **Local Treatment of Buboes.**—To prevent suppuration, treatment must be instituted as soon as they appear. Compresses, wet in a solution composed of half an ounce of muriate of ammonia, three drachms of the fluid extract of belladonna, and a pint of water, are beneficial, and should be continuously applied. The tumor may be scattered by painting it once a day with tincture of iodine.

5. **For Eruptions.**—The treatment of these should be mainly constitutional. Perfect cleanliness should be observed, and the sulphur, spirit vapor, or alkaline bath freely used. Good diet and the persistent use of alteratives will generally prove successful in removing this complication.

Recipe for Syphilis.—

Bin-iodide of mercury, 1 gr.

Extract of licorice, 32 gr.

Make into 16 pills. Take one morning and night.

LOTION.—

Bichloride of mercury, 15 gr.

Lime water, 1 pt.

Shake well, and wash affected parts night and morning.

For Eruptions on Tongue.—

Cyanide of silver, ½ gr.

Powdered iridis, 2 gr.

Divide into 10 parts. To be rubbed on tongue once a day.

For Eruptions in Syphilis.—A 5 per cent. ointment of carbolic acid in a good preparation.

BUBO.

Treatment.—
Warm poultice of linseed meal,
Mercurial plaster,
Lead ointment.

GLEET (Chronic Clap).

1. **Symptoms.**—When gonorrhœa is not cured at the end of twenty-one or twenty-eight days, at which time all [469]discharge should have ceased, we have a condition known as chronic clap, which is nothing more or less than gleet. At this time most of the symptoms have abated, and the principal one needing medical attention is the discharge, which is generally thin, and often only noticed in the morning on arising, when a scab will be noticed, glutinating the lips of the external orifice. Or, on pressing with the thumb and finger from behind, forward, a thin, white discharge can be noticed.

2. **Home Treatment.**—The diet of patients affected with this disease is all-important, and should have careful attention. The things that should be avoided are highly spiced and stimulating foods and drinks, as all forms of alcohol, or those containing acids. Indulgence in impure thoughts is often sufficient to keep a discharge, on account of the excitement it produces to the sensitive organs, thus inducing erections, which always do harm.

3. **General Treatment.**—The best injection is:
Nitrate of silver, ¼ grain.
Pure water, 1 oz.
Inject three or four times a day after urinating.

STRICTURE OF THE URETHRA.

Symptoms.—The patient experiences difficulty in voiding the urine, several ineffectual efforts being made before it will flow. The stream is diminished in size, of a flattened or spiral form, or divided in two or more parts, and does not flow with the usual force.

Treatment.—It is purely a surgical case and a competent surgeon must be consulted.

PHIMOSIS.

1. **Cause.**—Is a morbid condition of the penis, in which the glans penis cannot be uncovered, either on account of a congenital smallness of the orifice of the foreskin, or it may be due to the acute stage of gonorrhœa, or caused by the presence of soft chancre.

2. **Symptoms.**—It is hardly necessary to give a description of the symptoms occurring in this condition, for it will be easily diagnosed, and its appearances are so indicative that all that is necessary is to study into its cause and treat the disease with reference to that.

Treatment.—If caused from acute gonorrhœa, it should be treated first by hot fomentations, to subdue the swelling, when the glans penis can be uncovered. If the result of the formation of chancre under the skin, they should be treated by a surgeon, for it may result in the sloughing off of the end of the penis, unless properly treated.

[470]

Animal Magnetism.
WHAT IT IS AND HOW TO USE IT.
ILLUSTRATING MAGNETIC INFLUENCES.
ANIMAL MAGNETISM IS SUPPOSED TO RADIATE FROM AND ENCIRCLE EVERY HUMAN BEING.

1. **Magnetism Existing Between the Bodies of Mankind.**—It is rational to believe that there is a magnetism existing between the bodies of mankind, which may have either a beneficial or a damaging effect upon our health, according to the conditions which are produced, or the nature of the individuals who are brought in contact with each other. As an illustration of this point we might consider that, all nature is governed by the laws of attraction and repulsion, or in other words, by positive and negative forces. These subtle

forces or laws in nature which we call attraction or [471]repulsion, are governed by the affinity—or sameness—or the lack of affinity—or sameness—which exists between what may be termed the combination of atoms or molecules which goes to make up organic structure.

2. **Law of Attraction.**—Where this affinity—or sameness—exists between the different things, there is what we term the law of attraction, or what may be termed the disposition to unite together. Where there is no affinity existing between the nature of the different particles of matter, there is what may be termed the law of repulsion, which has a tendency to destroy the harmony which would otherwise take place.

3. **Magnetism of the Mind.**—Now, what is true of the magnet and steel, is also true—from the sameness of their nature—of two bodies. And what is true of the body in this sense, is also true of the sameness or magnetism of the mind. Hence, *by the laying on of hands*, or by the association of the minds of individuals, we reach the same result as when a combination is produced in any department of nature. Where this sameness of affinity exists, there will be a blending of forces, which has a tendency to build up vitality.

4. **A Proof.**—As a proof of this position, how often have you found the society of strangers to be so repulsive to your feelings, that you have no disposition to associate. Others seem to bring with them a soothing influence that draws you closer to them. All these involuntary likes and dislikes are but the results of the *animal magnetism* that we are constantly throwing off from our bodies,—although seemingly imperceptible to our internal senses.—The dog can scent his master, and determine the course which he pursues, no doubt from similar influences.

5. **Home Harmony.**—Many of the infirmities that afflict humanity are largely due to a want of an understanding of its principles, and the right applications of the same. I believe that if this law of magnetism was more fully understood and acted upon, there would be a far greater harmony in the domestic circle; the health of parents and children might often be preserved where now sickness and discord so frequently prevail.

6. **The Law of Magnetism.**—When two bodies are brought into contact with each other, the weak must naturally draw from the strong until both have become equal. And as long as this equality exists there will be perfect harmony between individuals, because of the reciprocation which exists in their nature.[472]

7. **Survival of the Fittest.**—But if one should gain the advantage of the other in magnetic attraction, the chances are that through the law of development, or what has been termed the "Survival of the Fittest"—the stronger will rob the weaker until one becomes robust and healthy, while the other grows weaker and weaker day by day. This frequently occurs with children sleeping together, also between husband and wife.

8. **Sleeping With Invalids.**—Healthy, hearty, vigorous persons sleeping with a diseased person is always at a disadvantage. The consumptive patient will draw from the strong, until the consumptive person becomes the strong patient and the strong person will become the consumptive. There are many cases on record to prove this statement. A well person should never sleep with an invalid if he desires to keep his health unimpaired, for the weak will take from the strong, until the strong becomes the weak and the weak the strong. Many a husband has died from a lingering disease which saved his wife from an early grave. He took the disease from his wife because he was the stronger, and she became better and he perished.

9. **Husband and Wife.**—It is not always wise that husband and wife should sleep together, nor that children—whose temperament does not harmonize—should be compelled to sleep in the same bed. By the same law it is wrong for the young to sleep with old persons. Some have slept in the same bed with persons, when in the morning they have gotten up seemingly more tired than when they went to bed. At other times with different persons, they have lain awake two-thirds of the night in pleasant conversation and have gotten up in the morning without scarcely realizing that they had been to sleep at all, yet have felt perfectly rested and refreshed.

10. **Magnetic Healing, or What Has Been Known as the Laying On of Hands.**—A nervous prostration is a negative condition beneath the natural, by the laying on of hands a person in a good, healthy condition is capable of communicating to the necessity

of the weak. For the negative condition of the patient will as naturally draw from the strong, as the loadstone draws from the magnet, until both become equally charged. And as fevers are a positive condition of the system "beyond the natural," the normal condition of the healer will, by the laying on of the hands, absorb these positive atoms, until the fever of the patient becomes reduced or cured. As a proof of this the magnetic healer often finds himself or herself prostrated after treating the weak; and excited or feverish after treating a feverish patient.

[473]
How to Read Character.
HOW TO TELL DISPOSITION AND CHARACTER BY THE NOSE.
WELL MATED.

1. **Large Noses.**—Bonaparte chose large-nosed men for his generals, and the opinion prevails that large noses indicate long heads and strong minds. Not that great noses cause great minds, but that the motive or powerful temperament cause both.

2. **Flat Noses.**—Flat noses indicate flatness of mind and character, by indicating a poor, low organic structure.

3. **Broad Noses.**—Broad noses indicate large passageways to the lungs, and this, large lungs and vital organs, and this, great strength of constitution, and hearty animal [474]passions along with selfishness; for broad noses, broad shoulders, broad heads, and large animal organs go together. But when the nose is narrow at the base, the nostrils are small, because the lungs are small and need but small avenues for air; and this indicates a predisposition to consumptive complaints, along with an active brain and nervous system, and a passionate fondness for literary pursuits.

4. **Sharp Noses.**—Sharp noses indicate a quick, clear, penetrating, searching, knowing, sagacious mind, and also a scold; indicate warmth of love, hate, generosity, moral sentiment—indeed, positiveness in everything.

5. **Blunt Noses.**—Blunt noses indicate and accompany obtuse intellects and perceptions, sluggish feelings, and a soulless character.

6. **Roman Noses.**—The Roman nose indicates a martial spirit, love of debate, resistance, and strong passions, while hollow, pug noses indicate a tame, easy, inert, sly character, and straight, finely-formed Grecian noses harmonious characters. Seek their acquaintance.

DISPOSITION AND CHARACTER BY STATURE.

1. **Tall Persons.**—Tall persons have high heads, and are aspiring, aim high, and seek conspicuousness, while short ones have flat heads, and seek the lower forms of worldly pleasures. Tall persons are rarely mean, though often grasping; but very penurious persons are often broad-built.

2. **Small Persons.**—Small persons generally have exquisite mentalities, yet less power—the more precious the article, the smaller the package in which it is done up,—while great men are rarely dwarfs, though great size often co-exists with sluggishness.

DISPOSITION AND CHARACTER BY THE WALK.

1. **Awkward.**—Those whose motions are awkward yet easy, possess much efficiency and positiveness of character, yet lack polish; and just in proportion as they become refined in mind will their movements be correspondingly improved. A short and quick step indicates a brisk and active but rather contracted mind, whereas those who take long steps generally have long heads; yet if the step is slow, they will make comparatively little progress, while those whose step is long and quick will accomplish proportionately much, and pass most of their competitors on the highway of life.[475]

2. **A Dragging Step.**—Those who sluff or drag their heels, drag and drawl in everything; while those who walk with a springing, bouncing step, abound in mental snap and spring. Those whose walk is mincing, affected, and artificial, rarely, if ever, accomplish much; whereas those who walk carelessly, that is, naturally, are just what they appear to be, and put on nothing for outside show.

194

3. **The Different Modes of Walking.**—In short, every individual has his own peculiar mode of moving, which exactly accords with his mental character; so that, as far as you can see such modes, you can decipher such outlines of character.

THE DISPOSITION AND CHARACTER BY LAUGHING.

1. **Laughter Expressive of Character.**—Laughter is very expressive of character. Those who laugh very heartily have much cordiality and whole-souledness of character, except that those who laugh heartily at trifles have much feeling, yet little sense. Those whose giggles are rapid but light, have much intensity of feeling, yet lack power; whereas those who combine rapidity with force in laughing, combine them in character.

2. **Vulgar Laugh.**—Vulgar persons always laugh vulgarly, and refined persons show refinement in their laugh. Those who ha, ha right out, unreservedly, have no cunning, and are open-hearted in everything; while those who suppress laughter, and try to control their countenances in it, are more or less secretive. Those who laugh with their mouths closed are non-committal; while those who throw it wide open are unguarded and unequivocal in character.

3. **Suppressed Laughter.**—Those who, suppressing laughter for a while, burst forth volcano-like, have strong characteristics, but are well-governed, yet violent when they give way to their feelings. Then there is the intellectual laugh, the love laugh, the horse laugh, the philoprogenitive laugh, the friendly laugh, and many other kinds of laugh, each indicative of corresponding mental developments.

DISPOSITION AND CHARACTER BY THE MODE OF SHAKING HANDS.

Their Expression of Character.—Thus, those who give a tame and loose hand, and shake lightly, have a cold, if not heartless and selfish disposition, rarely sacrificing much for others, are probably conservatives, and lack warmth and [476]soul. But those who grasp firmly, and shake heartily, have a corresponding whole-souledness of character, are hospitable, and will sacrifice business to friends; while those who bow low when they shake hands, add deference to friendship, and are easily led, for good or bad, by friends.

AN EASY-GOING DISPOSITION.

THE DISPOSITION AND CHARACTER BY THE MOUTH AND EYES.

1. **Different Forms of Mouths.**—Every mouth differs from every other, and indicates a coincident character. Large mouths express a corresponding quantity of mentality, while small ones indicate a lesser amount. A coarsely-formed mouth indicates power, while one finely-formed indicates exquisite susceptibilities. Hence small, delicately formed mouths indicate only common minds, with very fine feelings and much perfection of character.

2. **Characteristics.**—Whenever the muscles about the mouth are distinct, the character is correspondingly positive, and the reverse. Those who open their mouths wide and frequently, thereby evince an open soul, while closed [477]mouths, unless to hide deformed teeth, are proportionately secretive.

3. **Eyes.**—Those who keep their eyes half shut are peek-a-boos and eaves-droppers.

4. **Expressions of the Eye.**—The mere expression of the eye conveys precise ideas of the existing and predominant states of the mentality and physiology. As long as the constitution remains unimpaired, the eye is clear and bright, but becomes languid and soulless in proportion as the brain has been enfeebled. Wild, erratic persons have a half-crazed expression of eye, while calmness, benignancy, intelligence, purity, sweetness, love, lasciviousness, anger, and all the other mental affections, express themselves quite as distinctly by the eye as voice, or any other mode.

5. **Color of the Eyes.**—Some inherit fineness from one parent, and coarseness from the other, while the color of the eye generally corresponds with that of the skin, and expresses character. Light eyes indicate warmth of feeling, and dark eyes power.

6. **Garments.**—Those, who keep their coats buttoned up, fancy high-necked and closed dresses, etc., are equally non-communicative, but those who like open, free, flowing garments, are equally open-hearted and communicative.

THE DISPOSITION AND CHARACTER BY THE COLOR OF THE HAIR.

1. **Different Colors.**—Coarseness and fineness of texture in nature indicate coarse and fine-grained feelings and characters, and since black signifies power, and red ardor, therefore coarse black hair and skin signify great power of character of some kind, along with considerable tendency to the sensual; yet fine black hair and skin indicate strength of character, along with purity and goodness.

2. **Coarse Hair.**—Coarse black hair and skin, and coarse red hair and whiskers, indicate powerful animal passions, together with corresponding strength of character; while fine or light, or auburn hair indicates quick susceptibilities, together with refinement and good taste.

3. **Fine Hair.**—Fine dark or brown hair indicates the combination of exquisite susceptibilities with great strength of character, while auburn hair, with a florid countenance, indicates the highest order of sentiment and intensity of feeling, along with corresponding purity of character, combined with the highest capacities for enjoyment and suffering.[478]

4. **Curly Hair.**—Curly hair or beard indicates a crisp, excitable, and variable disposition, and much diversity of character—now blowing hot, now cold—along with intense love and hate, gushing, glowing emotions, brilliancy, and variety of talent. So look out for ringlets; they betoken April weather—treat them gently, lovingly, and you will have the brightest, clearest sunshine, and the sweetest, balmiest breezes.

5. **Straight Hair.**—Straight, even, smooth, and glossy hair indicate strength, harmony, and evenness of character, and hearty, whole-souled affections, as well as a clear head and superior talents; while straight, stiff, black hair and beard indicate a coarse, strong, rigid, straight-forward character.

6. **Abundance of Hair.**—Abundance of hair and beard signifies virility and a great amount of character; while a thin beard signifies sterility and a thinly settled upper story, with rooms to let, so that the beard is very significant of character.

7. **Fiery Red Hair** indicates a quick and fiery disposition. Persons with such hair generally have intense feelings—love and hate intensely—yet treat them kindly, and you have the warmest friends, but ruffle them, and you raise a hurricane on short notice. This is doubly true of auburn curls. It takes but little kindness, however, to produce a calm and render them as fair as a Summer morning. Red-headed people in general are not given to hold a grudge. They are generally of a very forgiving disposition.

SECRETIVE DISPOSITIONS.

1. A man that naturally wears his hat upon the top or back of the head is frank and outspoken; will easily confide and have many confidential friends, and is less liable to keep a secret. He will never do you any harm.

2. If a man wears his hat well down on the forehead, shading the eyes more or less, will always keep his own counsel. He will not confide a secret, and if criminally inclined will be a very dangerous character.

3. If a lady naturally inclines to high-necked dresses and collars, she will keep her secrets to herself if she has any. In courtship or love she is an uncertainty, as she will not reveal sentiments of her heart. The secretive girl, however, usually makes a good housekeeper and rarely gets mixed into neighborhood difficulties. As a wife she will not be the most affectionate, nor will she trouble her husband with many of her trials or difficulties.

[479]

Dictionary of Medical Terms.
Found in this and other works.

Abdomen—The largest cavity of the body, containing the liver, stomach, intestines, etc.

Abnormal—Unhealthy, unnatural.

Abortion—A premature birth, or miscarriage.

Abscess—A cavity containing pus.

Acetic—Sour, acid.

Acidity—Sourness.

Acrid—Irritating, biting.

Acute—Of short duration.

196

Adipose—Fatty.

Albumen—An animal substance resembling white of egg.

Alimentary Canal—The entire passage through which food passes; the whole intestines from mouth to anus.

Alterative—Medicines which gradually restore healthy action.

Amenorrhœa—Suppression of the menses.

Amorphous—Irregular.

Anæmia—Bloodlessness.

Anæsthetics—Medicines depriving of sensation and suffering.

Anatomy—Physical structure.

Anodyne—A remedy used for the relief of pain.

Ante-natal—Before birth.

Anteversion—Bending forward.

Antidote—A medicine counteracting poison.

Anti-emetic—That which will stop vomiting.

Antiseptic—That which will prevent putrefaction.

Anus—Circular opening or outlet of the bowels.

Aorta—The great artery of the heart.

Aphtha—Thrush; infant sore mouth.

Aqua—Water.

Areola—Circle around the nipple.

Astringent—Binding; contracting.

Auricle—A cavity of the heart.

Axilla—The armpit.

Azote—Nitrogen.

Bacteria—Infusoria; microscopical insects.

Bicuspid—A two-pointed tooth.

Bile—Secretion from the liver.

[480]

Bronchitis—Inflammation of the bronchial tubes which lead into the lungs.

Calculus—A stone found in the bladder, gall-ducts and kidneys.

Callous—A hard bony substance or growth.

Capillaries—Hair-like vessels that convey the blood from the arteries to the veins.

Carbonic Acid—The gas which is expired from the lungs.

Cardiac—Relating to the heart.

Catarrh—Flow of mucus.

Cathartic—An active purgative.

Caustic—A corroding or destroying substance.

Cellular—Composed of cells.

Cervix—Neck.

Cervix Uteri—Neck of the womb.

Chronic—Of long standing.

Clavicle—The collar bone.

Coccyx—Terminal bone of the spine.

Condiment—That which gives relish to food.

Congestion—Overfullness of blood vessels.

Contusion—A bruise.

Cuticle—The outer skin.

Dentition—Act of cutting teeth.

Diagnosis—Scientific determination of diseases.

Diarrhœa—Looseness of the bowels.

Disinfectant—That which cleanses or purifies.

Diaphragm—Breathing muscle between chest and abdomen.

Duodenum—The first part of the small intestines.

Dyspepsia—Difficult digestion.

Dysuria—Difficult or painful urination.

Emetic—Medicines which produce vomiting.
Enamel—Covering of the teeth.
Enema—An injection by the rectum.
Enteritis—Inflammation of the intestines.
Epidemic—Generally prevailing.
Epidermis—Outer skin.
Epigastrium—Region of the pit of the stomach.
Epilepsy—Convulsions.
Eustachian Tube—A tube leading from the side of the throat to the internal ear.
Evacuation—Discharging by stool.
Excretion—That which is thrown off.
Expectorant—Tending to produce free discharge from the lungs or throat.
Fallopian Tubes—Tubes from ovaries to uterus.
[481]
Fæces—Discharge from the bowels.
Fœtus--The child in the womb after the fifth month.
Fibula—The smallest bone of the leg below the knee.
Fistula—An ulcer.
Flatulence—Gas in the stomach or bowels.
Flooding—Uterine hemorrhage.
Fluor Albus—White flow; leucorrhœa; whites.
Flux—Diarrhœa, or other excessive discharge.
Fomentation—Warm or hot application to the body.
Friable—Easily crumbled or broken.
Friction—Rubbing with the dry hand or dry coarse cloth.
Fumigate—To smoke a room, or any article needing to be cleansed.
Function—The office or duty of any organ.
Fundament—The anus.
Fungus—Spongy flesh in wounds; proud flesh.
Fusion—To melt by heat.
Gall—Bile.
Gall-Stones—Hard biliary concretions found in the gall bladder.
Gangrene—The first stage of mortification.
Gargle—A liquid preparation for washing the throat.
Gastric—Of the stomach.
Gastritis—Inflammation of the stomach.
Gelatinous—Like jelly.
Genitals—The sexual organs.
Genu—The knee.
Genus—Family of plants; a group.
Germ—The vital principal, or life spark.
Gestation—Period of growth of child in the womb.
Gleet—Chronic gonorrhœa.
Glottis—The opening of the windpipe.
Gonorrhœa—An infectious discharge from the genital organs.
Gout—Painful inflammation of the joints of the toes.
Gravel—Crystalline sand-like particles in the urine.
Guttural—Relating to the throat.
Hectic—A fever which occurs generally at night.
Hemorrhage—A discharge of blood.
Hemorrhoids—Piles; tumors in the anus.
Hepatic—Pertaining to the liver.
Hereditary—Transmitted from parents.
Hernia—Rupture which permits a part of the bowels to protrude.
Hygiene—Preserving health by diet and other precautions.
[482]

198

Hyperæmia—Excess of blood in any part.
Hysteritis—Inflammation of the uterus.
Impregnation—The act of producing.
Incision—The cutting with instruments.
Incontinence—Not being able to hold the natural secretions.
Influenza—A disease affecting the nostrils and throat.
Infusion—The liquor in which plants have been steeped, and their medicinal virtues extracted.
Inhalation—Drawing in the breath.
Injection—Any preparation introduced into the rectum or other cavity by syringe.
Inspiration—The act of drawing air into the lungs.
Insomnia—Sleeplessness.
Involuntary—Against the will.
Introversion—Turned within.
Jaundice—A disease caused by the inactivity of the liver or ducts leading from it.
Jugular—Belonging to the throat.
Kidneys—Two organs which secrete the urine.
Labia—The lips of the vagina.
Laryngitis—Inflammation of the throat.
Larynx—The upper part of the throat.
Lassitude—Weakness; a feeling of stupor.
Laxative—Remedy increasing action of the bowels.
Leucorrhœa—Whites; fluor albis.
Livid—A dark colored spot on the surface.
Loin—Lower part of the back.
Lotion—A preparation to wash a sore.
Lumbago—Rheumatism of the loins.
Malaria—Foul marsh air.
Malignant—A disease of a very serious character.
Malformation—Irregular, unnatural formation.
Mastication—The act of chewing.
Masturbation—Excitement, by the hand, of the genital organs.
Matrix—The womb.
Meconium—The first passage of babes after birth.
Membrane—A thin lining or covering.
Menopause—Change of life.
Menstruation—Monthly discharge of blood from the uterus.
Midwifery—Art of assisting at childbirth.
Mucus—A fluid secreted or poured out by the mucous membrane, serving to protect it.

Narcotic—A medicine relieving pain and producing sleep.
Nephritis—Inflammation of the kidneys.
Neuralgia—Pain in nerves.
[483]
Normal—In a natural condition.
Nutritious—A substance which feeds the body.
Obesity—Excess of fat or flesh.
Obstetrics—The science of midwifery.
Oculus—The eye.
Œsophagus—The tube leading from the throat to the stomach.
Optic Nerve—The nerve which enters the back part of the eye.
Organic—Having organs.
Os—Mouth; used as mouth of womb.
Ostalgia—Pain in the bone.
Otitis—Inflammation of the ear.
Ovum—An egg.

199

Oxalic Acid—An acid found in sorrel, very poisonous.
Palate—The roof of the mouth.
Palliative—To afford relief only.
Palpitation—Unnatural beating of the heart.
Paralysis—Loss of motion.
Parturition—Childbirth.
Pathological—Morbid, diseased.
Pelvis—The bony cavity at lower part of trunk.
Pericardium—Sac containing the heart.
Perinæum—The floor of the pelvis, or space between and including the anus and vulva.
Peritonitis—Inflammation of lining membrane of bowels.
Placenta—After-birth.
Pleura—Membrane covering the lungs.
Pleurisy—Inflammation of the pleura.
Pregnancy—Being with child.
Prognosis—Prediction of termination of a disease.
Prolapsus—Falling; protrusion.
Prolapsus Uteri—Falling of the womb.
Prostration—Without strength.
Pruritis—A skin trouble causing intense itching.
Puberty—Full growth.
Pubes—External part of the organs of generation covered with hair.
Puerperal—Belonging to childbirth.
Pulmonary—Pertaining to the lungs.
Pulmonitis—Inflammation of the lungs.
Pus—Unhealthy matter.
Putrid—Rotten, decomposed.
Pylorus—Lower opening of the stomach.
Rectum—The lower portion of the intestines.
Regimen—Regulated habits and food.
[484]
Retching—An effort to vomit.
Retina—Inner coat of the eye.
Retroversion—Falling backward.
Rigor—Chilliness, convulsive shuddering.
Sacrum—Bone of the pelvis.
Saliva—Fluid of the mouth.
Salivation—Unnatural flow of saliva.
Sanative—Health-producing.
Sciatic—Pertaining to the hip.
Scrofula—A constitutional tendency to disease of the glands.
Scrotum—The sac which encloses the testicles.
Sedative—Quieting, soothing.
Semen—Secretion of the testes.
Sitz-bath—Bath in a sitting position.
Sterility—Barrenness.
Stimulant—A medicine calculated to excite an increased and healthy action.
Styptic—A substance to stop bleeding.
Sudorific—Inducing sweat.
Tampan—A plug to arrest hemorrhage.
Tonic—A medicine which increases the strength of the system.
Testicle—Gland that secretes the semen.
Therapeutic—Treatment of disease.
Tissue—The peculiar structure of a part.
Tonsils—Glands on each side of the throat.

Trachea—Windpipe. **Triturate**—To rub into a powder.

Tumor—A morbid enlargement of a part.

Ulceration—The forming of an ulcer.

Umbilicus—The navel.

Ureter—Duct leading from kidney to the bladder.

Urethra—Duct leading from the bladder.

Uterus—The womb.

Vagina—The passage from the womb to the vulva.

Varicose Veins—Veins dilated with accumulation of dark colored blood.

Vascular—Relating to the blood vessels.

Vena Cava—The large vein communicating with the heart.

Venous—Pertaining to the veins.

Ventricle—One of the lower chambers of the heart.

Viable—Capable of life.

Vulva—Outer lips of the vagina.

Womb—That organ of the woman which conceives and nourishes the offspring.

Zymotic—Caused by fermentation.

[485]